RC
454.4
.W4
1979

WITHDRAWN

Date

sudden death and psychiatric illness

sudden death and psychiatric illness

Martin H. Wendkos, M.D.
Jefferson Medical College (Psychosomatic Unit)
Thomas Jefferson University
Philadelphia, Pennsylvania

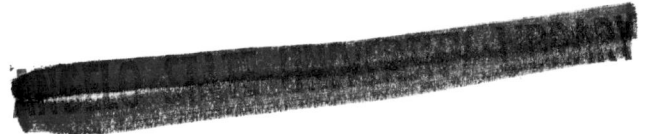

SP

SP MEDICAL & SCIENTIFIC BOOKS
a division of Spectrum Publications, Inc.
New York • London

Copyright © 1979 Spectrum Publications

All rights reserved. No part of this book may be reproduced in any form, by photostat, microform, retrieval system, or any other means without prior written permission of the copyright holder or his licensee.

SPECTRUM PUBLICATIONS, INC.
175-20 Wexford Terrace, Jamaica, N.Y. 11432

Library of Congress Cataloging in Publication Data

Wendkos, Martin H
  Sudden death and Psychiatric illness.

  Includes index.
  1. Psychology, Pathological—Complications and sequelae. 2. Sudden death. I. Title.
Rc454.4.W4   616.8'9'07   78-12854
ISBN 0-89335-069-9

*To a tireless
and highly dedicated
collaborator—my beloved wife*

Contents

Preface		—Daniel Lieberman, M.D.	
Chapter	1	Prologue.	1
Chapter	2	Terminology, Classification, and Definitions.	11
Chapter	3	Coronary Disease.	15
Chapter	4	Alcohol Abuse.	41
Chapter	5	Obstructive Asphyxia.	89
Chapter	6	Synsomnial Deaths.	103
Chapter	7	Postictal Fatalities.	123
Chapter	8	Fatal Megacolon in the Psychiatric Patient.	141
Chapter	9	Fatal Hyperpyrexia.	153
Chapter	10	Acute Exhaustive Mania.	165

Chapter 11 Wet Lung Syndrome in Narcotic Addicts.   177

Chapter 12 Myocardial Necrosis.   203

Chapter 13 Electrocardiographic Considerations.   229

Chapter 14 The Inherited Susceptibility to Sudden Death.   253

Chapter 15 Psychotropic Agents.   281

Appendix   317

    The Histopathologic Study of the Atrioventricular Node, The His Bundle and Its Branches.

    Tricyclic Antidepressant Poisoning: Therapeutic Aspects.

    Management of Acute Cardiac Arrest.

    Emergency Treatment of Alimentary Strangulation.

Preface

This well documented and very interesting book reflects an important trend in modern American medicine. The medical and surgical specialties are now beginning to recognize and accept the importance of psychological and social factors in the understanding of health and illness and in the prevention and treatment of all illness. In turn, those responsible for the care of psychiatric patients are beginning to seek more information from those whose major focus has been the treatment of somatic problems. This interaction has represented a gratifying development inasmuch as an improved understanding of genetics, physiology, biochemistry, and pathology must inevitably lead to the practice of holistic medicine—a goal which we all would like to achieve. Moreover, the recent acquisition of knowledge concerning brain biochemistry has contributed to the growth of psychiatry as a specialty and has extended the horizons for all those who deal with the various ailments which afflict mankind today.

The reintegration of psychiatry with the other medical specialties is helping to unveil the shroud of mystery and fear that often has surrounded psychiatric disorders and the patient with psychiatric disorders. Sudden death in the psychiatric patient is an unusual event and there is a great deal to learn about the ways an emotional disorder can favor such a catastrophe. In the years to come there is certain to be a growing interest in methods to avert the fatal consequences of organic illness and to recognize when the recovery of a patient must depend on a coordinated effort to deal successfully with the concomittant state of mind.

For example, the depressed patient with a myocardial infarction is much more likely to die of a second episode than the nondepressed patient. This important element of "the will to live" or, conversely, "the will to die" is an important factor that confronts the physician wherever he encounters illness and disease. Some people's ability to control physiologic events, either consciously or unconsciously, through various mental mechanisms has been documented and in some instances this power can be exercised to support the healing process. Thus, we have demonstrated that with the use of hypnotherapy in some burn patients, the pain is diminished and tissue healing is accelerated.

Correspondingly, along with the introduction during the present century of various psychopharmacologicals and other modalities, the outlook for the rehabilitation of psychiatric patients, regardless of the specific nature of their illness, has brightened considerably. Therefore, it is disarming, to say the least, when such a patient dies suddenly and unexpectedly. For this reason, the author of this book had deemed it important to familiarize psychiatrists— as well as all professionals responsible for the care of psychiatric patients— with the various elements and circumstances which may favor the occurrence of a sudden death. An ultimate derivative of this approach, it is hoped, will be an awareness of how such a tragedy can be prevented.

The author of this book is a clinician, teacher, internist, and cardiologist who has for many years worked with patients with psychiatric disorders in a consultant capacity. He has noticed that the same physiologic events affecting the general population affect people with psychiatric disorders. Using the tools available to him, his keen sense of observation, and his inquiring mind, he proceeded to study the phenomenon of sudden death in the psychiatric patient. The results of his study unwind like a fascinating novel. Enjoyable reading lies ahead.

        Daniel Lieberman, M.D.
        Professor
        Director, Division of Consultation/Liaison
            Psychiatry and Psychosomatic Medicine
        Jefferson Medical College
        of Thomas Jefferson University

CHAPTER 1

Prologue

Basically, the material in this monograph represents an overview of a variety of nonsuicidal sudden death syndromes and their relationship to the mortality of a selective sample of the population. In terms of its nature, this collective group can be defined simply as that separate subset of our society who require either short- or long-term psychiatric care. Moreover, it will be apparent that, throughout, the epidemiologic aspects of these sudden death syndromes have been emphasized; thus, along with this approach, there was a consistent attempt to identify the prodromal "risk factors" in each instance. Correspondingly, then, the data in this publication should prove to be especially meaningful to anyone concerned with the survivability of those afflicted with a psychiatric illness.

Traditionally, most sudden unexpected deaths in hospitalized psychotics have been linked to the disturbed behavior that the decedent had manifested prior to the time of death; in addition, such fatalities have been further subdivided on the basis of the findings disclosed by a postmortem examination. Thus, when these sudden deaths could not be explained by the autopsy findings (autopsy-negative deaths) they were ascribed, generally, to "lethal catatonia," a designation intended to signify that the fatality was due to an acute cardiac arrest resulting from an overwhelming but undefined physiologic derangement directly related in some manner to the bizarre behavior manifested by the decedent prior to the time of death.

More recently, however, it has become the mode to link certain autopsy-negative sudden deaths in psychiatric patients to the prior consumption of a psychotropic drug.[1-3,51] As far as can be determined, this sort of allegation has been based, first, on the recognition that such a drug, even in customary doses, can produce minor modifications of the T-wave in the electrocardiogram and, second, on the supposition that such a drug-induced wave form change should be considered an electrocardiographic hallmark of a myocardial aberration which would favor the occurrence of a cardioplegic ventricular arrhythmia. However, my own observations have indicated that, in semantic terms, it would be incorrect to view such a pharmacogenic electrocardiographic abnormality as an ominous finding. For this reason, there has been included in this monograph a lengthy discourse (see Chapter 14) concerning the various differences between electrocardiographic correlates of abnormal ventricular repolarization which indeed can be the forerunner of a life-threatening ventricular tachyarrhythmia and those benign electrocardiographic changes associated with the administration of customary doses of the major tranquilizers.

In connection with such an endeavor, a simplified eclectic approach instead of a reliance on basic electrophysiologic concepts of a theoretic nature has been adopted to validate the interpretation of the changes being discussed. Thus, the body of electrocardiographic data in this chapter should be understood easily by the reader who has even rudimentary perceptions concerning those electrocardiographic findings which may be diagnostically important but not necessarily prognostic of a sudden cardiac arrest. It is hoped that such clarifications will prove to be reassuring, particularly to those health professionals who, heretofore, may have been persuaded that a minor T-wave abnormality resulting from the administration of customary doses of antipsychotic drugs should be perceived as an alarming finding.

Actually, following my review of publications alleging that a life-threatening ventricular tachyarrhythmia in a mentally ill individual was due to prior consumption of a phrenotropic medication, it became evident that there was invariably an acceptable alternative explanation for the observed arrhythmia.[4] Thus, the results of such an analysis can be seen as a corroboration of the recent observations of Swett and Shader.[5] In their prospective study, which was conducted at the Massachusetts Mental Health Center, they monitored a random sample of 1932 consecutively admitted psychiatric patients in order to record the incidence of adverse reactions to psychotropic drugs. After they examined their data, they concluded that although "there were two sudden deaths in this group, neither of the decedents had received phenothiazines or tricyclic antidepressants and there was some doubt that drugs were related to the deaths."

Although all of the sudden deaths discussed in this monograph are the sort which have occurred in individuals who collectively could be identified by current standards as persons afflicted with some type of psychiatric illness, it was found that, for the most part, there were few precise correlations between the various sudden death syndromes and the nature of the underlying psychiatric disorder. The exceptions were the sudden death syndromes limited to social deviates addicted to either narcotic drugs, alcoholic beverages, or to both preparations (see Chapters 4 and 11); such a nonsologic distinction did not seem to be justified with respect to fatalities described in this monograph under the respective rubrics of Obstructive Asphyxia (see Chapter 5); Acute Exhaustive Mania (see Chapter 10); Synsomnial Deaths (see Chapter

6); Postictal Fatalities (see Chapter 7); Psychotogenic Megacolon (see Chapter 8); Myocardial Necrosis (see Chapter 12); Fatal Hyperpyrexia (see Chapter 9); Occlusive Coronary Artery Disease (see Chapter 3); or Psychotropic Agents (see Chapter 15).

Moreover, in connection with the preparation of this review of conditions responsible for sudden deaths in the psychiatrically ill, it became evident that the presence of segmental atherosclerotic stenosis of the epicardially located coronary arteries far exceeded all other causes of "natural" sudden deaths in patients with psychiatric disorders. Correspondingly, on the basis of such data, it can be construed that adult psychiatric patients resemble the remainder of the adult population in most westernized societies.[6-18,52] Moreover, for this reason, and because it is known that a sudden death often can be the earliest clinical expression of an underlying occlusive lesion of the extramural coronary arteries,[19-24] it is clear that certain reports which hitherto have alleged that a sudden death in the mentally ill was either inadequately explained or drug-related can hardly be considered to be reliable if the authors of such articles had provided postmortem data which were incomplete or, worse still, if they had indicated or implied that an autopsy had not been performed.

Admittedly, the thesis has been advanced that a routine autopsy examination often is not required in order to establish the cause of death but it should be explained that the proponents of such a position seemingly had not referred to fatalities which could be categorized as sudden or unexpected. Thus, it should be evident that there still is no reason to challenge the primacy of a postmortem examination in connection with efforts to determine which circumstance can be blamed for a "natural" sudden death. However, it must be recognized also that a cursorily performed autopsy cannot always be a reliable means of confirming or excluding occlusive coronary artery disease as the cause of the fatality.

In this connection, the observations of Schlesinger[25] and of others[26-29] are particularly noteworthy. These investigators showed, by the use of injection of colloidal suspensions in the extramural coronary arteries, that many occlusive coronary lesions in the exposed heart were overlooked even in well-staffed general hospitals in a large urban medical center, when the prosector failed to make a meticulous exploration of the caliber of all the extramural coronary arteries throughout their entire course.

Moreover, as recently as 1968, Leestma and Koenig,[2] who were concerned chiefly with sudden deaths in psychiatric patients, made the following comments in their paper:

"Before conclusions can be based upon the nonanatomic cause of death verdict of the pathologist, it is essential to be aware of the quality and extent of the autopsy. Thus, many pathologists in the course of a routine autopsy, examine organs in situ and do not completely dissect or remove them from the body. Often the larynx, brain, and spinal cord are left unexamined. In cases of food aspiration or diseases of the central nervous system which might have caused sudden death, these conditions would be missed in such an autopsy. However, when a reasonably careful postmortem examination has been performed, and when there is a lack of objective findings in a case of sudden death (in less than one hour), it has been the experience of most pathologists that the cause of such a death lies in the cardiovascular system. Such causes, which often leave little evidence of their presence, include very early acute myocardial infarction; air or fat embolism; cardiac arrhythmia; a sudden irreversible hypotension with cardiac arrest; and, in some cases, pulmonary thromboembolism. Thus, in such cases where postmortem information is scant, the determination of the cause of death will have to come from a careful scrutiny of what clinical facts are available; most germane would be information regarding the patient's prior health, drugs used, possible adverse reaction to these drugs, and many other clinical facts."[2]

Regrettably, however, Leestma and Koenig did not emphasize the importance of the family history in establishing the cause of sudden death. This consideration would seem to be an important factor inasmuch as detailed anamnestic data of this sort is crucial for identifying fatalities resulting from a condition discussed in this monograph under the rubric of the Inherited Susceptibility to Sudden Death (see Chapter 14).

The first description of genetically determined sudden deaths in patients with an established psychiatric disorder appeared in a report by Wilson and Reece in 1964.[30] The two decedents were homozygous relatively young twin adults who had been admitted to the hospital because of a schizophrenic reaction and whose deaths were both synsomnial and simultaneous; when the autopsies were performed, no findings were discovered that could account for these two fatalities.

Moreover, during my review of the electrocardiograms of two other unrelated phenothiazine-treated psychiatric patients whose subsequent sudden and unexpected deaths were unexplained even after an autopsy had been done, it was noted that there were changes in the premortem electrocardiograms which had been ascribed to a phenothiazine effect but which, in my opinion, resembled the sort of abnormality commonly associated with an inherited susceptibility to sudden death (see Chapter 14). Thus, this experience would seem to emphasize the need for circumspection in the interpretation of electrocardiograms in psychiatric patients.

It also would seem proper, in connection with this discussion concerning autopsy-negative sudden deaths, to explain that, for many years, pathologists who have been unable to find any evidence of organic heart disease or other meaningful abnormalities in the body of the decedent have contended that some such fatalities should be ascribed simply to a sudden physiologic derangement with respect to the heart, often induced by some emotional state.[31-45,53-56] Thus, Adelson, who discussed such "instantaneous physiologic deaths" in 1953[44] concluded not only that "abnormal neurological mechanisms" were involved, but also that the ultimate effect on the heart was an extreme degree of reflex cardiac inhibition. He stated: "deaths from inhibition are those sudden deaths which occur within a few seconds or not longer than 2 minutes after minor trauma or peripheral excitation of relatively simple and innocuous nature. Neither the trauma nor the nervous excitation are *ordinarily* in and of themselves sufficient to cause death directly. No pathological changes able to cause death are demonstrable at autopsy. There is thus a complete absence of pathological, traumatic, or toxic findings. An investigation of the circumstances surrounding death indicates that peripheral irritation or stimulation has probably initiated a fatal inhibitory reflex."[44]

It is also of interest that Adelson mentioned that "impingement of cold water on the nasal and postnasal mucus membrances after sudden immersion is a trigger mechanism for setting off the cardio-inhibitory reflex." Therefore, in this connection it would be an oversight not to allude to the views of Stewart Wolf regarding sudden death and the oxygen conserving diving reflex. In a brief article of his, which appeared in the American Heart Journal in 1966,[45] it was explained that "this reflex may be inhibited, facilitated, or even induced in response to symbolic stimuli, words, or events with emotionally charged significance to the individual concerned. On the other hand, during intense anxiety and fear, the reflex actually was facilitated, all of the changes resulting from it being accentuated."

The essential features of this reflex included bradycardia, decreased flow of blood to skin and viscera, increased arterial pressure, fall in blood pH, rise in lactic acid and other organic acids, and also a rise in the blood CO_2 and potassium level." He also mentioned that "sudden deaths occurring in civilized society are usually attributed to myocardial infarction, although often enough no necrosis of the myocardium is found. There is no means of proof in retrospect but one can reasonably suspect that a host of bizarre sudden deaths may be attributable to an overexuberant oxygen-conserving reflex." Moreover, even though extreme bradycardia is an important element of this oxygen conserving reflex, he acknowledged that the fatal cardiac mechanism might very well be ventricular fibrillation resulting from the combination of extreme bradycardia and an elevated serum potassium level in the presence of distinct metabolic and even respiratory acidosis.

Another interesting aspect of autopsy examinations which, seemingly, could contribute materially to an elucidation of certain mystifying sudden deaths in psychiatric patients is the refinement originally introduced by Lev in 1951[46] and subsequently used and modified by others[47-49] for the study of cardiac tissues. With the use of this method, these investigators had been able to demonstrate the presence of isolated pathology involving portions of the coronary microcirculation close to vital pacemaker sites as well as those areas of the heart in the immediate vicinity of the major branches of the specialized conducting system. Thus, their findings had been able to provide an explanation for certain sudden deaths which otherwise might have been considered to be mystifying fatalities. For this reason, it was deemed advisable to include in the Appendix of this monograph, a summary of the techniques this group of pathologists had employed.

There is also the possibility that even following gross examination of the exposed heart, the prosector may sometimes overlook certain accessible lesions which currently are recognized to be responsible for a sudden and unexpected death. These two lesions are, *first,* an unsuspected solitary occlusion of the left coronary artery near its emergence from the aorta (unassociated with any material arteriosclerotic changes elsewhere in the extramural coronary arterial circulation) and, *second,* a prolapsed or ballooning mitral valve.

The latter condition is an entity which currently can be recognized without too much difficulty while a person with this affliction still is alive, although it may be overlooked when the heart is adynamic, as it would be after the time of death. Moreover, inasmuch as it also has been established that a conspicuous U wave may be one of the findings in the premortem electrocardiogram of a decedent who has died suddenly because of a prolapsed mitral valve, it is conceivable that if phenothiazines, with their known predilection to alter the T-waves, had been consumed prior to the time of death, there would be a temptation on the part of those with only a rudimentary understanding of electrocardiographic interpretation to consider the cause of death in such an instance to be an adverse reaction to phenothiazine administration instead of the result of a mitral valve prolapse syndrome (see Chapter 14).

Finally, it should be explained that although this monograph is, essentially a review of the "risk factors" responsible for sudden deaths in persons with various disorders of the mind, it was deemed important to include also some guidelines with regard to the emergency management of a psychiatric patient who has collapsed suddenly while a health professional is nearby. Therefore, two sets of instructions regarding the procedures to be followed in such a situation have been placed in the Appendix of this monograph. One such item is a detailed outline of the Heimlich procedure which is considered generally the most effective emergency technique in instances of alimentary strangulation. The other item is a description of the essential principles of cardiopulmonary resuscitation in persons with an acute cardiac arrest. Hopefully, such additional information may ultimately make it possible to relabel cases of "fatal syncope" as instances of "thanatoid syncope." (see Chapter 2)

REFERENCES

1. Hollister, L.E. and Kosek, J.C. Sudden death during treatment with phenothiazine derivatives. J.A.M.A. 192:1035 (1965).
2. Leestma, J.E. and Koenig, K.L. Sudden death and phenothiazines: A current controversy. Arch. Gen. Psych. 18:137 (1968).
3. Fowler, N.O. et al. Electrocardiographic changes and cardiac arrhythmias in patients receiving psychotropic drugs. Am. J. Cardiol. 37:223 (1976).
4. Wendkos, M.H. (Unpublished observations).
5. Swett, C.P. and Shader, R.I. Cardiac side effects and sudden death in hospitalized psychiatric patients. Dis. Nerv. Sys. 38:69 (1977).
6. Helpern, M. and Rabson, S.M. Sudden and unexpected natural deaths: General considerations and statistics. New York. J. Med. 45:1197 (1945).
7. Epstein, F.H. The epidemiology of coronary heart disease: A review. J. Chronic Dis. 18:735 (1965).
8. Kuller, L. Sudden and unexpected non-traumatic deaths in adults: A review of epidemiological and clinical studies. J. Chronic Dis. 19:1165 (1966).
9. Kuller, L. et al. An epidemiologic study of sudden and unexpected deaths in adults. Medicine 46:341 (1967).
10. Burch, G.E. and De Pasquale, N.P. Sudden unexpected natural deaths. Am. J. Med. Sci. 249:86 (1965).
11. Pruitt, R.D. On sudden death. Am. Heart J. 68:111 (1964).
12. Myerburg, R.J. and Davis, J.H. The medical ecology of public safety I: Sudden death due to coronary heart disease. Am. Heart J. 68:586 (1964).
13. Wikland, B. Death from arteriosclerotic heart disease outside hospitals. Acta Med. Scand. 184:129 (1968).
14. Biorck, G. et al. Studies on myocardial infarction in Malmo 1935 to 1954: Morbidity and mortality in hospital material Acta Med. Scand. 159:253 (1957).
15. Bainton, C.R. and Peterson, D.R. Deaths from coronary heart disease in persons 50 years of age and younger: A community-wide study. New Eng. J. Med. 269:569 (1963).
16. Vedin, J.A. Sudden death: Identification of high risk groups. Am. Heart J. 86:124 (1973).
17. Vedin, J.A. et al. Mortality trends in Sweden 1951-1968 with special reference to cardiovascular causes of death. Acta Med. Scand. 515:76 (1971).
18. White, P.D. et al. A note on the discussion on non-traumatic sudden deaths by American and Soviet cardiologists in Moscow in May 1961. Am. Heart J. 64:842 (1962).
19. Moritz, A.R. and Zamcheck, N. Sudden and unexpected deaths of young soldiers: Diseases responsible for sudden deaths during World War II. Arch. Pathol. Lab. Med. 42:459 (1946).
20. Yater, W.M. et al. Comparison of clinical and pathologic aspects of coronary artery disease in men of various age groups: A study of 950 autopsied cases from the Armed Forces Institute of Pathology. Ann. Intern. Med. 34:352 (1951).
21. French, A.J. and Dock, W. Fatal coronary arteriosclerosis in young soldiers. J.A.M.A. 124:1233 (1944).

22. Spain, D.M. et al. Coronary atherosclerosis as a cause of unexpected and unexplained death: An autopsy study from 1949-1959 *J.A.M.A.* 174:384 (1960).
23. Adelson, L. Sudden death from coronary disease: The cardiac conundrum. *Postgrad. Med.* 30:139 (1961).
24. Goldstein, S. *Sudden Death and Coronary Heart Disease.* Futura Publishers, Mt. Kisco, New York (1974).
25. Schlesinger, M.J. An injection plus dissection study of coronary artery occlusions and anastamoses. *Am. Heart J.* 15:528 (1938).
26. Helwig, F.C. and Wilhelmy, E.W. Sudden and unexpected death from acute interstitial myocarditis. Report of 3 cases. *Ann. Int. Med.* 13:107 (1939).
27. Schlesinger, M.J. and Zoll, P.M. Incidence and localization of coronary artery occlusions. *Arch. Pathol. Lab. Med.* 32:178 (1941).
28. Allison, R.B. et al. Clinico-pathologic correlations in coronary arteriosclerosis: 430 patients with postmortem coronary angiography. *Circulation* 27:170 (1963).
29. Rodriguez, F.L. et al. Postmortem angiographic studies on the coronary arterial circulation: Incidence and topography of occlusive coronary lesions. *Am. Heart J.* 68:490 (1964).
30. Wilson, I.C. and Reece, J.C. Simultaneous deaths in schizoprenic twins. *Arch. Gen. Psych.* 11:377 (1964).
31. Moritz, A.R. Sudden death. *New Eng. J. Med.* 223:798 (1940).
32. Weiss, S. Instantaneous "physiologic" death. *New Eng. J. Med.* 223:793 (1940).
33. Markowitz, B. Sudden death: A neurocirculatory disturbance. *Am. J. Clin. Path.* 12:276 (1942).
34. Deadman, W.J. Sudden death. *Can. M.A.J.* 56:273 (1947).
35. Richter, C. On the phenomenon of sudden death in animals and man. *Psychosom. Med.* 19:190 (1957).
36. Yawger, N.S. Emotions as a cause of rapid and sudden death. *Arch. Neurol. Psych.* 36:875 (1936).
37. Gregg, D. The lethal power of the emotions. *Mental Hygiene* 20:30 (1936).
38. Weissman, A. and Hackett, T. Predilection to death. *Psychosom. Med.* 23:232 (1961).
39. Engel, G. Sudden and rapid death during psychological stress. *Ann. Int. Med.* 74:771 (1971).
40. Lown, B. et al. Basis for recurring ventricular fibrillation in the absence of coronary heart disease and its management. *New Eng. J. Med.* 294:623 (1976).
41. Wolf, S. Neural mechanisms in sudden cardiac death. *Trans. Am. Clin. Climatological Assoc.* 79:158 (1967).
42. Levitt, B. et al. Role of the nervous system in the genesis of cardiac rhythm disorders. *Am. J. Cardiol.* 37:1111 (1976).
43. Dimsdale, J.E. Emotional causes of sudden death. *Am. J. Psych.* 134:12 (1977).
44. Adelson, L. Possible neurological mechanisms responsible for sudden death. *J. Forensic Med.* 1:39 (1953).
45. Wolf, S. Sudden death and the oxygen conserving reflex. *Am. Heart J.* 71:840 (1967).
46. Lev, M. et al. A method for the histopathic study of the atrioventricular node bundle and branches. *Arch. Pathol. Lab. Med.* 52:73 (1951).
47. Shanklin, D.R. and Laite, M.B. Pickett-Sommer film strip technique. *Arch. Pathol. Lab. Med.* 75:91 (1963).
48. James, T.N. Pathology of small coronary arteries. *Am. J. Cardiol.* 20:679 (1967).
49. Schwartz, C.J. and Walsh, W.J. The pathologic basis of sudden death. *Progr. Cardiovasc. Dis.* 13:465 (1971).
50. James, T.N. et al. Observations on the pathophysiology of the long Q.-T. syndromes with special reference to the neuropathology of the heart. *Circulation* 57:1221 (1978).
51. Sydney, M.A. Ventricular arrhythmias associated with use of Thioridazine Hydrochloride in alcohol withdrawal. *Brit. Med. J.* 4:467 (1973).

52. Titus, J.L. et al. Sudden unexpected death as the initial manifestation of ischemic heart disease: Clinical and pathologic observations. *Am. J. Cardiol.* 29:294 (1972).
53. Lown, B. and Verrier, R.L. Neural activity and ventricular fibrillation. *New Eng. J. Med.* 294:1165 (1976).
54. Lown, B. et al Neural and psychologic mechanisms and the problem of sudden death. *Am. J. Cardiol.* 39:890 (1977).
55. Lown, B. and De Silva, R.A. Roles of psychologic stress and autonomic nervous system changes in provocation of ventricular premature complexes. *Am. J. Cardiol.* 41:979 (1978).
56. Goodfriend, M. and Wolpert, E.A. Death from fright: Report of a case and literature review. *Psychosom. Med.* 38:348 (1976).

CHAPTER 2

Terminology, Classifications, and Definitions

One traditional requirement in connection with the certification of any death has been to indicate not only its date but also the precise moment when the decedent was considered to be no longer alive. Clearly, then, data derived from a death certificate hardly can be utilized to differentiate between deaths which properly can be termed sudden from those not ordinarily perceived as such. Thus, any conclusion that a death was sudden must depend, actually, on an evaluation of the circumstances preceding the demise of the decedent.

Nevertheless, there are still no rigid guidelines which can indicate when a death should be designated a sudden one, even when it has been witnessed. Understandably, then, when the death has been unwitnessed, the decision to label it a sudden one can be more readily challenged.

For this reason, it has been my preference to differentiate between witnessed and unwitnessed sudden deaths. Thus, within such a context, an unwitnessed death properly can be considered to be sudden only on the basis of certain data available after the fact. Typical of such fatalities are those discussed in this monograph under the rubric of "Synsomnial Deaths" (Chapter 5).

On one hand, a death could be designated as sudden, though unwitnessed, if there were information that the decedent had been considered to be physically healthy prior to the conjectured time of death and that the fatality seemingly had occurred without any preceding prodromes or warnings. On the other hand, some unwitnessed deaths in almost moribund persons also can be considered a sudden life terminating event; such would include those fatalities which had been expected because the decedent had been known to be suffering already from a critical and prospectively fatal lingering illness, from an acute respiratory distress syndrome (see Chapter 11), or from an episode of status epilepticus (see Chapter 7).

Accordingly, although many unwitnessed deaths can be categorized as sudden fatalities, it would appear correct to add a qualifying term to indicate whether the death was not only sudden but unexpected as well. However, it should be emphasized that, in such instances, the death can be described as sudden only if the corpse was discovered only less than 24 hours after the decedent had last been seen alive. This qualification would comply with the guidelines established by the International College of Cardiology and the World Health Organization which not until 1970, had undertaken to establish suitable taxonomic criteria pertaining to the definition of a sudden death.[1]

With respect to witnessed sudden deaths, it must be acknowledged that there are those which properly can be designated as expected or unexpected, respectively; in these instances, the distinction would depend on the nature of the decedent's condition prior to the time of death. Moreover, an unexpected sudden death, whether witnessed or unwitnessed, sometimes also can prove to be mystifying as well. These are the unexpected sudden deaths for which there was no evident explanation despite the availability of reliable autopsy findings, toxicological studies, and detailed anamnestic data. (Chapter 1).

It is agreed generally that, in terms of frequency, occlusive coronary artery disease heads the list of conditions which can be responsible for sudden deaths (Chapter 10). Nevertheless, because they can differ in various ways, it has been suggested that coronary-related sudden deaths be described in a manner which would emphasize these distinguishing features. Thus, it has been advocated that in addition to their designation as witnessed or unwitnessed and expected or unexpected deaths, it would be proper to indicate whether an abruptly occurring witnessed coronary death should be designated sudden or instantaneous; in accord with this percept, it was recommended that when the attack of "fatal syncope" was unpreceded by warning symptoms, the fatality should be described as an instantaneous rather than a sudden death.[2]

Conceivably, then, such a novel terminology, with respect to coronary-related fatalities, would be applicable to other known cardiac states which, not infrequently, are responsible for sudden deaths. For example, either sudden or instantaneous deaths could result from the prolapsed mitral valve syndrome, various familial types of heart disease, the sick sinus syndrome, various myocardiopathies, various acquired lesions which lead to left ventricular hypertrophy, and a variety of congenital cardiac anomalies.

Since 1936, when Nathanson introduced the term,[3] "fatal syncope" has been the sobriquet usually employed to emphasize one of the chief clinical manifestations of a witnessed sudden death. Characteristically, it is accompanied by all the evidences of an acute cardiac arrest; thus, an attack of "fatal syncope" can be distinguished readily from that type of syncope commonly described as a simple faint. In 1973, Burch explained how the two differed in terms of their respective external features.[4]

As he indicated, "the patient who suddenly develops unconsciousness due to cardiac arrest often experiences a generalized flushing and warm or burning and tingling sensation of the skin of the entire body. He develops a marked redness or blush due to vasodilatation of the veins and other vessels of the skin and then suddenly falls unconscious. On the other hand, patients with the common forms of syncopal episodes gradually or relatively slowly become extremely pale to ashen grey, sweaty, weak, giddy, and then faint.

Occasionally, some persons have been observed to suddenly lose consciousness, clearly due to an acute cardiac arrest, and yet, even though death appears to be imminent, they will revive spontaneously. To differentiate such an incident from "fatal syncope" a suitable term would seem to be "thanatoid syncope"; therefore, in various places throughout this monograph, it has been employed to describe such a circumstance.

REFERENCES

1. Bulletin of the International Society of Cardiology, p. 9 (Winter 1970).
2. Friedman, M. et al. Instantaneous and sudden deaths. Clinical and pathological differentiation in coronary artery disease. *J.A.M.A.* 225:1319 (1973).
3. Nathanson, M.H. Pathology and pharmacology of cardiac syncope and sudden death. *Arch. Int. Med.* 58:685 (1936).
4. Burch, G.E. A sign of cardiac arrest. *Am. Heart J.* 86:138 (1973).

CHAPTER 3

Coronary Disease

Psychiatrists, pathologists, and internists who have been affiliated with psychiatric institutions have recognized for many years that atherosclerotic coronary artery disease always has been a major "risk factor" in relation to the occurrence of sudden deaths among adults whose principal disability was some form of mental illness. In this respect, then, psychiatric patients seem to resemble other civilians[1-18,85-87] or military personnel on active duty with the armed forces of the United States prior to 1948.[19-21]

EPIDEMIOLOGIC AND PATHOLOGIC ASPECTS

Moreover, data now are available to indicate that, in general, the number of such coronary-related sudden deaths in hospitalized psychiatric patients was inordinately high when a sequel of the coronary stenosis was an acute myocardial infarction. The data to support such a contention can be found in two reports.

In the article published in 1955 by Marchand[22] he described 51 authenticated cases of acute myocardial infarction among psychotics at the Bedford Massachusetts Administration Hospital, and he noted that the survival rate was quite low and also that sudden death was the primary manifestation of the acute myocardial lesion in 12 instances. The article by Hussar, appeared in 1962.[23] In this paper, he summarized his observations made at the Montrose New York Veterans Administration Hospital with respect to 66 fatalities ascribable to a confirmed acute myocardial infarction.

For the most part, in Hussar's sample, the nature of the psychiatric illness was a chronic schizoprenic reaction; in the remainder it was a chronic brain syndrome. However, this distribution could reflect the relatively dominant position of these two varieties of psychiatric ailments among the patients at that particular institution.

Furthermore, in this same connection, it is noteworthy that at a different neuropsychiatric facility of the Veterans Administration, my analysis of postmortem data pertaining to sudden deaths in a random group of elderly patients who had received long-term custodial care because of a chronic brain syndrome due to syphilitic disease of the central nervous system, had indicated that uniformly the cause of death was advanced atherosclerosis of the extramural coronary arteries sometimes, but not always, associated with an acute myocardial infarction.[24] Moreover, it is of interest that the pathologist was unable to demonstrate the presence of syphilitic cardiovascular disease in any of these particular decedents. Conceivably, this finding could be ascribed to the intensive penicillin therapy each had received during the early stages of the syphilitic infection.

In Hussar's series, there were 24 fatalities (36%) which could be classified as sudden deaths; thus, in 42, the terminal illness was more prolonged. These 24 sudden deaths which clearly were coronary related, had occurred between 1952 and 1959; consequently, it is evident that some had received phenothiazines prior to the time of death whereas others had not.

In connection with his review of these fatalities, Hussar also attempted to determine whether there was any relationship between the incidence of such coronary related sudden deaths and the consumption of the drugs the decedents had received prior to the time of death. Thus, he compared the incidence of non-sudden and sudden deaths among the 32 post-infarction fatalities observed between 1956 and 1959, which was the period when phenothiazines already were widely used at his institution. He found the ratio of the non-sudden variety to the sudden variety to be 20 to 12 and on this basis he concluded that phenothiazine therapy should not be viewed as a significant "risk factor" with respect to the occurrence of coronary-related sudden deaths associated with the presence of an acute myocardial infarction.

Other meaningful findings pertaining to the coronary-related sudden deaths in hospitalized psychotics were described by Hussar in subsequent publications which appeared in 1965[25] and in 1966.[26] Both of these reports were based on the results of an extensive retrospective cross-sectional study of fatalities in a large sample of chronic schizophrenics who had died seemingly from "natural causes." The ages of the decedents ranged from 40 to 83 years and the deaths which were analyzed had occurred in 29 United States Veterans Administration Hospitals during a 5 year period between 1954 and 1959.

The original sample comprised 1275 autopsied decedents but some of the protocols were discarded when it was discovered that suicide or some other type of violent act could account for the fatality (24 cases) and when the circumstances surrounding the deaths were not explained adequately (212 cases). Accordingly, there remained 1039 protocols suitable for analysis, inasmuch as these pertained to both sudden and non-sudden deaths which clearly were due to "natural causes."

However, of these 1039 fatalities due to "natural causes," only 321 properly could be categorized as sudden deaths (31%). Moreover, 343 of these 1039 fatalities proved to be coronary-related deaths (33%). On the other hand, inasmuch as 220 of these 343 fatalities due to coronary heart disease could be classified as sudden deaths, it was evident first, that 64% of the deaths ascribable to coronary heart disease actually were sudden and, second, that of all 321 sudden deaths due to "natural causes," 69% were linked to the presence of atherosclerotic coronary disease.

Thus, Hussar's survey with regard to the mortality of chronic schizophrenics makes it apparent that when sudden deaths from "natural causes" alone are under consideration, the underlying cause in most instances must be suspected to be a stenotic lesion involving the epicardially located branches of the coronary circulation.

Hussar had divided into three categories the anatomical changes in the hearts of 220 schizophrenics whose sudden deaths had been designated by him to be the result of coronary heart disease. One type of anatomical abnormality consisted of myocardial necrosis characteristic of an acute myocardial infarction; a second type of anatomical change consisted of a fresh thrombotic obstruction of an extramural coronary artery; another type of cardiac pathology which he identified with some of the coronary-related sudden deaths was termed by him "acute coronary insufficiency" and in conjunction with the use of such a designation, it was his intention to signify that the important finding at the necropsy was confined to the presence of a segmental luminal narrowing of either one or several extramural coronary arteries.

Furthermore, in this sample of 220 sudden coronary-related deaths, Hussar apparently was able to differentiate the incidence of deaths due to an acute lesion compared to the frequency of those fatalities which were ascribable to a chronic "angiophraxis"° of the extramural arteries. Thus, within this context, his data indicated clearly that the majority of these 220 coronary-related sudden deaths were linked to the presence of one or both of the two acute intercurrent complications such as an acute myocardial infarction with or without an associated acute coronary thrombosis or, conversely, an acute coronary thrombosis with or without an acute myocardial infarction; in 47 instances the autopsy revealed the presence of an acute myocardial infarction without an acute coronary thrombosis (21%) and in 50 instances both an acute myocardial infarction and an acute coronary thrombosis were present together, (23%).

°*Angiophraxix* is a coined word representing a synthesis of two Greek roots, namely *angio* (blood vessel) and *emphraxis* (blockage).

Conclusions

Collectively, then, the pathologic substrate of the 220 coronary-related sudden deaths in this large sample of psychiatric patients was an acute lesion in 139 (63%) and a progressive coronary stenosis without either an acute coronary thrombosis or an acute myocardial infarction in the remaining 81 instances (37%).

Myocardial Rupture

Another noteworthy aspect of Hussar's data was the demonstration that, in the sample of 220 coronary-related sudden deaths, there were an unusually large number ascribable to acute myocardial infarction complicated by myocardial rupture. Actually, this particular complication accounted for 46 fatalities; thus, it is evident that of the 97 sudden deaths linked to an acute myocardial infarction, a rent in the infarcted zone (cardiorrhexis), with its resulting acute cardiac tamponade, could be held responsible for a sudden death in 47% of these psychiatric patients who had developed an acute myocardial infarction. On the other hand, the results of earlier surveys based on autopsy data have indicated that the frequency of sudden deaths due to myocardial rupture in patients who had been under treatment for an acute myocardial infarction in the usual general hospital has ranged from 1% to 10%,[133-135] whereas, a more recent review by Bates et al[130] has shown that 4% to 24% of acute myocardial infarctions in a general hospital population will be followed by sudden death secondary to acute myocardial rupture. Accordingly, the inordinately high incidence of myocardial rupture reported by Hussar clearly emphasizes the dimensions of this complication among psychiatric patients with respect to sudden death due to "natural causes."

Moreover, inasmuch as a high incidence of fatal myocardial rupture has been observed among deteriorated patients in nursing homes,[131-132] it was suggested by Bates et al[130] that continued activity of chronic psychiatric patients after the occurrence of a clinically unrecognized acute myocardial infarction might possibly explain the inordinately high incidence of sudden death due to myocardial rupture in patients of this genre. This view seems to be supported also by the observations reported by Jetter and White as early as 1944[27] and by Marchand in 1955.[22]

The autopsy findings described by Jetter and White had indicated that of 22 consecutive instances of sudden death due to acute myocardial infarction in the insane, the terminal event in 16 of this number (72%) was a myocardial rupture. On the other hand, in connection with a survey conducted at the

Bedford, Massachusets Veterans Administration Hospital, Marchand has noted that among psychotic in-patients, there was also an excessive incidence of sudden death due to myocardial rupture; however, the incidence of this complication in his series was not as high as that reported by Jetter and White.

The findings Marchand had reported actually pertained to two separate patient samples. In one sample, which consisted of 51 confirmed causes of acute myocardial infarction, there were 12 sudden deaths (25.5%) and of these, 5 were proved by autopsy to be the result of myocardial rupture (42%). The other sample comprised 43 cases of sudden death due to a variety of "natural causes"; in order to make the data most meaningful, however, 9 of these cases were discarded because an autopsy had not been done following their deaths. Thus, of these 24 autopsied cases of sudden death due to "natural causes," the reason for the demise in 5 instances was found to be a myocardial rupture (21%).

In contrast, a report by Kavelman which appeared in 1960[28] seemed to indicate that myocardial rupture had occurred with almost equal frequency in psychotics and in nonpsychotics who had been hospitalized because of an acute myocardial infarction. The data which prompted this conclusion were derived from a retrospective study of postmortem protocols pertaining to 29 male psychotics and 62 male nonpsychotics who had "died within weeks of an acute infarction" at the Westminster Hospital in London, Ontario between 1949 and 1958. The 29 psychotics had been "certified to be mentally ill under the laws of the province of Ontario" and the 62 nonpsychotics had corresponded roughly to the male segment of the general hospital. However, in connection with his analysis of the postmortem findings pertaining to these two respective groups of decedents, Kavelman had not undertaken to separate those who had died suddenly from those whose deaths were not, in a strict sense, abrupt and unexpected. Thus, he had determined merely that whereas 4 of the 29 psychotics (14%) died because of a myocardial rupture, 12 of the 62 nonpsychotics (19%) had succumbed for the same reason.

It is equally noteworthy that Kavelman had not indicated the total number of sudden deaths among each of these two respective groups of patients; thus, he had been unable to compare adequately the frequency of myocardial rupture in relation to the incidence of sudden death in these two groups of decedents. Conceivably, if his computations had been confined to sudden death alone, he would have found that myocardial rupture had been a relatively more frequent cause of death in his sample of psychiatric patients who had suffered a fatal attack of acute myocardial infarction.

Moreover, it should be explained that Kavelman's data pertained only to patients who had been admitted to the hospital for treatment after an undesignated interval following the recognition that their illness was the result of an acute myocardial infarction. Thus, it is likely that inadvertently he had excluded from consideration not only those patients who had died suddenly before reaching the hospital but, even more particularly, those who had died suddenly because of an acute myocardial infarction alone or because of an acute myocardial infarction which had been followed by myocardial rupture. On the other hand, Kavelman's findings seem to imply that even though a sizeable number of psychiatric patients with acute myocardial infarction will die suddenly from a myocardial rupture, the frequency of sudden death from myocardial rupture should diminish in patients of this genre, provided appropriate treatment for the acute myocardial infarction is instituted promptly after its onset.

Observations made at the Coatesville Veterans Administration Hospital more than a decade ago[29] would seem to support such a hypothesis. The patient sample there consisted of a group of elderly psychotics with an electrocardiographically confirmed acute myocardial infarction. All but one of these patients had survived and the single fatality was the result of a myocardial rupture. However, it should be noted that with respect to these patients, the correct diagnosis was established very early in the course of the coronary-related illness and, as a consequence, there was a relatively short lag period between the onset of the myocardial infarction and their transfer to the medical service where they were promptly restricted to bed until the electrocardiographic and other laboratory findings had indicated satisfactory healing of the acute myocardial lesion.

Prevention

Perhaps, then, a diagnostic delay and, secondarily, a postponement of a program of enforced bed rest would explain the disproportionately high incidence of myocardial rupture in psychiatric patients which had been reported heretofore.

Thus, because acute myocardial infaction is the antecedent of acute myocardial rupture, it seems likely that a reduction in the mortality from acute myocardial rupture will be achieved in adults with psychiatric problems primarily when health professionals responsible for their care will come to realize that the classical features of acute myocardial infarction are observed only rarely in patients of this genre. It is therefore important to emphasize that the sudden appearance of any sign of physical discomfort in psychiatric patients or a sudden change in their behavior should prompt the attending physician to request, without unnecessary delay, those studies which can confirm or exclude the presence of an acute myocardial infarction.

Chest Pain as a Rare Symptom

Such a recommendation is especially germane inasmuch as it is a familiar experience that psychotics, unlike nonpsychotics, often will fail to complain of chest pain coincident with the onset of such a cardiac lesion; instead, they will develop other evidences of an acute intercurrent illness.

This aspect of acute myocardial infarction in hospitalized psychotics is discussed in some detail by Marchand in a paper which appeared in 1955.[22] His observations were confined to a patient sample consisting of 51 authenticated cases of acute myocardial infarction and a retrospective analysis of the clinical features in this group of psychotics at the Bedford, Massachusetts Veterans Administration Hospital showed that chest pain was the conspicuous symptom in only 7 instances (14%).

In 15 cases (30%) the leading manifestation was an episode of weakness, unsteadiness, or collapse and in 12 others (23%) the initial expression of the acute myocardial infarction was a sudden cardiac arrest. In the remainder, the symptomatic correlate was a sudden onset of dyspnea (4 cases); a sudden change in psychotic behavior (4 cases); an attack of vomiting or abdominal pain (3 cases).

Also in 1955, Lieberman[31] referred to experiences which coincided to some extent with those described by Marchand. In this report he mentioned that chest pain was a presenting symptom in only 3 of 56 hospitalized psychotics at the Northport New York Veterans Administration Hospital who had developed an acute myocardial infarction "confirmed either at autopsy or by unequivocal electrocardiographic tracings." He indicated also that in 4 of this sample of 56 psychotics with an acute myocardial infarction, a sudden change in the psychotic behavior was the clinical feature which often alerted the medical personnel at that institution to the possibility that the patient was developing an acute cardiac complication. Moreover, he noted an excessive mortality rate in these 56 psychotics (actually, 36 died but Lieberman did not indicate the number of these decedents whose demise was the result of a myocardial rupture). Included in his article was a description of the clinical course of one of the 56 patients who had survived the attack of acute myocardial infarction. Presumably, in this instance, the benign nature of the "attack" and the patient's recovery could be ascribed, at least in part, to the early detection of the myocardial lesion and therefore to the prompt institution of enforced bed rest.

Case Report. The patient in question was a 57-year-old man whose routine electrocardiograms in July of 1953 and in August of 1954 were normal. "On February 25, 1955, the psychiatric aid had observed that the patient suddenly became extremely quiet whereas prior to that date the patient had been delusional and, at times, hyperactive. Otherwise there was seemingly no significant change in the patient's condition. Coincident with this shift in behavior, his blood pressure was 155/85 and he did not complain of any discomfort. However, an electrocardiogram was requested immediately and this disclosed the presence of an acute anterolateral myocardial infarction. Accordingly, he was transferred without delay to the medical service where his ultimate recovery was unmarred by any complications."

In 1960, Sanen summarized the postmortem and clinical data pertaining to 50 psychotics at the Taunton Massachusetts State Hospital, whose deaths were related directly to a necropsy-confirmed acute myocardial infarction.[30] The ages of these decedents ranged from 53 to 93 years and the psychiatric diagnoses included chronic brain syndrome due to senile brain disease with psychosis (19 cases); chronic brain syndrome due to senile disease without psychosis (8 cases); schizophrenic reaction (9 cases); manic depressive psychosis (4 cases); involutional melancholia (2 cases); alcoholic psychosis (2 cases); paretic neurosyphilis (3 cases); miscellaneous mental disorders (3 cases).

Sanen did not indicate how many of these decedents had died suddenly but inasmuch as one had died of a myocardial rupture, 10 had developed "immediate shock," 2 had developed a "subsequent loss of consciousness" and 17 had "lapsed during the first 24 hours into pulmonary edema," it is likely that approximately 50% of these fatalities were sudden deaths. Nevertheless, prior to the time of death only four of these decedents had complained of chest pain. Among the remainder, 1 displayed fear of death, 2 complained of abdominal pain, and 14 developed one or more vomiting episodes.

Other manifestations included cyanosis (42 cases); breathlessness (36 cases); weak spells (32 cases); change in general behavior (32 cases); pallor (17 cases); orthopnea (17 cases); sweating (6 cases); singultus (6 cases); immediate drop in blood pressure (42 cases); low grade fever (21 cases). Moreover, in approximately one half of these decedents the physical examination of the heart had disclosed a cardiac arrhythmia, a gallop rhythm, or faint heart sounds.

Case Report. Sanen also described, in detail, the early symptoms and subsequent clinical course pertaining to one of his psychiatric patients who had developed a fatal attack of acute myocardial infarction; "the patient was a 58-year-old man with a diagnosis of the simple type of schizophrenia, who suddenly became cyanotic and gasped for air during the lunch hour in the cafeteria. The supervising aid rushed to the patient, surmising that he was suffocating from food lodged in his throat. The patient denied pain but remained in a state of respiratory difficulty and the ward physician also felt that there was an obstruction of the airway.

An immediate fluoroscopy was done but no foreign body was seen. Phys-

examination at the time revealed early pulmonary congestion, faint heart sounds, auricular fibrillation, and a blood pressure of 90/70. A tentative diagnosis of acute myocardial infarction was made. He was placed in an oxygen tent and digitalization was started. After a few hours he improved and was removed from the oxygen tent. When questioned at this time he again denied chest pain and requested that he be returned to his previous ward, claiming that he did not feel ill. The following night he was found dead in bed. A postmortem examination revealed severe coronary sclerosis with acute posterolateral myocardial infarction."

However, Marchand,[22] Lieberman,[31] and Sanen[30] have not been the only observers to comment on the infrequency of chest pain in psychiatric patients during an episode of acute myocardial infarction. Hussar, also, following his survey of patients with an acute myocardial infarction at the Montrose Veterans Administration Hospital noted that of "22 schizophrenic patients who suffered fatal fresh myocardial infarctions but did not die suddenly, the painless attack rate was 45%" and "of 20 schizophrenics who survived an attack of acute myocardial infarction, 50% were painless infarctions." Correspondingly, then, Hussar's data would seem to suggest that peri-infarction survivability among schizophrenics will not be determined by either the presence of such a symptom or its absence.

Moreover, in view of the observations of Marchand,[22] Lieberman,[31] and Sanen[30] already mentioned, it must be recognized that although it is customary to designate as a "silent" lesion any acute myocardial infarction unassociated with chest pain, it would be euphemistic to consider the usual athoracodynic acute myocardial infarction in psychiatric patients a truly "silent" entity, in a symptomatic sense. In this same connection, it should be noted also that although chest pain clearly occupies a relatively low position in the hierarchy of symptoms among psychiatric patients who have developed an acute myocardial infarction, there are not, as yet, any convincing data to indicate the extent to which this particular symptom is proportionately higher among members of the general population afflicted with a similar cardiac lesion. Thus, whereas Rosenman had noted that, in non-psychiatric persons, a "painless" acute myocardial infarction was almost never encountered,[32] Johnson et al had noted that "painlessness" was an attribute in 41% of 63 persons with this particular myocardial lesion.[33] Intermediate between these 2 extremes were the findings reported by others with respect to the prevalence of "painless" myocardial infarction in non-psychiatric groups of patients.[34-47]

PSEUDO-PNEUMONIC SYNDROME

However, it is recognized also that there are alternative symptoms which can be the clinical hallmark of an acute myocardial infarction. In this connection, Wendkos emphasized the presence of a "pseudo-pneumonic syndrome" in elderly psychotics which subsequently proved to be the predominant clinical feature associated with such an acute myocardial lesion.[29]

Manifestations

In these individuals, the first manifestations were a sudden development of pyrexia, cough, dyspnea, cyanosis, rales in the lungs, and disseminated pulmonary shadows in the teleoroentgenogram, and because of these findings, the illness at first was considered to be an acute pneumonic process. However, soon after these symptoms appeared, an electrocardiogram was obtained also and thereby the proper diagnosis was established. Correspondingly, it was evident that the respiratory symptoms and the radiologic findings were the result of discrete patches of pulmonary edema secondary to marginal "pump failure" incidental to the acute myocardial infarction and the fever in these instances was ascribed to the acute necrosis of the myocardium.

It is also noteworthy that with one exception, all the patients who exhibited this "cardio-pulmonary syndrome" made an uneventful recovery, presumably because, with the proper diagnosis having been made early, it was possible to institute, without delay, appropriate definitive treatment including enforced bed rest. Thus, such a favorable experience with respect to this group of elderly psychiatric patients would seem to confirm again how advisable it is to obtain, as soon as possible, a routine electrocardiogram whenever patients of this genre develop any type of acute illness regardless of the nature of its clinical manifestations.

Moreover, despite the current recognition that chest pain cannot be regarded as a reliable diagnostic clue with respect to acute myocardial infarction in psychiatric patients, it must be acknowledged that the "painlessness" of this entity in patients of this genre is a somewhat puzzling feature. However, it is uncertain whether there is as yet a satisfactory explanation for this aspect of coronary artery disease in psychiatric patients.

One hypothesis which has been advanced by Wolpert et al[48] would be to suppose that it was the treatment of the underlying psychiatric disorder which was responsible. Basically, it was their concept that the pain ordinarily associated with such a cardiac complication would not be likely to be perceived by patients of this genre if their appreciation of pain had been dulled already because of concurrent tranquilizer therapy. In addition, in accord with this premise, they postulated that a myocardial infarction in such patients would remain undetected not only during the acute phase of such a lesion but also later, when it had healed, unless periodic electrocardiograms would become a routine practice in institutions established for the care of the mentally ill.

ELECTROCARDIOGRAPHIC SURVEY

Thus, in order to test the validity of this hypothesis, Wolpert et al undertook an electrocardiographic survey of a large sample of psychiatric patients who, while receiving long-term phenothiazine therapy, had never developed, knowingly, an acute illness characterized by the sudden onset of chest pain. Altogether, they examined 1000 patients who seemed to be healthy except for the mental illness.

Patient Sample

The patient sample comprised both women and men; the ages ranged from 20 to 85 years. Most were chronic schizophrenics but a sizeable number also were suffering from the effects of a chronic brain syndrome.

Procedure

Each electrocardiographic study was made with the subject at rest and was evaluated by a cardiologist not directly associated with the study; in this way any possible bias with respect to the interpretation of these electrocardiograms was excluded. Afterward, when the electrocardiograms were diagnostic of a healed transmural myocardial infarction, the clinical charts of this "targeted" group of patients with an antecedent myocardial infarction were scrutinized very carefully.

The portions of these respective charts which were reviewed most closely were the ward and nursing notes. Special attention was paid to any mention of chest pain, dysrhythmia, shortness of breath, or other symptoms or signs suggestive of "cardiovascular involvement" prior to the time the electrocardiogram had been obtained. Also, the medical histories were thoroughly studied in order to establish the nature of any illnesses which preceded the admission of the patient to the hospital. Moreover, notations were made regarding the nature of the medications which had been administered during the hospitalization of those patients whose electrocardiograms "showed persistent unequivocal evidence of past infarctions."

Results

In this way, it was established that in only 2 of 324 surviving psychotics (0.6%) below the age of 50 years, there was unequivocal electrocardiographic evidence of an antecedent myocardial infarction whereas in 676 equally psychotic patients ranging in age from 50 to 85 years there were 24 such electrocardiographically determined myocardial lesions (3.5%). However, in the smaller patient sample (324 psychotics) the two healed infarcts could not be labeled a "silent" variety inasmuch as each was associated with either a past history of acute myocardial infarction or with some type of clinical manifestation ascribable to coronary artery disease.

On the other hand, with respect to the larger patient sample, comprising 676 patients it was found that 20 of the 24 electrocardiographically demonstrable healed myocardial infarctions properly could be classified as "silent" myocardial lesions, because, in these 20 instances, there was no recollection of any prior illness which would suggest an earlier attack of acute myocardial infarction and because the information in the clinical charts of these 20 patients did not indicate that the heart ever had been functionally impaired. Thus, in summary, the data disclosed by Wolpert's study have shown that, in their sample of 1000 surviving hospitalized psychotics, ranging in age from 20 to 85 years, the prevalence rate of "silent" myocardial infarction was 2% (20 cases).

The diagnostic categories, in psychiatric terms, with respect to the overall sample of 1000 subjects were not supplied, and so, the distribution of these 20 "silent" healed myocardial infarctions in relation to the nature of the underlying psychiatric disability could not be determined. However, their data did indicate that of the 20 "silent" healed myocardial infarcts, 12 were found in chronic schizophrenics, 4 in patients with a chronic brain syndrome due to chronic alcoholism and 4 in patients with a chronic brain syndrome associated with cerebral ateriosclerosis. Therefore, it is possible that the nature of the psychiatric handicaps in these respective 20 patients could account, in large part, for their inability to recall a previous illness which, at this onset, was characterized by the presence of chest pain of varying intensity.

This suggestion seems to be supported by the data in the recent article by Uretsky et al[47] concerning the prevalence of painless myocardial infarction in nonpsychiatric patients. In this publication, the authors explained that *typical* symptoms, even in cases of acute myocardial infarction are described with less frequency as persons become older and when their daily intake of alcohol, prior to the time of admission to the Coronary Care Unit, had exceeded 6 ounces of whiskey or other hard liquor.

Discussion

It is of interest that the observations of Uretsky et al[47] seem to agree with my published data[29] regarding the frequency and pathogenesis of the "pseudo-pneumonic syndrome" associated with acute myocardial infarction in elderly deteriorated schizophrenics. In this connection, it is noteworthy that Uretsky et al had found, likewise, that the older patients in their sample not only described atypical symptoms but also were more prone to develop "pneumonia" and "cardiogenic shock." Whereas my patients (with one exception) had made an uneventful recovery even though they had not been treated in a Coronary Care Unit, Uretsky et al had found that their older patients did not fare as well as the younger ones. Conceivably, this experience can be ascribed, at least in part, to the fact that, with respect to their older patients, there was a delay between the onset of their illness and the time they arrived at the unit where suitable treatment could be initiated.

It should be recognized, also, that despite the probable underestimation by Wolpert et al[48] of the incidence of healed myocardial infarctions disclosed in the course of their prospective investigation, their findings, at least, have made it clear that among any large sample of psychiatric patients, a sizeable number can be expected to be at "increased risk" of dying suddenly because of an underlying cardiac abnormality even though, prior to the time of death, its presence may have been unsuspected by either the patients or their attending physicians. The soundness of this view seems to have been confirmed by the results of the retrospective survey initiated by Hussar.[26] An analysis of such data, which were derived from a review of 1275 autopsy protocols submitted by a preselected group of neuropsychiatric facilities affiliated with the Veterans Administration, had indicated that there were 394 deaths in chronic schizophrenics which were ascribable to coronary heart disease and that 224 of this number (57%) could be categorized as sudden deaths. With respect to these 394 coronary related fatalities, the associated cardiac pathology was of an acute nature in 291 instances (77%). On the other hand, it was noteworthy that chronic pathology such as an old myocardial infarction was also present in the hearts of 216 of the 394 decedents (55%). Thus, since sudden deaths and a healed myocardial infarction were identified with almost equal frequency (57% and 55% respectively) in the 394 coronary-related deaths, it would seem correct to assume that the healed infarction had favored the occurrence of a sudden death in these instances.

Moreover, the demonstration by Hussar that, in chronic schizophrenics, the prospect of dying suddenly from a coronary-related illness is enhanced when a healed myocardial infarction already is present, is fully in accord with the observations of Wikland whose data pertained to coronary-related sudden deaths in a Scandinavian non-psychiatric population.[49] Correspondingly, then, a schizophrenic illness should not be regarded as an important "risk factor" with respect to either the pathogenesis of coronary arteriosclerosis or the occurrence of a coronary-related sudden death.

In addition, Hussar's postmortem data have been able to provide some insights regarding the frequency with which an acute myocardial infarct can be considered to be a "risk factor" in relation to the occurrence of sudden deaths in chronic schizophrenics. It will be recalled that his survey had demonstrated that of 224 coronary-related sudden deaths an acute myocardial infarction was present in 97 (43%); correspondingly, in relation to the 320 sudden deaths due to all sorts of "natural causes," an acute myocardial infarction was shown to be the proximate cause of death in 30%. Thus, as a precursor of sudden death, an acute myocardial infarction in his sample of chronic schizophrenics would seem to be approximately as important as it has been shown to be in nonpsychotic citizens of westernized societies.[7,9,12-14,50,49]

ARRHYTHMOGENIC CARDIAC ARREST: PATHOGENESIS

As far as can be determined, there are, aside from a catastrophic myocardial rupture, two main reasons an acute myocardial infarction represents an important "risk factor" in relation to the occurrence of a sudden death.

Cardiogenic Shock

Sometimes, as has been observed in both experimental animals[51,53] and in man[54-58,60] this type of lesion can be lethal when it induces an episode of cardiogenic shock (pump failure). In the human, the resulting hypotension exacerbates a marginal perfusion deficit through coronary arteries already stenosed by the atherosclerotic process and, as a consequence, there is a further deprivation of blood flow to the myocardium. This circumstance, then would render both the myocardial cells and conducting fibers of the heart even more hypoxic; concurrently, the internal environment of these structures would be altered thereby in a manner which would favor inhomogeneous dispersion of myocardial refractoriness.[59] At the same time, there would be functional changes with respect to automaticity in the Purkinje fibers[75-79] and impaired conduction through both the zone of acutely injured myocardium and the area of scar tissue in the region of any antecedent myocardial infarction, which may be present. The net effect, then, would be an increased firing of ectopic beats and their reentry through the ventricular myocardium.[68] Thus, in such a setting, there would exist all the elements which would favor the development of ventricular fibrillation and hence a sudden cardiac arrest.[68]

Excess Adrenomedullary Secretions

A contributory factor could be the reflex outpouring of adrenomedullary secretions,[65,66] a phenomenon which is known to constitute one of the responses to myocardial hypoxia accompanied by shock and hypotension. Undoubtedly, this brief description of the mechanisms involved does not provide a full explanation for the occurrence of such a lethal arrhythmia, but, in a monograph of this sort, there is no need for a more detailed discussion regarding pathogenesis during an episode of acute myocardial infarction with hypotension. If additional information is desired, there are excellent reviews and other publications concerned with the pathophysiology responsible for the occurrence of ventricular fibrillation.[68-72]

Other Mechanisms

The susceptibility of an acutely infarcted heart to an arrhythmogenic cardiac arrest even when it is unassociated with cardiogenic shock has been considered to be another reason a sudden death so often can be the sequel to an acute myonecrotic lesion in the heart. Moreover, this "vulnerability" to cardiac arrest in such a setting has been confirmed by experiences in coronary care units[73,74] and by suitable animal models.[61-63,75-77] In such instances a myocardial perfusion deficit would seem to play a lesser role in the initiation and maintenance of any ectopic activity. However, inasmuch as the infarction must represent a myocardial response directly or indirectly to a zonal type of myocardial hypoxia, the importance of this latter element in the genesis of an ectopic rhythm cannot be entirely dismissed.[77] Moreover, because inhomogeneous dispersion of refractoriness and impaired conduction characterize zones of acute myocardial injury,[79,64] it would be expected that such local tissue disturbances would tend to favor reentry of ectopic beats; the net effect, then, would be a level of "vulnerability" which would favor a cardiac arrest due to ventricular fibrillation.

It should be recognized also that, as in the case of an arrhythmogenic cardiac arrest related to the presence of cardiogenic shock, a contributory factor with respect to the genesis of ventricular fibrillation in persons with an acute myocardial infarction could be the adverse influence exerted by endogenously elaborated catecholamines on the marginally hypoxic and already disintegrated portion of the myocardium.[63,67,68,80-82,137-141]

However, in such instances, it could be the emotional response on the part of the infarcted patient toward his coronary-related illness,[81-84,120,123,124] as well as any shock-like state, which would be largely responsible for the sort of stimulation of the neuroendocrine apparatus apt to result in augmented release of pressor, "oxygen wasting" hormones such as epinephrine and norepinephrine.[127-128,111-113,119-120,123-125]

Emotional Stress

Considerations concerning the potentially lethal effects of "emotional stress" in persons confined to a coronary care unit because of an acute myocardial infarction have been discussed already in several publications[74,81,83,136] and, on the basis of such observations, it might be construed that, conversely, psychotics with such a cardiac lesion who are inherently apathetic may be less likely to die suddenly than nonpsychotics with the same condition.

Alternatively, it could be asked whether the acutely infarcted heart of an apathetic psychotic is not as "vulnerable" with respect to the development of an arrhythmogenic cardiac arrest than are psychiatric patients who before the occurrence of the myocardial infarction were in good contact with their surroundings. This sort of wording has been selected because, in current medical parlance, "increased vulnerability" of the heart to cardiac arrest implies that the threshold for the development of ventricular fibrillation has been appreciably lowered. Therefore, within such a context, this term has been invoked to describe the occurrence of any sudden cardioplegic ventricular arrhythmia.

With respect to the question regarding "vulnerability" of the heart and the severity of the psychiatric illness in terms of deterioration, it should be explained that there is not, as yet, sufficient evidence to indicate that the hearts of regressed psychiatric patients with coronary sclerosis and an acute myocardial infarction are indeed less "vulnerable" to cardiac arrest than their counterparts who, before the onset of a myocardial infarction, were less apathetic.

Nevertheless, my own observations[29] would seem to show that the prognosis is quite good when a regressed schizophrenic develops an acute myocardial infarction even when there is some degree of "pump failure" associated with such a cardiac lesion.

Summary

Moreover, inasmuch as it is known that an acute myocardial infarction frequently does not coincide with or precede a coronary-related sudden death,[7,11,14,85,86,15] numerous epidemiologic investigations have been undertaken in order to identify those "risk factors" which, seemingly, could enhance the likelihood of a cardiac arrest in the presence of chronic occlusive coronary artery disease. As a result of these efforts, a variety of such "risk factors" have been described. These include the presence of ventricular extrasystoles at rest or after exercise;[73,95-97] the numerous nonspychologic "risk factors" known to accelerate the process of coronary atherosclerosis[11,17,98,99,100,101] and a supposedly distinctive type of behavior.[102,126]

With regard to epidemiologic studies concerning the pathogenesis of sudden death related to atherosclerotic heart disease, the investigations of Wikland are particularly noteworthy.[8,49] His observations demonstrated that, in a large number of such incidents, a healed previous myocardial infarction seemed to be an important "risk factor" with respect to the occurrence of a sudden cardiac arrest among residents of one of the heavily populated cities in Sweden. Moreover, as far as he was able to determine, there were, frequently, no records in that community to indicate that the decedent either had been hospitalized or had been treated at home for a prior acute myocardial infarction; in addition, he observed that many of the decedents, prior to the time of death, had not complained of symptoms referrable to the heart.

ANGINA PECTORIS AS A RISK FACTOR

Thus, in view of the findings described separately by Wikland[49] and by Hussar[23,25,26] it would appear likely that, symptomatically, and in other respects, the mentally ill afflicted with arteriosclerotic vascular and myocardial disease need not be considered altogether different from adults in the general population who develop a sudden cardiac arrest linked to the presence of atherosclerotic coronary artery disease. On the other hand, Hussar's observations would imply that, in terms of the incidence of anginal prodromes in cases of sudden death due to atherosclerotic coronary artery disease, chronic schizophrenics are strikingly unlike nonpsychotics. Correspondingly, whereas it has been noted repeatedly that recurrent attacks of angina pectoris can precede the occurrence of coronary-related sudden deaths in the general population[103] Hussar stated that "a pre-infarction anginal syndrome was recorded only once in the 343 autopsied protocols containing clinical summaries of patients who died in coronary disease."

However, inasmuch as it is known that when they are diligently sought, anginal manifestations can be found to be present not uncommonly in psychotics with coronary arteriosclerosis, it is conceivable that Hussar's assertion was principally the result of a methodologic shortcoming inherent in his study rather than the result of a correct evaluation of the place of angina pectoris as a "risk factor" in relation to the coronary-related sudden deaths he had reviewed. As was evident, any statements Hussar had made with regard to anginal prodromes were based entirely on information submitted to him by the 29 Veterans Administration Hospitals participating in the study and, so, it should be clear that his conclusions depended on the quality and reliability of the anamnestic data he had received from such sources.

It would be important to know what criteria were employed by the interviewers who had excluded an anginal syndrome when the decedents had been interrogated prior to the time of death. If, for example, these interrogators had concentrated exclusively on the presence of chest pain following exertion in order to confirm a diagnosis of angina pectoris, it is likely that such a data gathering process alone could account for the almost total absence of anginal prodromes recorded in the charts of these decedents.

Experiences with psychotic anginal patients have indicated repeatedly that although they are not inclined to volunteer such a history, it can be demonstrated by other means that a diagnosis of "coronary insufficiency" is justified.[24] Actually, such a circumstance should not be a source of wonder, particularly since there are data to indicate that the development of an acute myocardial infarction may be unassociated with chest pain both in psychotics[22,31-42] and in those without a psychiatric handicap.[35-42]

Moreover, although chest pain may not be a conspicuous symptom in psychotics with angina pectoris, they may complain of a variety of other symptoms such as weakness, faintness, sweating, shortness of breath, or a tightness in the throat or arm during periods of increased physical activity. In addition, it has been observed that anger—even when this emotion is repressed—can "trigger" the appearance of one or more of such ischemogenic symptoms,[109] and it has been demonstrated by Lown et al[110] that repressed hostility may be responsible for recurrent episodes of life threatening ventricular tachyarrhythmias even in the absence of occlusive coronary artery disease.

Conceivably, then, overwhelming anger at the unconscious level might explain the occurrence, even during sleep, of a coronary-related sudden death in certain psychiatric patients whose extramural or intramural coronary arteries were or were not already stenosed.[121] The basis for this suggestion is the knowledge that when animals are mobilized for a fight, there is an outpouring of excessive quantities of adrenal medullary hormones[111,123] and the supposition that a comparable type of response would be produced by overt or repressed anger in man.[122-124,127-128] Thus, the net effect resulting from such a disturbance of affect when the myocardium is already marginally hypoxic because of coronary narrowing might be an arrhythmogenic cardiac arrest.

In this same connection, it is noteworthy that my analysis of the data published by Bogdanoff et al[112] has indicated that the production of anger in samples of normal adults was followed by an even greater heart rate-systolic blood pressure product than that resulting from induced anxiety. Thus, inasmuch as such data would seem to indicate that myocardial oxygen consumption is substantially increased by the development of emotional impulses in which anger is a major participant,[94] it is reasonable to suppose that when there are segmental occlusions in the extramural branches of the coronary circulation, augmented levels of underlying hostility could represent a meaningful "risk factor" with respect to the development of an arrhythmogenic cardiac arrest. Moreover, this view would seem to be supported by those experimental studies and clinical observations which repeatedly have demonstrated that increased catecholamine "traffic" along the neural pathways to the heart can lower, materially, the ventricular fibrillation threshold.[113]

Drug Effects

Coordinately, it has been observed that in adults with occlusive coronary artery disease, an injection of epinephrine often provoked a typical anginal episode[114] and, correspondingly, it has been noted that an infusion of isoproterenol frequently will be followed by the appearance of "typical ischemic" changes in the electrocardiograms of patients with angina pectoris.[115] Conversely, there is now a substantial body of data to indicate that the daily consumption of a preparation which blocks the beta-adrenoreceptors in the heart can reduce dramatically the severity of anginal symptoms in persons afflicted with arteriosclerotic heart disease.[116]

CATECHOLAMINES—CONCLUSIONS

Moreover, inasmuch as many observations implicitly emphasize the degree to which catecholamines can adversely affect the longevity of persons with chronic stenosing lesions involving the extramural coronary arteries, it is conceivable that the psychiatric patient with coronary arteriosclerosis is at increased risk of dying suddenly if high levels of hostility remain, persistently, an important part of his emotional disorder. Thus, within such a context, "Behavior Pattern A" which has been identified not only with the development of atherosclerotic coronary artery disease but also with its various clinical manifestations[102] actually might be linked, in large measure, to hostile elements within the emotional mosaic commonly termed the personality of man. Correspondingly, inasmuch as this type of behavioral manifestation, in some people, is perceived by Friedman, as well, to be an external counterpart of underlying hostility[126] and since the autonomic response to this sort of emotional infrastructure could be adrenergic augmentation[123] it is understandable why current efforts to prevent a sudden death at some later date in either anginal or post-infarction patients have emphasized the prospective benefits from long-term therapy with drugs which block the circulatory effects of beta adrenergic stimulation.[117,118]

REFERENCE

1. Helpern, M. and Robson, S.M. Sudden and unexpected natural deaths; general considerations and statistics. *N.Y. J. Med.* 45:1197 (1945).
2. Epstein, F.H. The epidemiology of coronary heart disease: a review. *J. Chronic Dis.* 18:735 (1965).
3. Kuller, L. Sudden and unexpected non-traumatic deaths in adults: A review of epidemiological and clinical studies. *J. Chronic Dis.* 19:1165 (1966).
4. Kuller, L. et al. An epidemiologic study of sudden and unexpected deaths in adults. *J. Medicine* 46:341 (1967).
5. Burch, G.E. and De Pasquale, N.P. Sudden unexpected natural deaths. *Am. J. Med. Sci.* 249:86 (1965).
6. Pruitt, R.D. On sudden death. *Am. Heart J.* 68:111 (1964).
7. Myerburg, R.J. and Davis, J.H. The medical ecology of public safety I: Sudden Death Due to Coronary Heart Disease. *Am. Heart J.* 68:586 (1964).
8. Wikland, B. Death from arteriosclerotic heart disease outside hospitals. *Acta Med. Scand.* 184:129 (1968).
9. Biorck, G. et al. Studies on myocardial infarction in Malmo, 1935 to 1954: Morbidity and mortality in a hospital material. *Acta Med. Scand.* 159:253 (1957).
10. Bainton, C.R. and Peterson, D.R. Deaths from coronary heart disease in persons 50 years of age and younger: A community-wide study. *New Eng. J. Med.* 269:569 (1963).
11. Vedin, J.A. Sudden death: Identification of high-risk groups. *Am. Heart J.* 86:124 (1973).
12. Vedin, J.A. et al. Mortality trends in Sweden 1951-1968 with special reference to cardiovascular causes of death. *Acta Med. Scand.* 515:76 (1971).
13. White, P.D. et al. A note on the discussion of non-traumatic sudden daths by American and Soviet cardiologists in Moscow in May 1961. *Am. Heart J.* 64:842 (1962).
14. Spain, D.M. et al. Coronary atherosclerosis as a cause of unexpected and unexplained death: An autopsy study from 1949-1959. *J.A.M.A.* 174-384 (1960).
15. Adelson, L. Sudden death from coronary disease: The cardiac conundrum. *Postgrad. Med.* 30:139 (1961).
16. Goldstein, S. *Sudden Death and Coronary Heart Disease.* Futura Publishers, Mt. Kisco, New York (1974).
17. Gordon, T. and Kannel, W.B. Premature mortality from coronary heart disease: The Framingham Study. *J.A.M.A.* 215:1617 (1971).
18. Anderson, T.W. and Le Riche, W.H. Ischemic heart disease and sudden death. 1901-1961. *B.J. Prev. Soc. Med.* 24:1 (1970).
19. Moritz, A.R. and Zamcheck, N. Sudden and unexpected deaths of young soldiers: Diseases responsibile for sudden deaths during World War II. *Arch. Path.* 42:459 (1946).
20. Yater, W.N. et al. Comparison of clinical and pathologic aspects of coronary artery disease in men of various age groups: A study of 950 autopsied cases from the Armed Forces Institute of Pathology. *Ann. Int. Med.* 34:352 (1951).

21. French, A.J. and Dock, W. Fatal coronary arteriosclerosis in young soldiers. *J.A.M.A.* 124:1233 (1944).
22. Marchand, W.E. Occurrence of painless myocardial infarction in psychotic patients. *New Eng. J. Med.* 253: 51 (1955).
23. Hussar, A.E. Effect of tranquillizers on medical morbidity and mortality in mental hospitals. *J.A.M.A.* 179:682 (1962).
24. Wendkos, M.H. (Unpublished data).
25. Hussar, A.E. Coronary disease in chronic schizophrenic patients: Clinico-pathologic study. *Circulation* 31:919 (1965).
26. Hussar, A.E. Leading causes of death in institutionalized chronic schizoprenic patients: A study of 1275 autopsied protocols. *J. Nerv. Ment. Dis.* 142:45 (1966).
27. Jetter, W.W. and White, P.D. Rupture of the heart in patients in mental institutions. *Ann. Int. Med.* 21:783 (1944).
28. Kavelman, D.A. Myocardial Rupture: A study of non-psychotic and psychotic patients. *Can. M.A.J.* 82:1105 (1960).
29. Wendkos, M.H. The recognition of acute myocardial infarction in the deteriorated elderly psychotic. *J. Am. Geriatrics Soc.* 11:511 (1963).
30. Sanen, F-J. Psychotic and senile patients with ischemic heart disease. *Geriatrics* 15:449 (1960).
31. Lieberman, A.L. Painless myocardial infarction in psychotic patients. *Geriatrics.* 10:579 (1955).
32. Rosenman, M.D. Painless myocardial infarction: A review of the literature and analysis of 220 cases. *Ann. Int. Med.* 41:1 (1954).
33. Johnson, W.J. et al. Unrecognized myocardial infarction. A Clinico-pathologic study. *Arch. Int. Med.* 103:253 (1959).
34. Margolis, J.R. et al. Clinical features of unrecognized myocardial infarction: Silent and asymptomatic. *Am. J. Cardiol.* 32:1 (1973).
35. Lindberg, H.A. et al. Totally asymptomatic myocardial infarction: An estimate of its incidence in the living population. *Arch. Int. Med.* 106:628 (1960).
36. Medalie, J.H. and Goldbourt, U. Unrecognized myocardial infarction: Five-year incidence, mortality, and risk factors. *Ann. Int Med.* 84:526 (1976).
37. Cohn, P.F. Severe asymptomatic coronary artery disease: A diagnostic, prognostic, and therapeutic puzzle. *Am. J. Med.* 62:565 (1977).
38. Babey, A.M. Painless acute infarction of the heart. *New Eng. J. Med.* 220:410 (1939).
39. Warner, H.R. Painless myocardial infarction. *Minn. Med.* 34:49 (1951).
40. Bruenn, H.G. et al. Notes on cardiac pain in coronary disease; Correlation of observations made during life with structural changes found at autopsy in 476 cases. *Am. Heart J.* 11:34 (1936).
41. Stokes, J. and Dauber, T.R. The "Silent Coronary": The frequency and clinical characteristics of unrecognized myocardial infarction in The Framingham Study. *Ann. Int. Med.* 50:1359 (1959).
42. Olin, H.S. and Hackett, T.P. The denial of chest pain in 32 patients with acute myocardial infarction. *J.A.M.A.* 190: 977 (1964).
43. Kennedy, J.A. The incidence of myocardial infarction without pain in autopsied cases. *Am. Heart J.* 14:703 (1937).
44. Rosenman, R.H. et al. Clinically unrecognized myocardial infarction in the Western Group Study. *Am. J. Cardiol.* 19:776 (1967).
45. Pollard, H.M. and Harvill, T.H. Painless myocardial infarction. *Am. J. Med. Sci.* 199:628 (1940).
46. Stroud, W.D. and Wagner, J.A. Silent or atypical coronary occlusion. *Ann. Int. Med.* 15:25 (1941).

47. Uretsky, B.F. et al. Symptomatic myocardial infarction without chest pain: Prevalence and clinical course. *Am. J. Cardiol.* 40:498 (1977).
48. Wolpert, A. et al. Silent myocardial infarction in a chronic psychotic population. *Dis. Nerv. Sys.* 32:280 (1971).
49. Wikland, B. Medically unattended fatal cases of ischemic heart disease in a defined population. *Acta Med. Scand.* (Suppl.) 524 (1971).
50. Fulton, M. et al. Sudden death and myocardial infarction. *Circulation* (Suppl. 4) 40:182 (1969).
51. Epstein, S.E. et al. Experimental acute myocardial infarction: Characterization and treatment of the malignant premature ventricular contraction. *Circulation* 47:466 (1973).
52. Braunwald, E. et al. Effects of drugs and of counterpulsation on myocardial oxygen consumption: Observations on the ischemic heart. *Circulation* (Suppl. 4) 39:220 (1969).
53. Libby, P. et al. The effects of practolol in the extent of myocardial ischemic injury following experimental coronary occlusion and its effects on ventricular function in normal and ischemic heart. *Cardiovasc. Res.* 7:167 (1973).
54. Hamosh, P. and Cohn, J.N. Left ventricular function in acute myocardial infarction. *J. Clin. Invest.* 50:523 (1971).
55. Wolk, M.J. et al. Heart failure complicating acute myocardial infarction. *Circulation* 45:1125 (1972).
56. Weber, K.T. et al. Left ventricular dysfunction following acute myocardial infarction: A clinico-pathologic and hemodynamic profile of shock and failure. *Am. J. Med.* 54:697 (1973).
57. Lassers, B.W. et al. Left ventricular failure in acute myocardial infarction. *Am. J. Cardiol.* 25:511 (1970).
58. Resnekov, L. Hemodynamic effects of acute myocardial infarction. *Med. Clin. North Am.* 57:243 (1973).
59. Han, J. Mechanisms of ventricular arrhythmias associated with myocardial infarction. *Am. J. Cardiol.* 24:800 (1969).
60. Walston, A. et al. Acute coronary occlusion and the "power failure" syndrome. *Am. Heart J.* 79:613 (1970).
61. Maling, H.M. and Moran, N.C. Ventricular arrhythmias induced by sympathomimetic amines in unanesthetized dogs following coronary artery occlusion. *Circ. Res.* 5:409 (1957).
62. Myers, R.W. et al. Beneficial effects of vagal stimulation and bradycardia during experimental acute myocardial ischemia *Circulation* 49:943 (1974).
63. Han, J. Adrenergic effects on ventricular vulnerability. *Circ. Res.* 14:516 (1964).
64. Wit, A.L. and Bigger, J.T. Possible electrophysiologic mechanisms involved in ventricular fibrillation. *Circulation* 51, 52 (Suppl. III) III-120; III-130 (1975).
65. Richardson, J.A. et al. Circulating epinephrine and norepinephrine in coronary occlusion. *Am. J. Cardiol.* 5:613 (1960).
66. Malliani, A. et al. A sympathetic reflex elicited by experimental coronary occlusion. *Am. J. Physiol.* 217:703 (1969).
67. Daggett, W.M. and Wallace, A.G. Vagal and sympathetic influences on ectopic impulse formation. In: *Mechanism and Therapy of Cardiac Arrhythmias*, L. Dreifus, W. Likoff, and J. Moyer, eds. Grune and Stratton, New York, p. 64 (1966).
68. Moe, G.K. et al. Factors responsible for the initiation and maintenance of ventricular fibrillation. In: *Sudden Cardiac Death*, B. Surawicz and E.D. Pellegrino, eds. Grune and Stratton, New York, p. 56 (1964).
69. Cranefield, P.F. Ventricular fibrillation. *New Eng. J. Med.* 289:732 (1973).
70. Hoffman, B.F. and Cranefield, P.F. The physiologic basis of cardiac arrhythmias. *Am. J. Med.* 37:670 (1964).

71. Cranefield, P.F. et al. Genesis of cardiac arrhythmias. *Circulation* 47:190 (1973).
72. Surawicz, B. Ventricular fibrillation. *Am. J. Cardiol.* 28:268 (1971).
73. Lown, B. and Wolf, M. Approaches to sudden death from coronary heart disease. *Circulation* 44:130 (1971).
74. Killip, T. Arrhythmia, sudden death, and coronary artery disease. *Am. J. Cardiol.* 28:614 (1971).
75. Han, J. Ventricular vulnerability during an acute coronary occlusion. *Am. J. Cardiol.* 24:857 (1969).
76. Waldo, A.L. and Kaiser, G.A. A study of ventricular arrhythmias associated with acute myocardial infarction in the canine heart. *Circulation* 47:1222 (1973).
77. Rogers, R.M. Vulnerability of canine ventricles to fibrillation during hypoxia and respiratory acidosis. *Chest* 63:986 (1973).
78. Schamroth, L. Genesis and evolution of ectopic ventricular rhythms. *Brit. Heart J.* 28:244 (1966).
79. Han, J. and Moe, G.K. Non-uniform recovery of excitability in ventricular muscle. *Circ. Res.* 14:44 (1964).
80. Kliks, B.R. et al. The influence of sympathetic tone on ventricular fibrillation threshold during experimental coronary occlusion. *Circulation* (Suppl. 2) 46:115 (1972).
81. Lown, B. Psychologic stress and threshold for repetitive ventricular response. *Science* 182:834 (1973).
82. Verrier, R.L. et al. Ventricular vulnerability during sympathetic stimulation: Role of heart rate and blood pressure. *Cardiovasc. Res.* 8:602 (1974).
83. Hackett, T.P. et al. Coronary care unit: An appraisal of its psychologic hazards. *New Eng. J. Med.* 279:1365 (1968).
84. Cassem, N.H. et al. Reactions of coronary patients to the CCU nurse. *Am. J. Nursing* 70:319 (1970).
85. Spain, D. Coronary atheromatous disease: Clinical and pathologic correlations. *Cardiovasc. Clin.* 4:No. 2: 53 (Ed. by A. Brest) F.A. Davis Company, Philadelphia, (1972).
86. Titus, J.L. et al. Sudden unexpected death as the initial manifestation of coronary heart disease: Clinical and pathologic observations. *Singapore Med. J.* 14:291 (1973).
87. Friedman, M. et al. Instantaneous and sudden deaths: Clinical and pathological differentiation in coronary artery disease. *J.A.M.A.* 225:1319 (1973).
88. Sakaibara, S. et al. An elevation of ventricular fibrillation threshold after surgical resection of infarcted myocardium. *Am. Heart J.* 74:381 (1967).
89. Page, D.L. et al. Myocardial changes associated with cardiogenic shock. *New Eng. J. Med.* 285:133 (1971).
90. Braunwald, E. and Maroko, P.R. The reduction of infarct size—an idea whose time for testing has come. *Circulation* 50:206 (1974).
91. Wolf, S. Emotions and the autonomic nervous system. *Arch. Int. Med.* 126:1024 (1970).
92. Henry, J.P. et al. Mental factors and cardiovascular disease: Psychosocial factors facilitating and inhibiting the influence of the neuroendocrine alarm responses upon the course of cardiovascular disease. *Psychiatr. Annals* 2:25 (1972).
93. Raab, W. et al. Sympathogenic origin and anti-adrenergic prevention of stress-induced myocardial lesions. *Am. J. Cardiol.* 8:203 (1961).
94. Raab, W. et al. Catecholamine-induced myocardial hypoxia in the presence of impaired coronary dilatability independent of external cardiac work. *Am. J. Cardiol.* 9:455 (1962).
95. Kotler, M.H. et al. Prognostic significance of ventricular ectopic beats with respect to sudden death in the late post-infarction period. *Circulation* 47:959 (1973).
96. Vismara, L.A. et al. Relation of ventricular arrhythmias in the late hospital phase of acute myocardial infarction to sudden death after hospital discharge. *Am. J. Med.* 59:6 (1975).

97. Chiang, B.W. et al. Relationship of premature systoles to coronary heart disease and sudden death in the Tecumseh Epidemiologic Study. *Ann. Int. Med.* 70:1159 (1969).
98. Epstein, F.H. Risk factors in coronary heart disease: Environmental and hereditary influences. *Israel J. Med. Sci.* 3:594 (1967).
99. Wilhelmsen, L. et al. Multivariate analysis of risk factors for coronary heart disease. *Circulation* 48:950 (1973).
100. Kannel, W.B. et al. Precursors of sudden coronary death: Factors related to the incidence of sudden death. *Circulation* 51:606 (1975).
101. Tibblin, G. et al. Risk Factors for myocardial infarction and deaths due to ischemic heart disease and other causes. *Am. J. Cardiol.* 35:514 (1975).
102. Friedman, M. and Rosenman, R.H. Association of specific overt behavior pattern with blood and cardiovascular findings: Blood cholesterol level, blood clotting time, incidence of arcus senilis and clinical coronary artery disease. *J.A.M.A.* 169:1286 (1959).
103. Reeves, T.J. et al. Natural history of angina pectoris. *Am. J. Cardiol.* 33:423 (1974).
104. Medalie, J.H. et al. Angina pectoris among 1000 men. *Am. J. Med.* 55:583 (1973).
105. Fulton, M. et al. Natural history of unstable angina. *Lancet* 1:860 (1972).
106. Wendkos, M.H. The anti-anginal effect of rapidly acting nitrates in subjects with ergot-induced angina. *Am. J. Med. Sci.* 253:39 (1967).
107. Kannel, W.B. The unrecognized myocardial infarction: 14 year follow-up experience in The Framingham Study. *Geriatrics* 25:75 (1970).
108. Brickner, R.M. Unexpected effect of rage on anginal pain. *Psychosom. Med.* 14:468 (1952).
109. Wendkos, M.H. and Wolff, K. Emotional correlates of angina pectoris, *J. Am. Geriatrics Soc.* 16:845 (1968).
110. Lown, B. et al. Basis for recurring ventricular fibrillation in the absence of coronary heart disease and its management. *New Eng. J. Med.* 294:623 (1976).
111. Russek, H.I. and Russek, L.G. Is emotional stress an etiologic factor in coronary heart disease? *Psychosomatics* 17:63 (1976).
112. Bogdonoff, M.D. et al. Cardiovascular responses in experimentally induced alterations of affect. *Circulation* 20:353 (1959).
113. Levitt, B. et al. Role of the nervous system in the genesis of cardiac rhythm disorders. *Am. J. Cardiol.* 37:1111 (1976).
114. Levine, S.A. *Clinical Heart Disease*, ed. 3. W.B. Saunders Co. Philadelphia (1948).
115. Krasnow, N. et al. Isoproterenol and cardiovascular performance. *Am. J. Med.* 37:514 (1964).
116. Warren, S.G. et al. Long-term propranolol therapy for angina pectoris. *Am. J. Cardiol.* 37:420 (1976).
117. Green, K.G. et al. Improvement in prognosis and myocardial infarction by long-term beta adrenoreceptor blockade using practolol: A multicenter international study. *Brit. Med. J.* 3:735 (1970).
118. Ross, J. Beta adrenergic blockade for prophylaxis against recurrent myocardial infarction and sudden death. *Ann. Int. Med.* 84:486 (1976).
119. Bergamaschi, M. et al. The role of beta adrenoceptors in the coronary and systemic hemodynamic responses to emotional stress in conscious dogs. *Am. Heart J.* 86:216 (1973).
120. Klein, R.F. et al. Emotional adjustment and catecholamine excretion during early recovery from myocardial infarction. *J. Psychosom. Res.* 18:425 (1974).
121. King, M.J. et al. Variant angina associated with angiographically demonstrated coronary artery spasm and REM sleep. *Am. J. Med. Sci.* 265:419 (1973).
122. Ax, A.F. The physiologic differentiation between fear and anger in humans. *Psychosom. Med.* 15:433 (1953).
123. Andrus, E.C. Emotional factors and cardiac function. *Biol. Psychiat.* 10:581 (1975).

124. Nestel, P.J. et al. Catecholamine secretion and sympathetic nervous system responses to emotion in man with and without angina pectoris. *Am. Heart J.* 73:227 (1967).
125. Von Euler, U.S. Quantitation of stress by catecholamine analysis. *Clin. Pharmacol. Therap.* 5:398 (1964).
126. Friedman, M. Modifying type-A behavior in heart attack patients. *Primary Cardiology* :9 (1978).
127. Eimadjian, F. et al. Excretion of epinephrine and norepinephrine in various emotional states. *J. Clin. Endocrinol.* 17:608 (1957).
128. Levi, L. The urinary output of adrenalin and noradrenalin during experimentally-induced emotional stress in clinically different groups. *Acta Psychotherap.* 11:218 (1963).
129. Friedberg, C.K. *Disease of the Heart*, ed. 3. Saunders. (1966).
130. Bates, R.J. et al. Cardiac rupture—challenge in diagnosis and management. *Am. J. Cardiol.* 40:429 (1977).
131. Zeman, F. and Rodstein, M. Cadiac rupture complicating myocardial infarction in the aged. *Arch. Int. Med.* 105:431 (1960).
132. Sigiura, M. at al. A clinico-pathological study on the cardiac rupture following myocardial infarction in the aged. *Jap. Heart J.* 9:265 (1968).
133. Mitchell, J.R.A. and Parish, D.J. Rupture of the heart. *Brit. Med. J.* 2:1626 (1960).
134. Friedman, S. and White, P.D. Rupture of the heart in myocardial infarction. *Ann. Int. Med.* 21:778 (1944).
135. Oblath, R.W. et al. Factors influencing rupture of the heart after myocardial infarction. *J.A.M.A.* 149:1276 (1952).
136. Nixon, P.G.F. et al. A sleep regimen for acute myocardial infarction. *Lancet* 1:726 (1968).
137. Han, J. et al. Adrenergic effects on ventricular vulnerability. *Circ. Res.* 14:516 (1964).
138. Hageman, G.R. et al. Cardiac dysrhythmias induced by autonomic nerve stimulation. *Am. J. Cardiol.* 32:823 (1973).
139. Vassalle, M. et al. On the sympathetic control of ventricular automaticity, the effects of stellate ganglion stimulation. *Circ. Res.* 23:249 (1968).
140. Maling, H.M. and Moran, N.C. Ventricular arrhythmias induced by sympathomimetic amines in unanesthetized dogs following coronary artery occlusion. *Circ. Res.* 5:409 (1957).
141. Harris, A.S. et al. The induction of arrhythmias by sympathetic activity before and after occlusion of a coronary artery in the canine heart. *J. Electrocardiol.* 4:34 (1971).

CHAPTER 4

Alcohol Abuse

Statistics regarding the mortality of alcohol addicts in westernized societies have clearly confirmed that, in general, those persons who belong to this subset of the population do not survive as long as non-alcholics.[1,2] However, there is also a meaningful body of data to indicate that the lives of alcoholics do not end abruptly solely because of vehicular or other types of accidents; actually, such data have shown that many alcholics die suddenly from "natural causes" as well.[3]

ALCOHOL-INDUCED FATTY LIVER SYNDROME

Most such fatalities have been found to be linked to alcoholic fatty liver disease, alcoholic myocardiopathy, and atherosclerotic coronary artery disease. Moreover, as far as can be determined, alcoholic fatty liver disease is the single medical complication which is both the result of an excessive consumption of alcoholic beverages and, at the same time, a leading cause of sudden death in alcoholics.

In the United States, the first investigator to clearly establish the importance of the alcohol-induced fatty liver syndrome as a cause of sudden death in alcoholics was Graham,[4] whose postmortem findings were described in 1944; however, the investigations of Kuller, reported between 1966 and 1972,[5,6] even more firmly drew attention to this relationship in persons of this genre. In his article, Graham described the clinical and post-mortem findings pertaining to 11 alcoholics in the Baltimore area, whose sudden deaths clearly were not the result of occlusive coronary artery disease. The anamnestic data pertaining to these decedents had indicated that up to the time of death they had been dipsomaniacs for several years and had not manifested any evidences of a serious illness other than unexplained syncopal attacks or convulsive episodes before the aprupt life-ending episode had occurred. However, detailed information with respect to only five of such decedents had been provided.

Postmortem Findings

Nevertheless, in these 11 instances, it was evident that the obvious pathologic substrate for the sudden death was a grossly enlarged and fatty liver; information regarding the respective weights of this organ was supplied in only five instances. Thus, Graham had observed that the heaviest of these five livers weighed 4000 gm whereas, in the remaining four livers, the average weight was 2680 gm and the lowest weight was 2350 gm. Microscopically, the only noteworthy finding in these livers was a marked degree of fatty metamorphosis within the hepatocytes.

It also was noted that the coronary arteries, in each instance, were remarkably free of atheromatous change; it should be explained, however, that the respective ages of these decedents were 27, 32, 34, 38, and 40 years. Another impressive autopsy finding with regard to these decedents was the absence of pulmonary edema or any other evidence of congestive failure; thus, it would be proper to surmise that the deaths of these five alcoholics were instantaneous.

Epidemiologic Surveys

The publications of Kuller[5,6] discussed the results of a much more extensive review of sudden deaths among alcoholics but the data he had studied were the findings derived from retrospective epidemiologic surveys conducted during 1964-1965 and again during 1970-1971 in and immediately around the Baltimore area.

Method

The methodology employed by him entailed an examination of the files in the Baltimore city and Maryland state health departments, a review of medical examiners reports, hospital records, and autopsy findings with respect to such decedents as well as the collection of anamnestic data which could indicate whether the decedents had been habitual consumers of alcohol prior to the time of death.

Samples

However, even though the samples of decedents before 1969 and after 1969 were identical in demographic and geographical terms there was one evident difference between them: the survey of sudden deaths during 1964-1965 was limited to fatalities in alcoholics 20-39 years of age whereas during 1970-1971 it pertained to sudden deaths in alcoholics 20-64 years of age. For this reason, the most meaningful observations which emerged from these epidemiologic studies seemed to be those which demonstrated the differences between these two respective samples of known alcoholics, when they were compared in terms of the numbers who had died suddenly either from alcoholic fatty liver disease or from atherosclerotic coronary artery disease.

Results

Actually, when the data pertaining to sudden deaths ascribable to only these two causes were examined, it was found that the total was 50 during the consecutive 12-months period in 1964-1965, whereas there were 296 during the consecutive 10-months period beginning in June 1970. Moreover, among the 50 sudden deaths during 1964 to 1965 there were 28 (58%) which were ascribable to alcoholic fatty liver disease and there were 22 (42%) which were the result of ischemic heart disease; by contrast, among the 296 sudden deaths during 1970-1971 there were 240 resulting from atherosclerotic coronary artery disease (81%) and 56 (19%) which were ascribable to the presence of steatosis of the liver.

Conclusions

It would seem correct to conclude that when an alcoholic dies suddenly from "natural causes" before the age of 40 years, such a fatality would be expected to result, for the most part, from the ill effects of alcohol-induced fatty changes in the liver, whereas the more usual cause of sudden death in older alcoholics is arteriosclerotic coronary artery disease. Nevertheless, these data would imply that when age considerations are disregarded, approximately one fifth of any large undifferentiated sample of urban alcoholics still can be expected to die suddenly as the result of alcoholic fatty liver disease.

Another interesting aspect of Kuller's investigations was his observation that a sudden death associated with fatty liver disease was not an event particularly likely to affect alcoholics who were heavily intoxicated. The evidence he cited in support of this view was of a dual nature: It was noted by him, first, that the blood alcohol levels were not excessive at the time the autopsies of such decedents were performed and, second, that the anamnestic data he had collected clearly indicated that the terminal collapse of these decedents had not occurred at the height of an alcoholic spree but, instead, only some days afterward.

Ethnic differences in alcohol sensitivity. In addition, my analysis of the data Kuller had reported in 1966[5] showed that of the 28 sudden deaths ascribable to a fatty liver, 16 (57%) occurred in men and 12 (43%) occurred in women. However, regardless of the sex of the decedents, 75% of these fatalities occurred in blacks. Thus, of the 16 men, 12 (75%) were black; again, of the 12 women, 9 (75%) were black.

Conceivably, these findings could be related to an ethnic difference in alcohol sensitivity[7] but it must be recognized also that such a racial difference in connection with sudden deaths as they related to alcoholic lipodystrophy of the liver could be dependent on other "risk factors" as well. These factors might include the nature of the alcoholic beverages which the blacks and the whites customarily had consumed during their respective lifetimes, as well as the differences between their nutritional habits. However, data pertaining to these characteristics were not provided. Moreover, it would have been important to exclude differences in duration of the drinking habit in these two racial groups, but Kuller discarded the information he had collected concerning this variable because he felt it to be insufficiently reliable.

Regardless of such considerations, it is an established fact that a sudden death in alcoholics often can be traced to a fatty liver or to coronary arteriosclerosis. However, relatively little data exists regarding the relative prevalence of these respective entities in surviving alcoholics. Therefore, it is important to discuss the observations of Ashley and her coworkers.[8]

Coronary Arteriosclerosis and Fatty Liver as Risk Factors

The subjects included in the study by Ashley et al[8] were a randomly selected group of alcoholics who had been admitted between April 1967 and July 1969 to the Medical Unit of the Addiction Research Foundation of Ontario, Canada. (This is an in-patient facility, which had been established for the treatment of persons with alcohol problems.) During this two-year period, 861 male alcoholics had remained there long enough to permit the attending personnel to collect a meaningful body of sociologic and medical data pertaining to each member of this sample.

Data Collection Methods

The medical data were obtained in two ways. First, a complete history was taken and a thorough physical examination was performed on every admission by the full time attending medical staff, and these procedures were supplemented by routine hematologic studies, urinalysis, chest x-ray, and liver function tests. Where indicated, additional roentgenographic, laboratory, and clinical diagnostic procedures and assessments were performed (e.g., gastrointestinal x-ray film series, gastroscopy, liver biopsy, electrocardiography.) Second, records that related to any previous hospital admissions were requested and, in most cases, were obtained. Thus, with respect to each member of this patient sample, it was possible to construct a long term medical profile.

Sample Description

Then, on the basis of the sociologic data, the overall sample was divided into two groups; one group, numbering 125, comprised "skid-row" alcoholics and the other group, numbering 736, comprised the "non-skid-row" variety. Age-wise, the two groups were comparable; the mean age of the "skid-row" subjects was 43.5 ± 9 years whereas with regard to the others, it was 45 ± 10.2 years.

By far, the leading medical complication in both groups was an enlarged and fatty liver; however, whereas the condition was present in 36% of the "skid-row" alcoholics, it was present in 52.3% of the others. Thus, such statistical data would indicate that, with regard to the Canadian alcoholic, there is an increased risk of developing a fatty liver but that the risk is slightly less if the alcoholic is a "skid-row" type of socially isolated individual. However, Ashley and her group were unable to determine whether, in Canada, more sudden deaths occurred in the "skid-row" type of alcoholic with fatty liver disease than occurred in the nonsocially-isolated alcoholic with a lipodystrophy of the liver.

Hypoglycemia as mechanism for syndrome

Moreover, because there is a recognition that fatty liver disease can be linked to sudden deaths in alcoholics, considerable interest has developed in data which might provide meaningful insights into the mechanisms possibly responsible for such an association.

In this connection, Graham, who was one of the first to report the occurrence of a series of sudden deaths due to a fatty liver syndrome, advanced the view that a hepatogenic type of hypoglycemia could be blamed for such fatalities.[4] In support of such a suggestion, he cited his own clinical observations as well as the data which had been reported by Brown and Harvey[10] and by Judd et al.[9]

In their paper, which appeared in 1934, Judd et al had described two cases of spontaneous hypoglycemia in association with marked fatty infiltration of the liver, the presence of which was confirmed by liver biopsy.[9] Moreover, neither patient died even though each had developed recurrent hypoglycemic attacks characterized by episodes of coma and epileptiform seizures.

The observations reported by Brown and Harvey in 1941[10] pertained to six alcoholics who drank denatured alcohol ("smoke") and then developed severe coma and bizarre neurologic symptoms. During the period of coma, all these patients were found to have severe hypoglycemia and, uniformly, the neurologic complications disappeared promptly following intravenous administration of glucose. A similar experience, in another group of alcoholics who also imbibed denatured alcohol, was mentioned in the paper by Tucker and Porter in 1942[11]

Hypoglycemia Episode as Potentially Fatal

However, Neame and Joubert whose report appeared in 1962[12] were among the first to present detailed data which not only demonstrated convincingly that an abrupt marked drop in the blood sugar level can occur in alcoholics with a fatty liver but also that, uncorrected, such a hypoglycemic episode can be followed rapidly by a fatal outcome. Their paper was based on an experience with 23 alcoholics who, over a consecutive ten months period had been admitted to the hospital because of the development of stupor following an alcoholic debauch. Throughout their hospitalization, numerous laboratory tests were performed but, inexplicably, the blood levels of such electrolytes as sodium, potassium, or magnesium were not measured.
Blood-sugar levels. In this group of alcoholics, a consistent finding was a low blood sugar level on admission; the values ranged from 9 to 49 mg%. The blood alcohol levels were either within normal limits or, if they were raised, they were not anywhere near the levels found in alcoholics who had become unconscious during an episode of acute alcoholic intoxication. All these patients, except one, received intravenous glucose promptly. The one who did not receive such an infusion never regained consciousness and died suddenly 18 hours after admission; two others were revived temporarily but ultimately succumbed.
Neurologic findings. Aside from stupor, five had manifested recurrent convulsions; other neurologic findings in the remainder included twitching of the extremities, facial palsy, hemiparesis, conjugate deviations of the eye, spasticity, hypotonia, abnormal deep tendon reflexes, clonus, and extensor plantar reflexes. In two patients, delirium tremens developed two days after admission. Although most of the patients were anicteric, the liver was palpable in

the majority. Apparently, electrocardiographic studies were not made a part of this investigation.

Dietary history. The dietary history and data pertaining to the consumption of alcohol in this sample of patients were reviewed and thus it was determined that, for a long time their diets were low in protein and fat and that they were chronic alcoholics who, periodically, went on alcoholic sprees, consuming native brews with a fairly heavy alcohol content. Moreover, most of the patients had not eaten for 12 to 24 hours prior to the drinking bout which immediately preceded their admission to the hospital. In seven cases, the interval between the end of the drinking bout and the onset of coma varied from 8 to 15 hours; the remaining 16 patients returned to bed in an intoxicated state and were in a coma when admitted to the hospital 12 to 24 hours afterward.

Liver biopsy findings. In all 20 patients who recovered, a liver biopsy had been performed and, with one exception, the findings confirmed the presence of fatty infiltration. In addition, necropsy findings were available for review with respect to the three patients who had died; in these instances, the only noteworthy abnormality was a fatty and enlarged liver.

Discussion

Moreover, when they emphasized that the hypoglycemic reaction among both the survivors and the decedents had been preceded by a reduced intake of important nutriments for many months and by a period of starvation for several days during the drinking spree, Neame and Joubert essentially had confirmed the validity of various other observations related to the pathogenesis of such a hypoglycemia. Thus, in their paper concerning alcohol-induced hypoglycemia, Marks and Medd[13] had mentioned that "most cases of post-alcoholic hypoglycemia have occurred in more or less chronically malnourished individuals." Equally meaningful, in this connection, are the data which have indicated that the consumption of alcohol is more likely to be followed by hypoglycemia if (as observed in experimental animals) food is withheld for a defined period before the alcohol is administered[14] and if (with respect to normal healthy human volunteers) the subject had been required to fast for a day or longer just before they were given moderate doses of an alcoholic beverage.[15,16]

Evidently, then, the deprivation of nutritional substrates required for the formation of glucose and liver glycogen represents an important "risk factor" with respect to the occurrence of hypoglycemic sudden deaths in alcoholics. Moreover, it has been shown by several investigators[15,17-21] that when an alcoholic develops a fatty liver and, in addition, by means of starvation, depletes liver glycogen stores, the required oxidation of any large quantities of alcohol would interfere, secondarily, with the maintenance of an adequate blood-sugar level dependent on gluconeogenesis. Hence, the presence of such biochemical and enzymatic derangements can account for the occurrence of a severe degree of hypoglycemia when, in someone with a fatty liver, there is a long period of dietary inadequacy in conjunction with overconsumption of various alcoholic beverages for long periods of time, particularly those beverages with a high alcohol content.

Fatal vs. symptomatic hypoglycemia. However, it must also be recognized that despite the intensive studies which have been undertaken with regard to the pathogenesis of alcohol-induced hypoglycemia,[15,17-21] the actual dimensions of the problem of fatal hypoglycemia in chronic alcoholics have been difficult to ascertain. In a recent review prepared by Seltzer[22] it was stated that until 1972, most instances of symptomatic hypoglycemia following the excessive consumption of alcoholic beverages represented a reversible rather than a fatal complication; actually, as far as Seltzer could determine, on the basis of a survey of the world literature, only 11% of alcoholics who had developed an alcohol-induced episode of hypoglycemia had died because of it. However, it should be explained that it is likely that there have been many hypoglycemic fatalities in alcoholics which have gone unrecognized and thus have been unreported as such. Consequently, it can be conjectured that although there are relatively few reports of hypoglycemic fatalities in alcoholics, such data do not provide an accurate estimate of the actual incidence of such deaths.

Hypoglycemia in development of myocardial necrosis. However, even if it is acknowledged that the risk of dying suddenly is enhanced by the occurrence of a lowered blood sugar level in alcoholics with fatty liver disease, there would still remain the need to explain the pathophysiology which could account for such hypoglycemia-induced fatalities. Thus it is of some importance that in one experimental study it was shown that hypoglycemia can favor the development of myocardial necrosis[24] and that there is a report which indicated that hypoglycemia seemed to be responsible for the occurrence of a life-threatening ventricular tachyarrhythmia in a patient with coronary artery disease[25]; however, a sizeable body of autopsy data has already demonstrated that when a sudden death was seemingly due to fatty liver disease, there was no evident myocardial abnormality and the coronary arteries were patent throughout their course.[4]

Thus, alternatively, it would seem proper to suggest that it is not only the hypoglycemia but also the compensatory release of catecholamines from the adrenal gland[26] and the accumulation of sympatheticomimetic aldehydes during the metabolism of ingested alcohol[27-29,31] which conceivably would create, within the myocardial structure, a set of disturbances likely to favor an arrhythmogenic sudden cardiac arrest (see Chapter 3).

An additional consideration is the possibility that disordered kinetics with respect to either the potassium or magnesium ion within the myocardium may contribute to the occurrence of such a cardioplegic ventricular arrhythmia in alcoholics with fatty liver disease. This proposition has been advanced inasmuch as it has been shown that potassium or magnesium loss will result in a material lowering of the ventricular fibrillation threshold in both experimental animals[32,33,38,39] and in man,[32,33,34,38,40-42,58-60] and because there is considerable evidence that the excessive consumption of alcoholic beverages can be followed by an inordinate loss of such essential electrolytes from the cellular or fluid compartments of the body.[42-57]

ANECDOTAL DATA

One of the first to demonstrate the conjunction of an electrolyte disturbance and the occurrence of major ventricular arrhythmias in alcoholics with a fatty liver were Scherf et al whose article appeared in 1967.[58]

Case Study No.1

The first of two such patients described by them was a 32-year-old black female who entered the hospital complaining of dizziness, tremor, numbness of the hands and feet, and shortness of breath. She had imbibed excessive amounts of alcohol for many years and had been on an alcoholic binge for one week preceding her hospitalization.

On separate occasions during the three years prior to this hospitalization, she had developed symptoms and signs of tetany associated with hyperventilation. The electrocardiograms during these prior admissions were normal.

On the day of this admission, the patient vomited repeatedly and passed several watery stools. When examined, she was breathing rapidly and had carpopedal spasms. Positive Chvostek and Trousseau signs were elicited. The pulse was found to be irregular at a rate of approximately 170 per minute. During the next hours the arterial blood pressure fluctuated widely between extremes of 180/110 and 60/0. Chest x-rays revealed a cardiac shadow normal in size and configuration.

The patient developed generalized convulsive seizures five times following hospitalization. Because of her serious clinical condition, several antiarrhythmic and vasopressor drugs were administered intravenously.

About 12 hours after her admission to the hospital, a low serum potassium concentration (2.9 mEq per liter) was reported and, accordingly, potassium chloride was administered intravenously. Despite the presence of a marked cardiac irregularity, repeated examinations did not reveal any evidence of organic heart disease. It is noteworthy that serum magnesium levels were not obtained.

On admission, the electrocardiographic tracings revealed multifocal ventricular extra systoles and runs of ventricular tachycardia. The T-waves following normal sinus beats were scarcely visible and, in lead I there were huge U waves which appeared even larger when a long pause preceded the sinus beat. Multiple extrasystoles occurred whenever the first ectopic beat appeared superimposed early on the downslope of the U wave.

Following the intravenous infusion of the potassium chloride, there were fewer groups of extra systoles and during the cycles of normal rhythm, distinct T-waves were visible and the Q-T interval was 0.40 seconds; U waves were not present at this time. On the following day, after the patient had recovered completely, there was a normal QRS-T complex and a PR interval of approximately 0.11 seconds; the U waves were not evident and the T-waves were normal.

Thus, in this instance, the findings not only indicated the presence of a life-threatening ventricular arrhythmia secondary to hypokalemia but, in addition, the symptomatology and electrocardiographic findings suggested that there may also have been a hypomagnesiumemia, which could have been confirmed if a serum magnesium level had been obtained. This experience also emphasizes the need to be alert to the possibility that life-threatening arrhythmias in alcoholic patients may be secondary to either magnesium loss or to potassium loss and that immediate treatment of such an electrolyte disturbance must be instituted if a sudden arrhythmogenic cardiac arrest is to be avoided.

Case Study No. 2

Except for one important difference, the findings reported by Scherf et al with respect to their patient, were similar to those in an article by Mullican and Fisch which was published in 1964.[60] The patient described by Mullican and Fisch was an alcoholic with a ventricular arrhythmia unassociated with a lowered serum potassium level; nevertheless, the arrhythmia was abolished by the administration of potassium salts.

In this instance, it was suspected that the arrhythmia was due to potassium loss inasmuch as there was in the electrocardiogram a huge enlargement of the U wave during the post extrasystolic cardiac cycle, a phenomenon which Scherf et al had observed in the electrocardiograms of the two hypokalemic alcoholics described in their report. Thus, the experience reported by Mullican and Fisch serves to emphasize that, sometimes, enlargement of the U wave in the electrocardiogram can be a more important clue to the presence of potassium depletion than the measurement of the serum potassium level (see Chapter 14). Moreover, the recognition that the electrocardiographic features of potassium loss do not always correlate with serum potassium values, affirms the need to disregard the potassium level in selecting the appropriate antiarrhythmic preparation whenever the findings in the electrocardiogram of an alcoholic indicate the presence of both a ventricular arrhythmia and an enlargement of the U wave. In 1970, Nevins and Lyon reported the occurrence of a sudden death in a hypokalemic alcoholic with a fatty liver.[59] Their patient was a 35-year-old woman who was hospitalized because of weakness, anorexia, nausea, and dyspnea of several days duration. She had lost 70 pounds in the preceding eight months because of heavy alcohol ingestion and poor dietary habits. She had been hospitalized six months previously because of epigastric pain radiating to the back; at that time, there was evidence of muscle wasting and hepatomegaly. One month later, she was readmitted with similar complaints but after three days she signed out against advice.

At the time of her final admission to the hospital she appeared emaciated and somewhat dehydrated. Vital signs were normal except for sinus tachycardia of 128 per minute and her respiratory rate was 28 per minute. There were no other cardiorespiratory abnormalities. There was enlargement of the liver and slight epigastric tenderness and the remainder of the physical examination did not disclose any significant abnormalities. The chest x-ray showed a small infiltrate at the right costophrenic angle but the remainder of the lung fields was clear and there was no cardiomegaly. The electrocardiographic findings indicated a sinus tachycardia with minor nonspecific S-T depressions and a prolonged Q-T interval.

The significant laboratory findings on the day of admission included a marked lowering of the carbon dioxide combining power, a lowering of the serum potassium level varying between 2.8 and 3.1 mEq per liter, a lowering of the serum calcium level and a lowering of the serum phosphorous level.

Treatment included infusions of sodium bicarbonate and potassium chloride; 30 hours after admission and shortly after being checked by the nurse, she suddenly developed cardiac and respiratory arrest and died.

Postmortem Findings

A postmortem examination was performed and this disclosed the following: the heart weighed 220 gm and was unremarkable except for a flabby consistency. However, on microscopic examination of the heart, it was found that there was marked hydropic vacuolar degeneration most prominent in the subendocardium. Some fibers were enlarged and others atropic and some were undergoing myocytolysis. There was also moderate separation of muscle fiber groups in the heart consistent with interstitial edema. The liver was enlarged and weighed 1930 gm and there was severe fatty metamorphosis of this organ.

Cause of Death

The pathologist considered his microscopic findings in the heart to be the result of the decedent's basic electrolyte disorder and he also suspected that the sudden cardiac arrest was the result of a lethal ventricular arrhythmia secondary to the underlying electrolyte disturbance. In this instance, the electrolyte disturbance was considered to be secondary to renal tubular dysfunction associated with alcoholism, starvation, and potassium loss. An alcoholic myocardiopathy was excluded because of the lack of cardiac hypertrophy or enlargement.

In their final evaluation of this patient's illness and death, the authors concluded that both could be ascribed to complex interactions of multiple end-organ failure and metabolic derangements resulting from alcoholism and malnutrition.

Discussion

The data from the cases reported by Scherf et al,[58] Mullican and Fisch,[60] as well as by Nevins and Lyon[59] would point to the likely conclusion that, in these three instances, the arrhythmias (clearly evident in two and conjectured to be a preterminal event in the third) were part of an alcoholic fatty liver syndrome. Thus, it would not be unrealistic to suspect that the infrastructure of these arrhythmias was a hypoglycemic reaction which, as has been mentioned already, can be an important clinical correlate of fatty liver disease during a period of prolonged alcoholic intoxication. Correspondingly, it can be supposed that, to a material degree, the arrhythmias can be related to a hypoglycemia-induced compensatory release of catecholamines and lowering of the serum potassium level.

Acetaldehyde Excess As A Fundamental Risk Factor

Inasmuch as the data pertaining to these three respective patients had indicated that all had consumed excessive quantities of alcohol before they were admitted to the hospital, it would seem proper, additionally, to postulate that their respective hearts had been exposed to excessive accumulations of acetaldehyde,[27,28,29,31] which is not only the major metabolite of alcohol,[29,31] but also a substance with a marked sympatheticomimetic property.[29-31,61-62,205] Correspondingly, this view would assign to acetaldehyde excess an important position in the hierarchy of "risk factors" which could account for a life-threatening ventricular tachyarrhythmia in problem drinkers with an alcohol-related steatosis of the liver.

Effects of Disulfiram

The thesis that acetaldehyde excess is a fundamental feature of the sudden death syndrome in alcoholics with a fatty liver obtains some support from the data in reports which described sudden deaths in alcoholics soon after disulfiram (Antabuse) was introduced to discourage the overconsumption of alcoholic beverages.[63-67] However, although the interaction of that compound with alcohol results in a marked augmentation of acetaldehyde levels within the body,[68-75] it should be explained also that my examination of the autopsy findings which were included in those reports[63-67] has disclosed that almost without exception the only noteworthy pathology was an enlarged and fatty liver.

The following conglomeration of events would seem to be the fundamental mechanisms with respect to the occurrence of a sudden death in disulfiram-treated alcoholics, afflicted with a fatty metamorphosis of the liver: (a) there is an impairment of carbohydrate metabolism characterized by a lowering of the blood sugar level ultimately due, in large measure, to defective hepatic gluconeogenesis; (b) secondary to this disruption of carbohydrate metabolism there is a reflex elevation of the catecholamine levels and an alteration of ionic kinetics involving principally the potassium cation; (c) concurrently, as a result of the disulfiram-alcohol interaction, there is an augmented over-accumulation of acetaldehyde in the body; (d) because of reduced effectiveness of the acetaldehyde dehydrogenase which ordinarily (in a normal healthy functioning liver) serves to metabolize acetaldehyde, there is a reduced effectiveness with respect to the removal of acetaldehyde; (e) the myocardial cells become exposed to the sympatheticomimetic actions of both the reflexly elaborated catecholamines and the accumulated acetaldehyde; (f) within such a setting, there is a lowering of the ventricular fibrillation threshold of the heart and ultimately an abrupt cardiac arrest. Thus, within this context, the problem drinker with a clinically detectable fatty liver must be perceived as a person at increased risk of dying suddenly if the treatment program is to include the administration of a substance like disulfiram.

Effects of Phenothiazine Derivatives and other Cerebrotropic Drugs

In addition, there have been allegations that certain drugs other than disulfiram also should be listed as "risk factors" in the occurrence of sudden death in alcoholics. These alleged pharmacogenic fatalities have been sudden deaths which have been linked to the administration of phenothiazine-derivatives, to a concurrent addiction to narcotic substances such as heroin (see Chapter 12); and to overdoses of propoxyphene. It is also suspected that even customary doses of a monoamine oxidase inhibitor may be responsible, sometimes, for a sudden death in alcoholics with fatty liver disease.

In the medical literature, there are reports which occasionally mention the triad of phenothiazine therapy, sudden death, and alcohol-related steatosis of the liver. In retrospect, my examination of such data has indicated that there was reason to suppose it was the combination of alcohol abuse and a large fatty liver, rather than the drug, that was responsible for any of these fatalities. Possible exceptions were the two deaths reported by Kaplan.[84]

Effects of Promazine

In his article, which appeared in 1959, Kaplan had described the sudden deaths of two middle-aged female alcoholics, aged 53 years and 33 years. These two patients had been admitted to the hospital because they had been on a drinking spree for several days prior to admission. When they were admitted, neither was agitated; however, both women were confused and semicomatose. Each received an intramuscular injection of a customary dose of promazine and, in each instance, a fatal irreversible episode of profound hypotension followed the administration of the drug; this untoward reaction occurred within one half hour after the injection. The autopsy data pertaining to these two decedents did not indicate that any pathology existed other than an enlarged fatty liver, and, in one instance, the liver weighed 6000 gm.

Moreover, investigators at Yale University[8] have suggested that "promazine should be regarded as a dangerous drug in severely ill patients with delirium tremens if they do not respond favorably to the drug within a short time." However, these investigators also found that "promazine may produce a more rapid response than paraldehyde in alcoholic patients with mild withdrawal symptoms."

Somewhat different experiences were reported by Lynch et al.[86] In their article, these investigators indicated that promazine was both harmless and beneficial when it was used to manage highly disturbed acutely intoxicated alcoholics. They described the favorable effects of this drug in 51 alcoholics who had been admitted to a neuropsychiatric unit because of an alcoholic psychosis following a heavy drinking bout. Routinely, each such patient received, at the time of admission, 100 mg of promazine intravenously and, soon afterward, the same dose intramuscularly; during the next 24 hours, 100 mg of promazine was administered intramuscularly every six hours for 4 doses. Subsequent doses were administered perorally but these were prescribed only if the agitation and delirium persisted. Moreover, following such a program of drug therapy in this type of setting, no untoward effects were noted.

In 1956, an equally favorable experience was reported by Mitchell[88] and by Fazekas, et al[87] with regard to the use of intramuscular promazine in alcoholics who exhibited all the features of an acute alcohol-related psychotic state. In 1958 Figurelli,[89] who had used promazine to control the agitation of a large sample of alcoholics with delirium tremens, also confirmed that this phenothiazine derivative was helpful in reducing the mortality and morbidity customarily associated with this type of psychotic manifestation. Moreover, all these authors[86-89] and others[117-118] had noted that, in customary doses, promazine had not produced any serious hypotensive reaction.

Effects of Chlorpromazine

In contrast with the reports of Albert et al in 1954[92] and Mitchell in 1955,[91] which had indicated that in patients with delirium tremens, chlorpromazine produced beneficial effects without any observable adverse manifestations, the article by Rea et al[90] described a single fatality due to a hypotensive reaction following the administration of nonexcessive doses of chlorpromazine to an alcoholic who was in the hospital because of an episode of delirium tremens. However, Rea et al also noted that other alcoholics with delirium tremens who were treated with chlorpromazine had survived and had not developed any serious adverse reactions to the drug. Regrettably, no autopsy data were included in the publication of Rea et al and so the precise cause of death with respect to the single fatality they had encountered was not established with any degree of accuracy.

Effects of Propoxyphene

It has been shown by Sturner and Garriott[93] that even if the overconsumption of alcohol alone may be compatible with survival, the prospect of a sudden death in an alcoholic is enhanced if an overdose of propoxyphene is consumed along with the alcoholic beverage. This conclusion was based on the results of toxicologic studies during 1970 and 1971 in 12 decedents who, prior to the time of death, had been residents of Dallas County, Texas.

By currently accepted standards, the dose of propoxyphene that these victims had swallowed was not considered to be inordinately high. Thus, with respect to this feature, these 12 sudden deaths ascribable to the combined effects of alcohol and propoxyphene, resembled previously reported sudden deaths that were due to the combined effects of alcohol and barbiturates.[94] Three of the 12 victims were below 30 years of age. During the same period of time in that particular geographic area, there were 10 sudden deaths which proved to be due merely to an overdose of propoxyphene which had been either swallowed or injected intravenously.

Monoamine Oxidase Inhibitors

Conceivably, under certain circumstances, a different sort of drug also may increase the risk of a sudden death in problem drinkers. One such example would be monoamine oxidase inhibitors which customarily are prescribed for patients who exhibit evidences of a depressive reaction. Thus, since many alcoholics tend to evidence depressive reactions, some of them (although inadvisably) may be treated with such a preparation. It is only in the group of alcoholics who habitually drink sizeable quantities of wine or beer containing tyramine in substantial amounts that a monoamine oxide inhibitor could produce a life-threatening reaction, such as the possible catastrophic hypertensive response known to result from the concurrent consumption of both a monoamine oxidase inhibitor, and certain cheeses or other foods containing this particular precursor of catecholamine elaboration in the body.[95-98]

Another conceivable adverse and possibly life-threatening response to a monoamine oxidase inhibitor is one which would be limited to one subtype of chronic alcoholic. This is the sort of problem drinker who also is afflicted with a steatosis of the liver and is generally malnourished because of poor dietary habits. Thus, when such a person remains drunk for several days in succession, the presence of the diseased liver will favor the development of a complicating life-threatening hypoglycemic reaction[13,23] and, in such a setting, the consumption of either customarily prescribed or excessive amounts of a monoamine oxidase inhibitor may exacerbate the hypoglycemia and reduce even more the prospect of survival.

Within this context, a monoamine oxidase inhibitor can be perceived as a possible additional "risk factor" with respect to the occurrence of a sudden death in alcoholics with a fatty liver syndrome. Moreover, it should be explained that the prospects of a worsening of the hypoglycemic reaction in persons of this genre is based on observations which indicate that monoamine oxidase inhibitors potentiate the action of insulin and thereby lower blood sugar levels.[99,100]

FAT EMBOLISM SYNDROME

In addition, it should be recognized that, despite the attention already given to the prospect of a link between a "biochemical lesion" and the occurrence of a sudden death in alcoholics with a fatty liver, there may be other factors which, conceivably, might account for sudden deaths in this particular subset of problem drinkers. In this connection, it seems appropriate to suggest that fat embolism, with a resulting wet lung syndrome, sometimes may be the underlying cause for such fatalities.[86]

The view that fat embolism to the lungs could be responsible for some sudden deaths in patients of this genre was a thesis which was advanced by Scuderi as early as 1941.[102] At that time, however, no meaningful data were provided by him to support such a contention. Ten years later, this possibility was reaffirmed by Hartroft and Ridout[103] who adopted this position on the basis of observations in rats with a fatty metamorphosis of the liver induced by the feeding of a choline-deficient diet.

With the use of this experimental model, these investigators were able to show that, histologically, one of the important findings was the formation of fatty cysts within the hepatocytes and the rupture of these cysts into sinusoids and biliary canaliculi. Moreover, they were able to demonstrate the presence of hepatic fat in embolic form in the lungs, kidneys, and brains of these animals and therefore they surmised that the same phenomenon may be of significance as a cause of sudden death in patients with alcoholic fatty livers.

Scoring Intravascular Lipid Deposits

In 1954, Durlacher et al[104] reported that by scoring the extent of the intravascular lipid deposits in the lungs of 25 alcoholics with alcoholic liver disease, they were able to demonstrate that, "in 5 instances, the quantity of fat in the pulmonary vessels was as great or greater than that seen in acute deaths due to pulmonary fat embolism following fractures," even though with respect to these five cases, there was no history of trauma and there were no evidences of injury at the time of the necropsy. Thus, Durlacher et al averred that the cause of death in these five alcoholics with fatty liver disease was the presence of pulmonary intravascular fatty emboli released from the fatty liver. However, Durlacher et al did not state whether or not the weight of the affected lungs was increased; they also omitted any reference to the degree of pulmonary edema or hemorrhagic consolidation in the lung which may have been present.

Conflicting Studies

Subsequently, in 1958, Holler et al[105] reported that they could not confirm the findings described by Durlacher et al.[104] Holler et al processed blocks of tissues removed from 14 autopsied alcoholics who had died suddenly "without any demonstrable cause of death other than a fatty liver." They carefully examined frozen sections of the pulmonary tissue. It was necessary "to cut the lung sections at 40 micra to prevent any distortions when they were mounted; also, all sections were stained with Sudan IV and Erlich's hematoxylin taking particular care not to leave tissue in 70% alcohol long enough to dissolve out any fat. Significance was attributed only to intravascular sudanophilic material, the extent of which was scored from 1+ to 4+, with 3+ representing intravascular fat in every field and 4+ in every visible arteriole."

In summing up their findings, Holler et al stated that, "intravascular fat was seen in only 4 instances and in no instance did it exceed 2+ in extent." As controls, they processed in the same fashion the lung sections from two fracture cases with known fat embolism. The histologic findings in these two instances confirmed that the extent of intravascular fat could be graded as 4+ in accord with the classification they had adopted. Thus, although they conceded that fatty particles may migrate from the parenchyma of a fatty infiltration of the liver, they also concluded that their findings indicated that the sudden deaths of the 14 alcoholics with a fatty liver could not be ascribed to fat embolism.

In the following year, Lynch et al[86] challenged the position adopted by Holler et al. Thus, like Durlacher et al,[104] Lynch et al emphasized the frequency of extensive occlusions by fatty emboli in the capillaries of the lungs of alcoholics whose deaths were linked to the presence of a large fatty liver. In their investigation of 40 fatalities attributed to an alcoholic fatty liver, they found in 31 instances, evidence of extensively distributed fatty emboli in the lungs. In 14 of these cases the brain also was examined; and in 12 of these instances, fatty emboli were present in the lung as well.

Lynch et al also observed that when they conducted histologic studies of the livers of alcoholics with fatty emboli to the lungs, they usually found that fused and ruptured fatty cysts were in communication with the hepatic sinusoids; accordingly, they discounted any suggestion that the fatty intravascular occlusions in the lung represented locally deposited material derived from circulating blood lipids. Moreover, following microscopic examination of pulmonary tissue obtained from 250 consecutively autopsied decedents, they were able to detect a sizeable number of fatty emboli in the lungs in 58 instances; of these, the conditions preceding death were severe trauma (37 cases), acute pancreatitis (2 cases), and alcoholic fatty liver (19 cases).

It should be explained, however, that although it is common for fatty emboli in the lungs to be linked to the deaths of alcoholics with fatty livers, there is some dispute regarding the importance of these emboli in relation to such fatalities if, in conjunction with this type of embolization, the usual pathologic correlates of the pulmonary disorder (which currently is subsumed under the rubric of the "adult respiratory distress syndrome")[106-108] are not present. Thus, within such a context, it would seem proper to exclude fatty emboli as a cause of death if the autopsy findings do not conform with the changes generally considered to be characteristic of this entity.

Animal Experiments

Within the restrictions of such a formulation, Cotev et al[110] evaluated the results of a series of animal experiments undertaken to determine the effects produced by the intravenous infusion of a fat cell suspension during a variety of circumstances. Following such a procedure, the animals were sacrificed and any changes in the lungs were carefully described.

Findings

The gross findings which Cotev et al considered to be especially meaningful included a rubbery consistency of the lungs, increased weight of the lungs, scattered subpleural petechial hemorrhages, and frothy hemorrhagic fluid exuding from cut surfaces.

The microscopic findings they viewed as corroborative of an "adult respiratory distress syndrome" consisted of intravascular fat emboli, focal or widespread interstitial and intra-alveolar edema and hemorrhages; large or small areas of focal or diffuse atelectasis and compensatory emphysema; thrombotic occlusion of pulmonary vessels of various sizes, often admixed with fat emboli; and leukocytic stasis or thrombi.

When they designed experiments which employed stress-producing interventions (induced hypovolemia or prolonged compression of a limb) in conjunction with the infusion of the adipose material, they obtained evidence to suggest that the entry of fatty cellular material into the circulation from any site in the body could lead to such pulmonary changes only if, simultaneously, a certain degree of shock or stress also had been present. As these investigators explained, "in evaluating the degree of generalized pulmonary damage it was observed that fat cell injections, together with induced hypovolemia or ischemic tourniquet-induced shock, significantly brought about the severest alterations while the administration of fat cells alone resulted in only a moderate degree of damage."[110]

Cotev et al ascribed the intravascular coagulation to the liberation of thromboplastin from pulmonary embolized fat cells, and, in this regard, their views are in accord with those of other investigators who, similarly, have attempted to evaluate the pathologic features of the fat embolism syndrome.[101,109,116] Moreover, Cotev et al, like Carlson and Liljendahl[115] attributed the hemorrhagic exudate and intracapillary endothelial changes to the toxic effects of free fatty acids released locally within these vessels upon lipolysis of the fatty emboli. However, the results of experiments conducted by Reidbord[111] would seem to invalidate any alleged nexus between such capillary changes and the presence of free fatty acids. Nevertheless, it seems quite clear that there are now sufficient human and animal data to suggest that a fatty liver in an alcoholic sometimes might be the underlying cause for a fatal variety of "adult respiratory distress syndrome,"[106-108,114] secondary to the lodgement of fatty emboli in the pulmonary circulation.[137]

DELIRIUM TREMENS

Two other alcohol-related entities which, separately, can be responsible for sudden deaths in chronic alcoholics are delirium tremens and an alcoholic myocardiopathy. However, most observers would agree that sudden deaths in alcoholics with delirium tremens are likely to be the result of a co-existing "biochemical lesion" whereas sudden deaths linked to an alcoholic myocardiopathy are prone to be due to an abrupt cardiac arrest which occurs when there is an advanced degree of myocardial pathology.

Furthermore, the differences between these two alcohol-related entities, in terms of sudden deaths, is emphasized by the rarity of an alcoholic myocardiopathy in alcoholics who have succumbed during the withdrawal phase of an alcoholic debauch.[120]

ALCOHOL ABUSE 61

Postmortem data associated with fatal delirium tremens

Generally, the important findings during the postmortem examination have consisted of cerebral edema, intracerebral degeneration of cells and an increase of glia associated with some round cell infiltration; sometimes, the liver will be enlarged and fatty or it may show evidences of marked cirrhosis.[119,122,126] Although the incidence of fatalities ascribable to delirium tremens is still uncertain, it has been estimated that the mortality rate may be as high as 10% or 15%.[120-124] However, it is likely that a better understanding of its underlying mechanisms ultimately may lead to a marked reduction of sudden deaths from this particular complication, which has been defined as an acute psychotic syndrome characterized by tremors, hallucinations, and delirium.[126]

Hyperactivity and "Restraint Stress"

It has been suggested that the hyperactivity characteristic of this disorder may be an element which favors the occurrence of a sudden death; but, in the absence of any associated serious biochemical alterations, it is unlikely that in patients of this genre, such an element can be blamed for a sudden unexpected death. However, it has been observed that "many a patient with delirium tremens has died suddenly while struggling against bodily restraints."[126] Thus, in this respect, the alcoholic with delirium tremens resembles patients exhibiting the usual features of lethal catatonia (see Chapter 11).

Effects of Hyperpyrexia

There is some evidence to indicate that hyperpyrexia, when it is not the result of any infection, may be a possible forerunner of sudden death in alcoholics with delirium tremens; such a correlation has been reported by Thompson et al[125] and by Tavel et al.[125]

Thompson et al described the findings with respect to two fatalities and implied, despite the omission of autopsy data, that both were ascribable to a variety of fatal hyperpyrexia and postulated that, in these two instances, the fever was secondary to the presence of cerebral edema with hypothalamic malfunction. As they noted, in one of these decedents "the temperature was

40.1° C. but 20 minutes before he was found dead, his temperature had decreased to 38.9°C." Moreover, 30 minutes before the second patient died suddenly, his temperature was 37.9° C. but earlier that day it was 38.7° C.

Hyperpyrexia and "Calming Drugs"

These same authors also speculated that drug therapy (paraldehyde) may have contributed to these two sudden deaths; they made this suggestion, however, only because they had observed, in their large sample of alcoholics with delirium tremens, that a variety of adverse reactions followed the administration of "calming preparations" such as paraldehyde or diazepam when the recipients of these drugs exhibited the febrile phase of this particular alcohol withdrawal syndrome.

This concept, that hyperpyrexia and "calming drugs" when combined can be considered joint "risk factors" in relation to the occurrence of sudden deaths in alcoholics with delirium tremens, is supported also by data reported by Cutshall.[120] However, he did not provide any autopsy data and, hence, it is uncertain whether a fatal fatty-liver syndrome could have been a contributory "risk factor" with respect to his sample of phenothiazine-treated alcoholics whose primary illness was an episode of delirium tremens. However, he did indicate that although appropriate sedatives were effective in controlling convulsions and reducing hallucinations, the administration of such drugs may be followed by fatalities in patients with severe liver disease and delirium tremens.

Other Studies

Equally noteworthy are the data provided by Leevy et al.[126] Their patient sample comprised 66 living alcoholics who had been admitted to the hospital for the treatment of an episode of delirium tremens and, in conjunction with their investigation, these authors obtained, routinely, a liver biopsy and a battery of liver function tests. In this manner, they were able to establish an array of meaningful correlations, some of which seem to be related to the triad of sudden death, lipodystrophy of the liver and delirium tremens.

Thus, it was determined in their group of patients with delirium tremens that the histologic findings following liver biopsy were compatible (a) with normal liver structure in 19 instances (30%); (b) with focal inflammation in 4 instances (6%); (c) with fatty metamorphosis in 20 instances (30%); (d) with portal cirrhosis in 23 instances (34%). Moreover, although hyperpyrexia without infection (temperature 104°F or over) was observed in patients with normal, fatty, or cirrhotic livers, the relative incidence of this febrile state could not be correlated with the status of the liver in terms of its pathology. Thus, in the overall sample of these 66 patients, 13 (20%) were hyperpyrectic; but among these 13 febrile patients, a concurrent finding was cirrhosis of the liver in 54% of the sample, a normal liver in 23% of the sample, and a fatty liver also in 23% of the sample.

Conclusions

Thus, it is evident that in 15% of the 66 patients, there was both hyperpyrexia and some form of alcoholic liver disease. Moreover, inasmuch as no deaths were reported in this patient sample, this finding could mean that if the combination of hyperpyrexia and alcoholic liver disease does, indeed, increase the risk of a sudden death, an additional "risk factor" supposedly should be present if such a fatality is to occur in alcoholics with delirium tremens.

Although the role of "calming drugs" has been considered to be such a possible additional risk factor it also is conceivable that a possible supplementary risk factor could be the presence of an associated "biochemical lesion" such as a lowered concentration of potassium or magnesium.

There is now, in the literature, a sizeable body of data to indicate not only that deficits of one or the other of these electrolytes commonly accompany any severe alcohol withdrawal syndrome[128,130,133,134] but, also, that such electrolyte deficits can favor the occurence of a life-threatening ventricular tachyarrhythmia.[32,33,35,37,38,40]

TRIAD OF DELIRIUM TREMENS, POTASSIUM DEPLETION, AND CARDIAC ARRHYTHMIAS

At the time alcoholics with a fatty liver are admitted to the hospital because of an episode of delirium tremens, a basic requirement should be to obtain measurements of the serum electrolyte levels and electrocardiographic studies in order to exclude the need for prompt and aggressive therapy with potassium or magnesium salts in conjunction with the use of other suitable measures customarily employed in the management of such patients.

Conceivably, it was the lack of adherence to such a proposed plan of action which may have accounted for the ultimate and untimely sudden death of an alcoholic with delirium tremens which was described by Sydney in a report which appeared in 1973.[83] In this instance, the decedent was a 41-year-old male alcoholic who, developed delirium tremens after alcohol withdrawal. He was given haloperidol (20 mg daily) and thioridazine (up to 600 mg daily). However, two days later he collapsed and was found to be in ventricular fibrillation; he was defribrillated and transferred to the Cardiology Unit of the Royal Infirmary in Manchester, England. Presumably, only after the development of this episode of ventricular fibrillation, it was discovered that the patient's serum potassium level was 2.6 mEq per liter and that the pH value was 7.32. Apparently, a determination of the serum magnesium level was not requested. Thus, after the presence of hypokalemia was established, the patient "continued to have numerous ventricular ectopic beats with runs of ventricular tachycardia and fibrillation. He was given potassium chloride in 5% dextrose intravenously, 10 mEq per hour with intravenous lidocaine at 1 to 4 mg per minute and defibrillated as necessary. After 48 hours the rhythm stabilized and when the serum potassium level became 4.7 mEq per liter, the infusion was stopped. Unfortunately, he remained unconscious and after four days he died. Necropsy showed terminal bronchopneumonia, a fatty liver, and an area of necrosis in the posterior myocardium without any evidence of coronary artery occlusion."

A survey of Vetter et al[128] has provided additional meaningful data with respect to the hazards of the triad of delirium tremens, potassium depletion, and cardiac arrhythmias.The patient sample studied by these investigators consisted of 50 consecutively admitted alcoholics, none of whom died subsequently. Shortly after these patients were admitted to the hospital, the serum levels of potassium, sodium, carbon dioxide, and chloride were determined and an electrocardiogram was obtained. The results were reported promptly and any patients found to be potassium depleted were admitted promptly to the medical service where appropriate amounts of potassium chloride solutions were administered intravenously without delay. Moreover, in these 50 patients several follow-up electrocardiograms were made and particular attention was given to the following items: (a) conduction defects, (b) ectopic contractions, (c) S-T segment displacements, (d) T-wave abnormalities, (e) U-wave enlargement.

Potassium Depletion

As a result of such a screening procedure, Vetter et al found that nine patients (18%) were severely depleted of potassium (serum potassium values ranged from 1.5 to 2.5 mEq per liter); that 23 patients (46%) were moderately depleted (serum potassium values ranged from 2.6 to 3.4 mEq per liter); that in 10 patients (20%) the serum potassium levels ranged from 3.5 to 3.9 mEq per liter; that in eight patients, the serum potassium levels were normal, the values ranging from 4.0 to 4.5 mEq per liter.

Electrocardiographic Findings

Abnormalities of rhythm, conduction, and repolarization were present in the electrocardiograms of 38 patients (76%); in 16 of the patients, arrhythmias, conduction defects, or ectopic contractions occurred; in the remaining 22 patients only repolarization abnormalities were present. Abnormalities of rhythm and conduction included premature atrial, nodal, and ventricular beats, atrial fibrillation, paroxysmal atrial tachycardia, wandering atrial pacemaker, incomplete right bundle branch block, and ventricular tachycardia. All but 2 of the 16 patients also had repolarization abnormalities. Abnormal rhythms were present in 4 of the 9 severely depleted patients (45%), in 10 of the 23 moderately depleted patients (44%), in 1 of the 10 low normal patients (10%), and in 1 of the 8 normal patients (12.5%). The patients with arrhythmias in the last two groups were moderately acidotic and therefore the levels may not accurately reflect the degree of potassium depletion. Eighteen of the 22 patients with only repolarization abnormalities were severely or moderately depleted of potassium; in the remaining 4, the plasma potassium level was either a low normal or normal value.

The electrocardiographic repolarization abnormalities (depressed S-T segment, low T-waves, and prominent U waves) which were observed in 36 of the 50 patients were abolished following potassium repletion. It also should be noted that when intravenous administration of glucose and water was used to correct dehydration and to provide calories, serious ventricular arrhythmias developed. Thus, such an experience corroborated the observations of Kunin and his co-workers[34] who found that despite the administration of 20 or even 40 mEq per hour of potassium chloride in 250 ml of 5% glucose solution to potassium-depleted patients, the level of serum potassium would fall temporarily and at this juncture arrhythmias would supervene.

Role of Magnesium Depletion

Moreover, it should be explained that in addition to articles pertaining to the triad of alcoholism, potassium depletion, and life-threatening tachyarrhythmias, there also can be found, in the medical literature, several publications which have described the occurrence in alcoholics of life-threatening ventricular tachyarrhythmias which were due, not to a deficit of potassium alone but, instead, to a depletion of magnesium as well as potassium. However, so far, it has been possible to locate only five reports which have confirmed the presence, in alcoholic patients, of ventricular arrhythmias linked to a deficit of both cations.[40,42,83,143,204]

Case study. One such alcoholic who had been studied by Loeb et al[40] was a 29-year-old woman who had been admitted to the hospital because of convulsions which developed after she had been drinking excessive amounts of alcoholic beverages continuously for several weeks. Clearly, she was malnourished, but alert, cooperative, and in no apparent distress. Blood pressure was 110/60, the pulse rate was 90 per minute and regular; the temperature was normal. Examination of the heart revealed findings consistent with minimal aortic regurgitation but the remainder of the physical examination was unremarkable."

On admission, the hemoglobin value was 8.7 gm and levels of blood glucose, urea nitrogen, albumin, globulin, protein-bound iodine, and amylase were normal. The concentration of serum potassium was 3.5 mEq; the serum sodium value was 126 mEq; the serum chloride value was 89 mEq; and the serum calcium level was 9.6 mg. However, there was definite evidence of hypo-magnesemia; the serum magnesium concentrations were 0.3 mEq on admission, 0.6 mEq the following day, and 0.7 mEq six days later.

Serial electrocardiograms, made soon after admission, indicated the presence of bigeminal rhythm, mutifocal ventricular complexes, and ventricular fibrillation terminating spontaneously in sinus rhythm. It was noted that the Q-T interval lengthened progressively (presumably, this interpretation referred to enlargement of the U wave) prior to the appearance of bigeminy but returned to a near normal duration (disappearance of U-wave enlargement, presumably) immediately following several transient episodes of ventricular fibrillation. Although these brief periods of ventricular fibrillation were unaccompanied by clinical sequelae, longer episodes were observed during which the patient lost consciousness and developed clonic convulsions. Although each episode appeared to terminate spontaneously, the possibility of a single fatal episode prompted the treating physician to institute artificial cardiac pacing as a means of controlling the rhythm. A bipolar pacing catheter was inserted without difficulty and pacing from the right ventricle appeared to be effective in preventing further episodes of ventricular fibrillation.

Recovery was uneventful and prior to discharge, myocardial biopsy was performed at open operation which revealed only minimal edema of the myocardium on light microscopy. When last seen, the patient felt well, cardiac findings were unchanged and the electrocardiogram showed a normal Q-T interval. At that time the serum magnesium concentration was 1.0 mEq.

Regrettably, in this instance, repletion therapy with magnesium salts was not instituted before the implantation of the artifical cardiac pacemaker. In all likelihood, if this had been done, the need for the implanted pacemaker would have been obviated.

It is also conceivable that infusions of potassium salts would have abolished the arrhythmia, even though the serum potassium level was only slightly low. There are several reasons for this suggestion: First, enlargement of the U wave was visible in the electrocardiographic "clips" which accompanied the text of the article by Loeb et al; this U-wave enlargement was seen in electrocardiograms made during interarrhythmic periods and it also was evident during the post extrasystolic cycles whenever a bigeminal rhythm was present. Second, several studies have shown that, in the presence of hypomagnesemia, there is usually a concurrent disorder of potassium ion transport in the myocardial cell.[41,42,135,136] Third, other investigators have demonstrated that arrhythmias associated with hypomagnesemia can be corrected by the administration of potassium salts[135,136]. Fourth, the experience of Mullican and Fisch[60] has indicated that, in an alcoholic, potassium repletion therapy can abolish major ventricular arrhythmias associated with a normal potassium level in the serum and an enlargement of the U wave in the electrocardiogram.

The hypomagnesemic chronic alcoholic discussed in the review by Iseri et al[42] was a 54-year-old woman who was admitted to the hospital on September 7, 1973 for acute alcohol withdrawal symptoms following a heavy drinking bout lasting 4 weeks. While being transferred to the Intensive Care Unit, accompanied by a portable monitor and defribrillator, acute ventricular fibrillation developed. She was counter-shocked immediately and given injections of 150 mg lidocaine and 250 mg of procaine amide, followed by an infusion of lidocaine. Sinus rhythm was maintained for 12 hours with gradually decreasing rates of lidocaine infusion. Then, without warning, the patient had several episodes of ventricular fibrillation for which she required countershock eight times in 3 hours, despite two injections of lidocaine and two injections of procaine amide.

Blood for determination of serum magnesium was drawn and 10 cc of 20% magnesium sulphate was injected intravenously over a 1-minute period. As a result, the recurrent episodes of ventricular fibrillation were abolished. Later, the serum magnesium level was reported to be 1.39 mEq; the normal level is sightly above 2 mEq/L.

Magnesium Depletion Therapy. The patient was then given 5 gm more of magnesium sulphate by slow infusion over 4 hours; she was weaned off lidocaine and continued to receive oral quinidine as before. Supplementary potassium chloride was given to counteract a rapidly developing associated hypopotassemia. The serum magnesium level 24 hours later was reported to be 2.13 mEq (a normal level). No further arrhythmias occurred and she was discharged from the hospital 10 days later.

Thus, in this instance, there must have been a combined deficit of magnesium and potassium, with the latter becoming recognized only after magnesium repletion therapy was instituted. Conceivably, then, despite the hypomagnesemia it would have been preferable to infuse a potassium solution at the outset, with the expectation, in view of the known interplay between the kinetics of the magnesium and potassium cations[135] that although the primary effect would have been a correction of the potassium loss, the secondary result would have been a restoration of normal magnesium balance.

An alternative plan could have been the simultaneous administration of both a solution of potassium and of magnesium. In this connection, it should be noted that, as yet, there is no fixed schedule with respect to the doses of magnesium which should be used for repletion purposes.

Chesley and Tepper[141] maintained a serum magnesium level of 5 mEq for 5 hours by giving 3 gm of magnesium sulphate intravenously followed by 10 gm of magnesium sulphate intramuscularly. They observed, also, that 2 gm given rapidly into the vein will raise serum magnesium to 5 mEq with a fall to normal in 15 minutes. Pritchard[142] found that 4 gm given intravenously will raise the level up to 9 mEq with a fall to normal in 40 minutes. Flink[143] has recommended a loading dose of 6 gm (49 mEq) given intravenously in 3 hours, followed by 10 gm by slow infusion during the first 24 hours and, for the next three days, 6 gm every 24 hours. The method advocated by Iseri et al (reference) would be to infuse intravenously over a period of 60 seconds, 10 to 15 cc of a 20 percent solution of magnesium sulphate and to follow this dose with 500 cc of 2 percent magnesium sulphate given by means of a slow intravenous drip over a period of 6 hours; in an adult, this dose was considered to be safe and effective. Also, these authors recommended that when there are frequent recurrences of arrhythmias in hypomagnesemic adults, maintenance doses of magnesium, administered by infusion, should be continued; the maintenance dose they suggested was 500 cc of 2 percent magnesium sulphate infused over a 24 hour period.

STRUCTURAL CARDIAC ABNORMALITIES

In the preceding sections of this chapter, considerable attention has been given to the matter of sudden cardiac arrests in alcoholics, which were not linked, primarily, to the presence of an underlying structural cardiac abnormality. To deal properly with this aspect of the sudden death issue in problem drinkers requires that consideration be given to fatalities related directly to either ischemic heart disease or to an alcoholic myocardiopathy.

Occlusive Disease of Coronary Circulation

In terms of "naturally-caused" sudden deaths in alcoholics, it has been fairly well established that the condition which is most often responsible for such fatalities is occlusive disease of the coronary circulation (See Chapter 10). Consequently, it is clear that, in this respect, alcoholics do not differ materially from the general population in industrialized societies.[6, 144-146] Inasmuch as the methodical large scale survey conducted by Ashley et al[8] has demonstrated that, in surviving middle-aged alcoholics, the major physical affliction is atherosclerotic heart disease, it can be anticipated that, for many years to come, most sudden deaths due to "natural causes" in alcoholics above 30 years of age will be the resuult of this type of cardiovascular abnormality. This view also would conform with the findings revealed by earlier epidemiologic studies.[6]

In connection with their investigation, Ashley et al[8] divided a large sample of alcoholics into two broad categories (based on sociologic considerations) and, with the adoption of this procedure, they were able to make comparisons between 125 "skid-row" alcoholics and 736 alcoholics who were not socially isolated. Although most of the members of the "skid-row" group were regular cigarette smokers and 91% of the others were equally habituated to the use of tobacco in this form, their study showed that there were significant differences between the two groups in terms of the incidence of atherosclerotic coronary artery disease, hypertension, and obesity.

Findings

In the sample of "skid-row" alcoholics they had examined, they found evidences of coronary heart disease in 4%, the presence of hypertension in 4%, and obesity in 0.8% whereas, in the other type of alcoholic, these respective items were observed in 8.8%, 14%, and 3.5%. Moreover, in view of such data, it is evident that the non-"skid-row" alcoholic—who is the prevalent type of problem drinker in industrialized societies—possesses, to a higher degree than the "skid-row" alcoholic, that combination of "risk factors" most likely to be the forerunner of a coronary-related sudden death.[145]

A Fatal Triad in Alcoholics with Coronary Disease

It has been noted also that there is a subset of sudden deaths due to occlusive coronary artery disease in alcoholics which can be ascribed to a distinctive syndrome. It is one which is characterized by the conjunctive presence of alcoholic fatty liver disease, coronary arteriosclerosis, and acute alcoholism in chronic alcoholics. Such a syndrome has been described by Heggtveit.[147]

Case Study No. 1

One of their decedents was a 35-year-old man who suddenly collapsed and died while riding on a bus. His body was removed to a hospital where an autopsy was performed. At the same time, a sample of blood was removed in order to measure the level of circulating alcohol; this proved to be 500 mg%. The postmortem examination disclosed the presence of segmental atherosclerotic narrowing of the major coronary arteries but, in addition, the liver was found to be infiltrated heavily with fat.

Discussion. Thus, in this instance, it is uncertain whether it was the coronary sclerosis or the fatty liver which should have been blamed for the sudden death. On the other hand, it is conceivable that, because of the conjunction of a high blood alcohol level and the steatosis of the liver, it was a "biochemical lesion" such as excessive accumulation of acetaldehyde which could have been responsible for the development of a cardioplegic ventricular arrhythmia in a heart already impaired as a result of a marginal degree of myocardial ischemia. As has been established already, this particular metabolite of alcohol undergoes incomplete degradation when, because of a fatty metamorphosis of the liver, there is a reduced availability of acetaldehyde dehydrogenase;[31] moreover, acetaldehyde is known to be a substance which, in large amounts, can lower the ventricular fibrillation threshold.[61, 64]

Case Study No. 2

The other decedent "dropped dead" unexpectedly at home. After his body was removed to a nearby hospital, an autopsy was performed and a sample of blood was removed for an alcohol level determination. The noteworthy pathologic findings included marked atherosclerotic disease of the extramural coronary arteries, cardiac hypertrophy (heart weight was 430 gm) and a large fatty liver; the blood alcohol level in this instance was 240 mg%. Supposedly, the mechanism already suggested to explain the sudden death of the first of these two fatalities would pertain to this decedent, as well.

Alternative Hypothesis

However, the proposition which Heggtveit advanced to account for these two sudden deaths was of a different sort entirely. In his view, it was primarily an exaggerated degree of myocardial ischemia induced by the heavy alcohol intake which could be inculpated. Within this context, he envisaged, in each instance, the occurrence of three concurrent events during the bout of heavy drinking which preceded, presumably, these two respective fatalities. Thus, it was his concept that there was, on the one hand, a reduction of coronary blood flow due to a diversion of blood to the periphery secondary to "the potent vasodilating effect of alcohol on the peripheral arteriolar bed" and, simultaneously, an alcohol-related coronary vasoconstriction along with an alcohol-induced "pronounced increase in oxygen consumption by the myocardium."

Clearly, this alternative hypothesis is equally attractive, especially since there are some experimental data which have demonstrated that, indeed, one of the acute effects of alcohol is to increase myocardial oxygen consumption.[148,150,151,155,157]

Anginal Syndrome

Perhaps, too, it was this effect on myocardial oxygen consumption which could account for the nexus between the consumption of alcoholic beverages and the occurrence of the anginal syndrome, at rest, which was observed by Fernandez et al in an alcoholic with demonstrable atherosclerotic coronary artery disease.[149]

Case Study

In this instance, the patient was a 47-year-old man whose first anginal symptoms consisted of recurrent nocturnal attacks of pain in the jaw which regularly aroused him from his sleep. These pains occasionally radiated to the anterior chest and generally they persisted for 1 to 2 hours. Then, a few weeks later, the symptoms changed mainly with respect to their time of onset and the nature of the trigger which provoked the pain. Thus at this time, the patient had observed that the pain "now appeared only in the early evening and only if he drank beer or whiskey before dinner."
Test Results. Subsequently, it was found that after a graduated exercise test on a bicycle ergometer (100 watts during the forenoon), no S-T segment changes appeared in the electrocardiogram and no pains in the jaw or chest developed. However, when he was attached to a cardiac monitor and was given 24 ounces of beer before dinner, it was observed that 2½ hours after he had consumed this beverage there were S-T segment displacements in the electrocardiogram associated with the occurrence of pains in the jaws; morever, the S-T segment changes disappeared concurrently with a gradual subsidence of these anginal pains.

Coronary arteriography was performed in this patient on the following morning and this revealed 90% stenosis of the main left circumflex artery and 50% to 75% stenosis of the proximal left anterior descending artery. In addition, left ventriculography revelaed a hypokinetic inferior wall. Then, in the afternoon of that same day, aortocoronary saphenous vein bypass grafts to the circumflex and anterior descending arteries were performed. The post operative course was uneventful and following his discharge from the hopsital, he remained asymptomatic even after the ingestion of alcoholic beverages.

Furthermore, the results of several systematic studies have demonstrated repeatedly that evidences of myocardial ischemia will be accentuated in known anginal patients, following the consumption of alcoholic beverages. Thus, Conway reported in 1968[150,157] that although the administration of "3 to 4 whiskies" to five anginal patients 1 hour prior to a measured amount of exercise did not reduce the amount of work required to induce an episode of angina pectoris "the ethanol did induce ischemic S-T segment after exercise for the first time in one of these five patients and greater S-T segment depression after exercise in another member of this patient sample."

Group Study

Essentially similar data accrued from a comparable study reported in 1976 by Orlando et at[151] but some of their test subjects also were chronic alcoholics.

Patient sample. Altogether, their patient sample consisted of 12 men with a mean age of 52.6 ± 6.1 years "who had classic stable exertional angina pectoris and angiographic evidence of severe coronary artery disease with 75% or greater narrowing of at least one major coronary vessel." All 12 subjects had a normal left ventricular ejection fraction and no clinical evidences of congestive heart failure or cardiomegaly at the time of this study. Five subjects drank less than 1 ounce of ethanol daily, five subjects drank 1 to 2 ounces of ethanol daily, and two subjects drank more than 2 ounces of ethanol daily. None of the patients were hypokalemic and all were instructed to desist from the use of nitroglycerin on the day the various tests were performed.

Procedure. On three successive study mornings, venous blood was drawn from each subject and analyzed for an ethanol level. Afterward, simultaneous leads II and V_5 were recorded with an electrocardiograph while the subject was first supine and then sitting upright on the bicycle ergometer. The resting blood pressure was then measured with a mercury sphygmomanometer with the subject sitting upright on the bicycle. Each subject then exercised upright on the ergometer with a progressive workload until the onset of angina pectoris; the duration of exercise required to induce such an episode was recorded with a stop watch.

Furthermore, an electrocardiogram was recorded at the onset of angina with the subject in the upright position and then, with the subject supine, 1, 2, 3, 4, 5 and 6 minutes after the onset of such exercise-induced angina pectoris. Fifteen minutes after completion of the exercise electrocardiograms, simultaneous leads II and V_5 were recorded with the subject supine and then sitting upright on the bicycle ergometer. The heart rate and blood pressure were measured with the patient sitting upright, as well.

Each subject then drank, in a double-blind, randomized study, one drink every 12 minutes for a total of five drinks. Ten minutes after the fifth drink was consumed, simultaneous leads II and V_5 were recorded with the subject supine and then sitting upright on the bicycle ergometer; at this time the heart rate and blood pressure were also measured. After this procedure was completed, venous blood was drawn for an ethanol level. After the patient had exercised on the bicycle ergotometer until the onset of angina pectoris, the duration of exercise required to induce the anginal symptoms was measured with a stop watch. Simultaneously, the blood pressure and heart rate were measured. Successive electrocardiograms over a 15-minute period were again obtained in the manner already described. Thereafter, the data derived from this investigation were statistically analyzed using Student's t-test for correlated means.

Results. The following significant differences were observed: a significant increase in resting heart rate developed after 2 or 5 ounces of ethanol; a significant increase in resting systolic blood pressure was evident after 2 or 5 ounces of ethanol; a significant increase in resting diastolic blood pressure was present after 2 ounces of ethanol. Additionally, there were: at rest, a significant increase in the product of heart rate times systolic blood pressure after 2 or 5 ounces of ethanol; a significant shortening in the duration of exercise required to provoke an attack of angina pectoris after the administration of 2 or 5 ounces of ethanol; a significant increase in maximal post-exercise ischemic S-T segment depression after the consumption of 2 or 5 ounces of ethanol.

Conclusions. The findings of this study properly were interpreted by Orlando et al to indicate that when a predetermined stress sufficient to produce an episode of angina pectoris remained the same, the consumption of 2 or 5 ounces of whiskey prior to the time of the stressful procedure increased myocardial oxygen consumption and induced more myocardial ischemia.

Moreover, aware that others had shown that myocardial depression will result from the consumption of alcoholic beverages.[155,158,174,169,170,171] Orlando et al posited that such effects might be ascribed to an alcohol-induced reduction of left ventricular performance and, as a consequence, a further decline in myocardial perfusion through already stenosed extramural coronary arteries. However, these investigators seemed to favor the view that their data meant that the lowered anginal threshold after alcohol was due primarily to an alcohol-induced augmentation of myocardial oxygen consumption.

Thus, it should be apparent that there is now a sufficient body of evidence to indicate that when alcoholics with atherosclerotic coronary artery disease persistently consume alcoholic beverages, they are, in effect, increasing the prospect of an abrupt cardiac arrest. Correspondingly, despite some traditional beliefs regarding the virtues of alcohol consumption for patients with coronary-related symptoms, the much more prudent practice would seem to be to proscribe the use of any alcoholic beverages once the diagnosis of atherosclerotic heart disease has been established.

Prinzmetal Angina

In all likelihood, a similar recommendation would be advisable with respect to the management of individuals afflicted with the Prinzmetal variant form of angina pectoris. This view is based on data which indicate that some patients with this type of cardiac disorder can die suddenly and unexpectedly.[152] It is also based on knowledge that although certain persons with arteriographic evidence of occlusive coronary artery disease may not develop an anginal episode after exercise, the consumption of an alcoholic beverage will produce characteristic anginal pains and, simultaneously, the transient S-T segment elevation which is the electrocardiographic hallmark of the Prinzmetal syndrome.[149]

Atherosclerotic Coronary Lesions in Cirrhotic Patients

Still incompletely understood, in terms of its implications, is the negative correlation in alcoholics with respect to atherosclerotic coronary disease and the presence of cirrhosis of the liver. Several observers[153,154] have confirmed the infrequency of atherosclerotic lesions in the hearts of cirrhotic patients. However, inasmuch as such data (for the most part) were dependent on findings during postmortem examinations, the lack of coronary artery disease in these instances cannot be viewed as a particularly favorable circumstance. Moreover, as would be expected, there has been much speculation regarding the manner whereby alcoholic cirrhosis of the liver could reduce the likelihood of atheromatous deposits in the coronary vessels. So far, a satisfactory explanation has not been forthcoming but it is suspected that the process of retardation of atherosclerotic vascular changes in the heart could be dependent on an ill-defined effect on estrogen metabolism or blood coagulation, or both.[154]

Alcoholic Myocardiopathy

Although ischemic heart disease represents a cardiovascular entity which is an important cause of sudden death in alcoholic patients,[6] it is not the only type of cardiac affliction in patients of this genre which can be responsible for such fatalities. Another variety is the one which presumably is due solely to overconsumption of alcoholic beverages and hence is termed an alcoholic myocardiopathy.

Generally, in alcoholics with an alcoholic myocardiopathy, death is not an explosive event but rather the termination of a period of gradually progressive cardiac decompensation due to the pump failure which inevitably must follow the structural myocardial changes characteristic of this type of organic heart disease.[159-169] Thus, although in a certain sense the terminal event in patients with an alcoholic myocardiopathy is an abrupt cardiac arrest, such a catastrophe is not unexpected and it follows a period of invalidism resulting from a progressive diminution of the myocardial reserve.

At an early state of this form of heart disease, the myocardial lesions can heal as long as the patient desists completely from the use of any alcoholic beverages. The continued use of alcohol, once evidences of alcoholic myocardiopathy supervenes, will be followed by progressive structural changes in the myocardium and, inevitably, will be followed by the hemodynamic changes which ultimately will favor the development of a sudden irreversible life-threatening ventricular tachyarrhythmia.

Until now, it has been difficult to locate precise data pertaining to the incidence of alcoholic myocardiopathy in relation either to the overall population or to those who properly can be classified as chronic alcoholics. One estimate has suggested, on the supposition that 12% of the adult population in an industrialized society consume excessive amounts of alcohol, that 1% of this number eventually will exhibit clinical evidences of an alcoholic myocardiopathy if alcohol abuse remains a way of life.[159] However, inasmuch as many instances of alcoholic myocardiopathy are unrecognized as such, it is likely that the mortality rate from alcoholic myocardiopathy is higher than is generally realized.

Conclusions of Studies

In this connection, the observations of Alexander[164] and others[161, 166] are particularly noteworthy. These investigators (who have conducted a number of meaningful studies concerning the nature of alcoholic myocardiopathy) have adopted the position, on the basis of a large body of experiential data, that there are many fatalities resulting from congestive heart failure in general hospitals which, erroneously, have been attributed to arteriosclerotic coronary artery disease when, actually, the underlying cause was an unsuspected alcoholic myocardiopathy. However, even if it is assumed that a sizeable number of deaths from "heart disease" should be linked to an alcoholic myocardiopathy, it still is uncertain how many sudden deaths are traceable to this alcohol-related entity. Admittedly, Laurie has stated that in Australia the leading cause of non-violent sudden deaths in chronic alcoholics is an alcoholic myocardiopathy[176] but it should be recognized that in his paper he did not explain precisely how this conclusion was reached. Nevertheless, it is conceivable that such an entity can be responsible for more sudden deaths in alcoholics than had formerly been supposed.

Clinical Features

According to various investigators,[161,163,168] the diagnosis of an alcoholic myocardiopathy need not depend entirely on the findings of the pathologist, inasmuch as it is now known that there are certain clinical features which should alert one to its presence.

Generally, the earliest symptom is post exertional dyspnea and cough. However, at this stage of the disease, the alcoholic rarely seeks medical advice or hospitalization because, commonly, such symptoms are dismissed as the result of smoking—a habit which almost invariably accompanies the excessive consumption of alcohol. Therefore, it is more likely that the alcoholic with an alcoholic myocardiopathy will not be identified in the hospital until there are more classical evidences of myocardial failure such as edema of the legs, swelling of the abdomen, and orthopnea.

Associated physiologic changes. Hemodynamic studies have demonstrated that the classical changes associated with alcoholic mycardiopathy are a low cardiac output and an impairment of left ventricular performance.[168-170] Clinically, evidences of cardiac enlargement usually are present and auscultation of the heart frequently will disclose an atrial or ventricular gallop or an arrhythmia of some type.

Associated ECG Changes. Various electrocardiographic changes are also associated with an alcoholic myocardiopathy but none are particularly specific. Early in the course of an alcoholic myocardiopathy, the only noteworthy electrocardiographic abnormality can be a distortion of the T-wave and, accordingly, some authors have adopted the view that even minor T-wave changes in the routine electrocardiogram of an alcoholic without cardiac symptoms, hypertension, cardiac enlargement, or adventitious cardiac sounds should be interpreted to signify the onset of an alcoholic myocardiopathy.[177] [,178] However, the validity of such an interpretation is highly questionable.

Discussion. In the course of an unpublished study[203] which involved an electrocardiographic screen of chronic alcoholics supposedly free of organic heart disease, it was found that in a substantial number, even during a drinking-free interval, there were variable minor malformations of the T-waves resembling those which experience has shown to be expressive autonomic dysfunction[179-181,] or some nonorganic disorder[182-186,188,190-192] Therefore, aware that most alcoholics have an underlying emotional disturbance of variable severity, and since emotional states are known to alter, in varying degrees, the configuration of the T-waves,[179,180,184,185] it seems that minor T-wave anomalies in the electrocardiogram of an alcoholic should not be interpreted to be a substantiation of the diagnosis of alcoholic myocardiopathy unless there are additional findings to justify such a conclusion[181,206]

Moreover, it is now evident that there are no recognizable risk factors which can warn when a patient with an alcoholic myocardiopathy is likely to die suddenly. As far as can be determined, a sudden death related to an alcoholic myocardiopathy tends to occur under a variety of circumstances. Thus, it could occur when the myocardial reserve has diminished to the point at which continued myocardial contractility is no longer possible. It could also result from an embolus to the lung or brain—an event which is a known possibility inasmuch as intraventricular mural thrombosis is not an infrequent feature of alcoholic myocardiopathy.[159,164] Finally, because of the underlying chronic alcoholism with its attendant cationic deficits, it is conceivable that a sudden cardiac arrest could result not only from the structural changes in the heart but also from a electrolyte-related and catecholamine induced superadded physiologic disorder of the myocardium which, in turn, would facilitate the development of a life-threatening ventricular tachyarrhythmia.[172,173]

Although the myocardial pathology of alcoholic myocardiopathy has been clarified by various investigators,[159,163,196,197] it must be recognized that the findings which they have described represent the changes associated with only an advanced stage of the disease. Thus, the pathologic data published by Alexander[164] would seem to be more meaningful inasmuch as he had the opportunity to obtain myocardial biopsies in connection with his studies of alcoholic myocardiopathy in surviving alcoholics.

Electron Microscopic Findings

Alexander considered the results of electron microscopy to be more revealing than the findings disclosed by light microscopy. His description of the changes he observed under the electron-microscope consisted of the following: (a) destruction and fragmentation of muscle elements into short segments arranged in more or less haphazard fashion; (b) swollen, damaged, mitochondria; (c) evacuation of mitochondrial contents leaving mitochondrial ghosts; (d) enlargement of the nuclei and dilatation of the sarcoplasmic reticulum; (e) abundant deposits of glycogen without increased distribution of lipid material; (f) absence of inflammatory cells. Moreover, he was impressed by the resemblance of such changes to those produced experimentally in animals deficient in potassium and magnesium.[193-195]

However, the results of electron microscopic examinations by Hibbs et al[196] of postmortem material in alcoholics did not entirely agree with the findings reported by Alexander. The changes these investigators considered to be most noteworthy were the following: (a) swelling of the endoplasmic reticulum; (b) degenerative changes in the myofibrils; (c) increased numbers of lipofuscin granules and lysosome-like bodies; (d) large numbers of lipid droplets; (e) mitochrondrial swelling; (f) alterations of the mitochondrial cristae; and (g) the formation of dense intramitochondrial inclusions.

Postmortem Histochemical Findings

In addition, in order to comprehend more clearly the pathogenesis of the alterations discernable by electron microscopy, this same group of investigators undertook a postmortem tissue study which employed specialized histochemical stains.[197] Seven of the decedents had died from progressive congestive heart failure, refractory to the usual measures employed in such a situation and one had died suddenly from multiple emboli after cardiac compensation had been restored. Nevertheless, the changes observed in the heart of the single decedent who died suddenly were not different from the findings in the hearts of the remainder.

A detailed description of the results of such histochemical studies can be found in their publication and need not be summarized here. However, it is important to mention that they found that although the cardiac changes, in the aggregate, only partially resembled the sort which have been identified with myocardial ischemia or infarction, these changes could be likened to the nature of the myocardial responses induced by catecholamine excess[198]. Thus, it can be speculated that accumulations of acetaldehyde (an important metabolite of alcohol and a substance known to possess sympatheticomimetic properties)[30] may be a meaningful element in the hierarchy of risk factors with respect to the pathogenesis alcoholic myocardiopathy.

In this connection, it is noteworthy that other observers[171] have also suggested but for different reasons that such an alcohol-induced "biochemical lesion" may be partially responsible for the development of a myocardiopathy in persons addicted to alcohol. Furthermore, inasmuch as most chronic alcoholics are heavy smokers[8,203] and because nicotine is known to possess sympatheticomimetic properties,[158] the smoking habit may be considered a possible additional "risk factor" in either the development of an alcoholic myocardiopathy or, conceivably, the occurrence of a life-threatening ventricular tachyarrhythmia, as well.

Gross Physiologic Findings

In instances of alcoholic myocardiopathy, the usual gross findings consist of dilatation of the cardiac chambers, hypertrophy of the ventricles, and scattered areas of intramural fibrosis throughout the myocardium;[159] sometimes, in both ventricles, there are patches of endocardial fibroelastosis with overlying mural thrombi, which can be the source of emboli to the lungs and elsewhere.[159,163,164] However, there is no general agreement with respect to the condition of the coronary arteries in such hearts. Some authorities have discerned very few abnormalities in such vessels[165] whereas others[199-200] have described narrowing of the lumen of the intramural microvascular branches and thickening of their walls. Nevertheless, as yet, it has never been suggested that alcoholic myocardiopathy should be classified as a coronary-related entity.

Pathogenesis

Most observers who have studied the pathogenesis of alcoholic myocardiopathy have claimed that it is a form of heart disease which can be correlated, to a large extent, with the excessive consumption of alcoholic beverages.[160,162] This view is also supported by the results of a unique study by Myerson.[201] In this investigation, skeletal muscle biopsies were performed in a group of alcoholic patients who, after a prolonged drinking spree, developed a skeletal muscle myopathy characterized by marked myoglobinuria, severe muscle tenderness, and increased blood levels of serum glutamic oxaloacetic transaminase and creatine phosphokinase. Examination of the biopsied muscle, during the acute phase of the alcohol-induced complication disclosed severe intracellular edema and destruction of mitrochondrial and myofibrils, changes which generally are observed in the hearts of alcoholics whose death was attributed to an alcoholic myocardiopathy. Therefore, the findings derived from this investigation can be construed to be indirect evidence that overindulgence in alcoholic beverages can be linked, to some extent, to the pathogenesis of alcoholic myocardiopathy.

Moreover, somewhat comparable observations have been reported by Seneviratne[202] with respect to skeletal muscle changes in alcoholics. On the other hand, in his report, there are also described a variety of cardiac abnormalities which suggest that, simultaneously, both the myocardium and the voluntary muscles had been affected by the myonecrotic process. Thus, the author of this article had postulated that the clinical phenomena and anatomical changes he had described were part of a diffuse myopathic syndrome etiologically related to the overconsumption of alcoholic beverages.

Clearly, there is a voluminous amount of data which has been published with respect to the interaction between alcohol and the heart, yet there is still no consensus regarding the pathogenesis of alcoholic myocardiopathy.[159] Nevertheless, it is acknowledged that a certain percentage of problem drinkers who habitually drink excessive amounts of beer or "hard liquor" will die suddenly as a result of a myocardiopathy linked to the overconsumption of alcoholic beverages.

REFERENCES

1. Tashiro, M. and Lipscomb, W.R. Mortality experience of alcoholics. *Quart. J. Stud. Alc.* 24:203 (1963).
2. Nicholls, P. et al. Alcoholics admitted to four hospitals in England. II: General and cause specific mortality. *Quart. J. Stud. Alc.* 35:841 (1974).
3. Schmidt, W. and de Lint, J. Causes of death of alcoholics. *Quart. J. Stud. Alc.* 33:171 (1972).
4. Graham, R.L. Sudden death in young adults in association with fatty liver. *Bull. Johns Hopkins Hospital* :16 Vol. 74 (1944).
5. Kuller, L. et al. Sudden and unexpected deaths in young adults. *J.A.M.A.* 198:248 (1966).
6. Kuller, L. et al. Epidemiology of sudden death. *Arch. Int. Med.* 129:714 (1972).
7. Wolff, P.H. Ethnic differences in alcohol sensitivity. *Science* 175:449 (1972).
8. Ashley, M.J. et al. Skid row alcoholism: A distinct sociomedical entity. *Arch. Int. Med.* 136:272 (1976).
9. Judd, E.S. et al. Spontaneous hypoglycemia: Report of 2 cases associated with fatty metamorphosis of the liver. *Am. J. Surg.* 24:345 (1934).
10. Brown, T.M. and Harvey, A.M. Spontenous hypoglycemia in "smoke" drinkers. *J.A.M.A.* 117:12 (1941).
11. Tucker, H. and Porter, W.B. Hypoglycemia following alcoholic intoxication. *Am. J. Med. Sci.* 204:559 (1942).
12. Neame, P.B. and Joubert, S.M. Post-alcoholic hypoglycemia and toxic hepatitis. *Lancet* 2:893 (1961).
13. Marks, V. and Medd, W.E. Alcohol-induced hypoglycemia. *Brit. J. Psychiat.* 110:228 (1964).
14. Clark, W.C. et al. Production of hypoglycemia by solox and by ethanol. *Quart. J. Stud. Alc.* 22:365 (1961).
15. Freinkel, N. et al. Studies on the pathogenesis and clinical features of "alcoholic hypoglycemia." *J. Clin. Invst.* 41:1359 (1962).
16. Field, J.P. and Williams, H.E. Mechanism of ethanol-induced hypoglycemia. *J. Clin. Invest.* 41:1357 (1962).
17. Freinkel, N. et al. Alcohol hypoglycemia. IV: Current concepts of its Pathogenesis. *J. Diabetes* 14:350 (1965).

18. Lieber, C.S. Liver adaptation and injury in alcoholism. *New Eng. J. Med.* 288:356 (1973).
19. Freinkel, N. et al. Alcohol hypoglycemia II: A postulated mechanism of action based on experiments with rats liver slices. *J. Clin. Endocr.* 25:76 (1965).
20. Madison, L.L. et al. Ethanol induced hypoglycemia. II: Mechanism of suppression of hepatic gluconeogenesis. *Diabetes* 16:252 (1967).
21. Madison, L.L. Ethanol-induced hypoglycemia. *Adv. Metab. Dis.* 3:85 (1968).
22. Seltzer, H.S. Drug induced hypoglycemia: a review based on 473 cases. *Diabetes* 21:955 (1972).
23. Lundquist, F. Influence of ethanol on carbohydrate metabolism. *Quart. J. Stud. Alc.* 32:1 (1971).
24. Libby, P. et al. The effect of hypoglycemia on myocardial ischemic injury during acute experimental coronary artery occlusion. *Circulation* 51:621 (1975).
25. Chase, P.H. et al. Hypoglycemic cardiac arrhythmia in early diabetes mellitus. *New York State J. Med.* :3647 Vol. 62 (1962).
26. Goldfien, A. et al. Plasma epinephrine and norepinephrine levels during insulin-induced hypoglycemia in man. *J. Clin. Endocrin.* 21:296 (1961).
27. Majchrowicz, E. and Mendelson, J.H. Blood concentrations of acetaldehyde and ethanol in chronic alcoholics. *Science* 168:1100 (1970).
28. Truitt, E.B. Blood acetaldehyde levels after alcohol consumption by alcoholic and non-alcoholic subjects. In: *Biological Aspects of Alcohol* M.K. Roach et al., eds. University of Texas Press, p. 212 (1971).
29. Truitt, E.B. and Duritz, G. The role of acetaldeldehyde in the actions of ethanol. In: *Biochemical Factors in Alcoholism* R.P. Maikel, ed. Pergamon Press, p. 61 (1967).
30. Eade, N.R. Mechanism of sympathomimetic action of aldehydes *J. Pharmacol. Exp. Ther.* 127:29 (1959).
31. Korsten, M.A. et al. High blood acetaldehyde levels after ethanol administration: Difference between alcoholics and non-alcoholic subjects. *New Eng. J. Med.* 292:386 (1975).
32. Surawicz, B. Role of electrolytes in etiology and management of cardiac arrhythmias. *Progr. Cardiovasc. Dis.* 8:364 (1966).
33. Fisch, C. Relation of electrolyte disturbances to cardiac arrhythmias. *Circulation* 47:408 (1973).
34. Kunin, A.S. et al. Decrease in serum potassium concentrations and appearance of cardiac arrhythmias during infusion of potassium with glucose in potassium-depleted patients. *New Eng. J. Med.* 266:228 (1962).
35. Redleaf, P.D. and Lerner, I.J. Thiazide-induced hypokalemia with associated major ventricular arrhythmias: Report of a case and comment on therapeutic use of bretylium. *J.A.M.A.* 206:1302 (1968).
36. Curry, P. et al. Ventricular arrhythmias and hypokalemia. *Lancet* 2:231 (1976).
37. Daniell, H.W. Arrhythmia in hypokalemia. *New Eng. J. Med.* 284:1385 (1971).
38. Surawicz, B. Arrhythmias and electrolyte disturbances. *Bull. N.Y. Acad. Med.* 43:1160 (1967).
39. Penna, M. et al. Effects of adenosine triphosphate and potassium chloride on ventricular fibrillation induced by lack of substrates. *Circ. Res.* Vol. 10 page 642 (1962).
40. Loeb, H.S. et al. Paroxysmal ventricular fibrillation in two patients with hypomagnesemia: Treatment by transvenous pacing. *Circulation* 37:210 (1968).
41. Chadda, K.D. et al. Hypomagnesemia and refractory cardiac arrhythmia in a nondigitalized patient. *Am. J. Cardiol.* 31:98 (1973).
42. Iseri, L.T. et al. Magnesium deficiency and cardiac disorders. *Amer. J. Med.* 58:837 (1975).
43. Heaton, F.H. et al. Hypomagnesemia in chronic alcoholism. *Lancet* 2:802 (1962).
44. Sullivan, J.F. et al. Magnesium metabolism in alcoholism. *Amer. J. Clin. Nutr.* 13:297 (1963).

45. Fankushen, D. et al. Significance of hypomagnesemia in alcoholic patients. *Amer. J. Med.* 37:802 (1964).
46. Martin, H.E. et al. Electrolyte disturbances in acute alcoholism with particular reference to magnesium. *Amer. J. Clin. Nutr.* 7:191 (1959).
47. Martin, H.E. and Bauer, F.K. Magnesium studies in the cirrhotic and alcoholic. *Proc. Royal Soc. Med.* 55:912 (1962).
48. Flink, E.B. et al. Magnesium deficiency after prolonged parenteral fluid administration and after chronic alcoholism complicated by delirium tremens. *J. Lab. Clin. Med.* 43:169 (1954).
49. Mendelson, J.H. et al. Effects of alcohol ingestion and withdrawal on magnesium states of alcoholics: Clinical and experimental findings. *Ann. N.Y. Acad. Sci.* 162:918 (1969).
50. Jones, J.E. et al. Magnesium balance studies in chronic alcoholism. *Ann. N.Y. Acad. Sci.* 162:934 (1969).
51. Sullivan, J.F. et al. Serum magnesium in chronic alcoholism *Ann. N.Y. Acad. Sci.* 162:947 (1969).
52. Hilden, T. and Svendsen, T.L. Electrolyte disturbances in beer drinkers. *Lancet* 2:245 (1975).
53. Iakawa, J.K. et al. Alternations in body potassium content in cirrhosis of liver. *Gastroenterology* 24:437 (1953).
54. Sereny, G. et al. The effect of alcohol withdrawal on electrolyte and acid-base balance. *Metabolism* 15:896 (1966).
55. Lim, P. and Jacob, E. Magnesium status of alcoholic patients. *Metabolism* 21:1045 (1972).
56. Mendelson, J.H. et al. Experimentally-induced chronic intoxication and withdrawal in alcoholics: Serum magnesium and glucose. *Quart. J. Stud. Alc.* Supplement #2, p. 108 (1964).
57. Ogata, M. et al. Electrolytes and osmolality in alcoholics during experimentally-induced intoxication. *Psychosom. Med.* 30:463 (1968).
58. Scherf, D. et al. Ectopic ventricular tachycardia, hypokalemia, and convulsions in alcoholics. *Cardiologia* 50:129 (1967).
59. Nevins, M.A. and Lyon, L.J. Sudden death and metabolic derangements in alcoholism with malnutrition. *J. Med. Soc. New Jersey.* 69:155 (1972).
60. Mullican, W.S. and Fisch, C. Postextrasystolic alternans of the U wave due to hypokalemia. *Am. Heart J.* 68:383 (1964).
61. Asmussen, E. et al. The pharmacological action of acetaldehyde on the human organism. *Acta Pharmacol. Toxicol.* 4:311 (1948).
62. Nelson, E.E. Pressor response to acetaldehyde and its potentiation by cocaine. *Proc. Soc. Exper. Biol. Med.* 62:23 (1943).
63. Kumar, M.A. and Sheth, U.K. The sympathomimetic action of acetaldehyde on isolated atria. *J. Arch. Int. Pharmacodyn Ther.* 137:188 (1962).
64. James, T.N. and Bear, E.S. Effects of ethanol and acetaldehyde on the heart. *Am. Heart J.* 74:243 (1967).
65. Jacobsen, E. Deaths of alcoholic patients treated with disulfiram (tetraethylthiuram disulphide) in Denmark. *Quart. J. Stud. Alc.* 13:16 (1952).
66. Andreani, G. and Castelleti, V.G. Dangers and complications in the treatment of chronic alcoholism with tetraethylthiuram disulphide. *Psichiat. Neuropat.* 81:319 (1953).
67. Klapetek, J. Death of a person treated with tetraethylthiuram disulphide (Antabuse). *Lek. Listy.* 8:250 (1953).
68. Becker, M.C. and Sugarman, G. Death following "test drink" of alcohol in patients receiving antabuse. *J.A.M.A.* 149:568 (1952).
69. Jones, R.O. Death following the ingestion of alcohol in an antabuse-treated patient. *Canad. M.A.J.* 60:609 (1949).

70. Alha, A.R. et al. Disulfiram-alcohol intoxication: Investigation of five fatal cases and the chemical determination of disulfiram and blood acetaldehyde. *Acta Pharmacol. Toxicol.* 13:277 (1957).
71. Hald, J. et al. The sensitizing effect of tetraethylthiuram disulphide (Antabuse) to ethyl alcohol. *Acta Pharmacol. Toxicol.* 4:285 (1948).
72. Lester, D. and Greenberg, L.A. The role of acetaldehyde in the toxicity of tetraethylthiuram disulphide and alcohol. *Quart. J. Stud. Alc.* 11:391 (1950).
73. Thimann, J. Review of new drug therapies in the treatment of alcoholism, *New Eng. J. Med.* 244:939 (1951).
74. Ferguson, J.K.W. Antabuse (Editorial). *Canad. M.A.J.* 60:295 (1949).
75. Hald, J. and Jacobsen, E. A drug sensitizing the organism to ethyl alcohol. *Lancet* 2:1001 (1948).
76. Hald, J. and Jacobsen, E. The formation of acetaldehyde in the organism after ingestion of antabuse (tetraethylthiuram disulphide) and alcohol. *Acta Pharmacol Toxicol.* 4:305 (1948).
77. Larsen, V. The effect in experimental animals of antabuse (tetraethylthiuram disulphide) in combination with alcohol. *Acta Pharmacol. Toxicol.* 4:321 (1948).
78. Jacobsen, E. and Martenson-Larsen, O. Treatment of alcoholism with tetraethylthiuram disulphide (antabuse) *J.A.M.A.* 139:918 (1949).
79. Reinert, R.E. and Hermann, C.G. Unexplained deaths during clorpromazine therapy. *J. Nerv. Ment. Dis.* 131:435 (1960).
80. Greiner, A.C. and Nicolson, G.A. Pigment deposition in viscera associated with prolonged chlorpromazine therapy. *Canad. M.A.J.* 91:627 (1964).
81. Hollister, L.E. and Kosek, J.C. Sudden death during treatment with phenothiazine derivatives. *J.A.M.A.* 192:1035 (1965).
82. Moore, M.T. and Book, M.H. Sudden death in phenothiazine therapy: A clinicopathologic study of twelve cases. *Psychiat. Quart.* 44:389 (1970).
83. Sydney, M.A. Ventricular arrhythmias associated with use of thioridazine hydrochloride in alcohol withdrawal. *Brit. Med. J.* 4:467 (1973).
84. Kaplan, N.M. Hypotension as a complication of promazine therapy. *Arch. Int. Med.* 103:219 (1959).
85. *Special Report: Psychopharmacology Program of the National Institute of Mental Health*, Washington, D.C., page 41 (1965).
86. Lynch, M.J.G. et al. Fat embolism in chronic alcoholism *Arch. Path.* 67:68 (1959).
87. Fazekas, J.F. et al. Management of acutely disturbed patients with promazine (Sparine). *J.A.M.A.* 161:46 (1956).
88. Mitchell, E.H. Treatment of acute alcoholism with promazine (Sparine) *J.A.M.A.* 161:44 (1956).
89. Figurelli, F.A. Delirium tremens. *J.A.M.A.* 166:747 (1958).
90. Rea, E.L. et al. Hypotensive action of chorpromazine. *J.A.M.A.* 156:1249 (1954).
91. Mitchell, E.H. Chlorpromazine in treatment of acute alcoholism. *Am. J. Med. Sci.* 229:363 (1955).
92. Albert, S.N. et al. Use of chlorpromazine in the treatment of acute alcoholism. *M. Ann. Dist. of Col.* 23:245 (1954).
93. Sturner, W.Q. and Garriott, J.C. Deaths involving propoxyphene: A study of 41 cases over a two-year period. *J.A.M.A.* 223:1125 (1973).
94. Fisher, R.S. et al. Quantitative estimation of blood barbiturates in blood by ultraviolet spectrophotometry. II: Experimental and clinical results. *Am. J. Clin. Path.* 18:462 (1948).
95. Davies, B.E. Tranylcypromine and cheese. *Lancet* 2:691 (1963).
96. Bethune, H.C. et al. Vascular crises associated with monoamine oxidase inhibitor. *Am. J. Psych.* 121:245 (1963).

97. Horwitz, D. et al. Monoamine oxidase inhibitors, tyramine and cheese. *J.A.M.A.* 188:1108 (1964).
98. Blackwell, B. et al. Hypertensive interactions between monoamine oxidase inhibitors and foodstuffs. *Brit. J. Psychiat.* 113:349 (1967).
99. Cooper, A.J. and Ashcroft, G. Potentiation of insulin hypoglycemia by monoamine oxidase inhibitor antidepressant drugs. *Lancet* 1:407 (1966).
100. Van Praag, H.M. and Leijnsf, B. The influence of some antidepressives of the hydrazine type of glucose metabolism in depressed patients. *Clin. Chim. Acta* 8:466 (1963).
101. Berrigan, T.J. et al. Fat embolism. Roentgenographic-pathologic correlation in 3 cases. *Am. J. Roentgen. Rad. Ther. Nuc. Med.* 96:967 (1966).
102. Scuderi, C.S. Fat embolism: A clinical and experimental study. *Surg. Gyn. Obs.* 72:732 (1941).
103. Hartroft, W.S. and Ridout, J.H. Escape of lipid from fatty hepatic cysts into biliary and vascular systems. *Am. J. Path.* 27:951 (1951).
104. Durlacher, S.H. et al. Sudden death due to pulmonary fat embolism in persons with alcoholic fatty liver. *Am. J. Path.* 30:633 (1954).
105. Holler, J.C. et al. On the significance of fatty embolism as a cause of sudden death in alcoholics. *South. Med. J.* 51:380 (1958).
106. Fishman, A.P. Shock lung. A distinctive non-entity. *Circulation* 47:921 (1973).
107. Pontoppidan, H. et al. Acute respiratory failure in the adult. *New Eng. J. Med.* 287:690 (1972).
108. Bergofsky, E.H. The adult acute respiratory insufficiency syndrome following non-thoracic trauma: The lung in shock. *Am. J. Cardiol.* 26:619 (1970).
109. Weisz, G.M. and Steiner, E. The cause of death in fat embolism. *Chest* 59:511 (1971).
110. Cotev, S. et al. The role of hypovolemic stress in the production of fat embolism in rabbits. I: Morphologic alterations of the lungs. *Chest* 69:523 (1976).
111. Reidbord, H.E. Pulmonary fat embolism: An ultrastructural study. *Arch. Pathol.* 98:122 (1974).
112. Soloway, H.B. and Robinson, E.F. The coagulation mechanism in experimental pulmonary fat embolism. *J. Trauma.* 12:630 (1972).
113. Bruecke, P. et al. The pathophysiology of pulmonary fat embolism. *J. Thorac. Cardiovasc. Surg.* 61:949 (1971).
114. Wilson, J.W. Leucocyte sequestration and morphologic augmentation in the pulmonary network following hemorrhagic shock and related forms of stress. *Adv. Microcirculation* 4:197 (1972).
115. Carlson, L.A. and Liljindahl, S.O. Lipid metabolism and trauma. *Acta. Med. Scand.* 173:787 (1963).
116. Wilson, J.W. Pulmonary disease and the microcirculation, in: *The Microcirculation in Clinical Medicine* R. Wells, ed. Academic Press p. 181 (1973).
117. Gruenwald, F. et al. A comparative study of promazine and trifluoperazine in the treatment of acute alcoholism. *Dis. Nerv. Sys.* 21:32 (1960).
118. Hart, W.T. A comparison of promazine and paraldyhde in 175 cases of alcohol withdrawal. *Am. J. Psych.* 118:323 (1961).
119. Goldberg, M. and Thompson, C.M. Acute fatty metamorphosis of the liver. *Ann. Int. Med.* 55:416 (1961).
120. Cutshall, B.J. The Saunders-Sutton syndrome: An analysis of delirium tremens. *Quart. J. Stud. Alc.* Vol. 26 :423 (1965).
121. Travel, M.E. et al. A critical analysis of mortality associated with delirium tremens. *Am. J. Med. Sci.* 242:18 (1961).
122. Chafetz, M.E. Alcoholism and alcoholic psychoses, In: *"Comprehensive Textbook of Psychiatry,"* A.M. Freedman, H.I. Kaplan, and B.J. Sadock, eds. Williams and Wilkins, Baltimore, Maryland, p. 1341 (1975).

123. Lundquist, G. Delirium tremens. A comparative study of pathogenesis, course, and prognosis. *Acta Psychiat. Neur. Scand.* 36:443 (1961).
124. Victor, M. Significance of cardiac arrhythmias observed during alcohol withdrawal. *J.A.M.A.* 236:1063 (1976).
125. Thompson, W.L. et al. Diazepam and paraldehyde for treatment of severe delirium tremens. *Ann. Int. Med.* 82:175 (1975).
126. Leevy, C.M. et al. Hepatic abnormalities in alcoholics with delirium tremens. *Quart. J. Stud. Alc.* 14:563 (1953).
127. Krystal, H. The physiological basis of treatment of delirium tremens. *Am. J. Psych.* 116:137 (1959).
128. Vetter, W.R. et al. Hypokalemia and electrocardiographic abnormalities during acute alcohol withdrawal. *Arch. Int. Med.* 120:536 (1967).
129. Becker, C.E. Significance of cardiac arrhythmias observed during alcohol withdrawal. *J.A.M.A.* 236:1062 (1976).
130. Wolfe, S.M. and Victor, M. The relationship of hypomagnesemia and alkalosis to alcohol withdrawal symptoms. *Ann. N.Y. Acad. Sci.* 162:973 (1969).
131. Weaver, W.F. and Burchell, H.B. Serum potassium and the electrocardiogram in hypokalemia. *Circulation* 21:505 (1960).
132. Seelig, M.S. Electrographic patterns of magnesium depletion appearing in alcoholic heart disease. *Ann. N.Y. Acad. Sci.* 162:906 (1969).
133. Randall, R.E. et al. Magnesium depletion in man. *Ann. Int. Med.* 50:257 (1959).
134. Mendelson, J. et al. Serum magnesium in delirium tremens and alcoholic hallucinosis. *J. Nerv. Ment. Dis.* 128:352 (1959).
135. Seller, R.H. et al. Digitalis toxicity and hypomagnesemia. *Am. Heart J.* 79:57 (1970).
136. Webb, S. and Schade, D.S. Hypomagnesemia as a cause of persistent hypokalemia. *J.A.M.A.* 233:23 (1975).
137. Bellet, S. The electrocardiogram in electrolyte imbalance. *Arch. Int. Med.* 96:618 (1955).
138. Surawicz, B. et al. Polarity and amplitude of the U wave of the electrocardiogram in relation to that of the T-wave. *Circulation* 15:90 (1957).
139. Surawicz, B. and Lepeschkin, E. The electrocardiographic pattern of hypopotassemia with and without hypocalcemia. *Circulation* 8:801 (1953).
140. Bashour, T. et al. U-wave alternans and increased ventricular irritability. *Chest* 64:377 (1973).
141. Chesley, L.C. and Tepper, I. Some effects of magnesium loading, upon renal excretion of magnesium and certain other electrolytes. *J. Clin. Invest.* 37:1362 (1958).
142. Pritchard, J.A. Use of magnesium ion in management of eclamptogenic toxemias. *Surg. Gyncol. Obstet.* 100:131 (1955).
143. Flink, E.B. Therapy of magnesium deficiency. *Ann. N.Y. Acad. Sci.* 162:901 (1969).
144. Reader, R. and Wynn A. The increasing mortality from coronary heart disease in men 1950 to 1962. *Med. J. Aust.* 2:740 (1966).
145. Vedin, J.A. et al. Sudden death: Identification of high risk groups. *Am. Heart J.* 86:124 (1973).
146. Tibblin, G. et al. Risk factors for myocardial infarction and death due to ischemic heart disease and other causes. *Am. J. Cardiol.* 35:514 (1975).
147. Heggtveit, H.A. Alcohol and the heart. *Am. Heart J.* 69:422 (1965).
148. Ganz, V. The acute effect of alcohol on the circulation and on the oxygen metabolism of the heart. *Am. Heart J.* 66:494 (1963).
149. Fernandez, D. et al. Alcohol-induced Prinzmetal variant angina. *Am. J. Cardiol.* 32:238 (1973).
150. Conway, N. Hemodynamic effects of ethyl alcohol in patients with coronary heart disease. *Brit. Heart J.* 30:638 (1968).

151. Orlando, J. et al. Effect of ethanol on angina pectoris Ann. Int. Med. 84:652 (1976).
152. Shubrooks, S.J. et al. Variant angina pectoris: Clinical and anatomic spectrum and results of coronary bypass surgery. Am. J. Cardiol. 36:142 (1975).
153. Howell, W.L. and Manion, W.C. The low incidence of myocardial infarction in patients with portal cirrhosis of the liver. A review of 639 cases of cirrhosis of the liver from 17,731 autopsies. Am. Heart J. 60:341 (1960).
154. Hirst, A.E. et al. The effect of chronic alcoholism and cirrhosis of the liver on atherosclerosis. Am. J. Med. Sci. 249:143 (1965).
155. Regan, T.J. et al. Depression of cardiac function and altered myocardial metabolism after ethanol. Ann. Int. Med. 60:709 (1964).
156. Mc Cloy, R.B. et al. Effects of acetaldehyde on the systemic, pulmonary, and regional circulations. Cardiovasc. Res. 8:216 (1974).
157. Conway, N. Hemodynamic effects of ethyl alcohol in coronary heart disease. Am. Heart J. 76:581 (1968).
158. Grollman, A. The action of alcohol, caffeine, and tobacco on the cardiac output (and its related function) of normal men. J. Pharmacol. Exp. Therap. 39:313 (1930).
159. Parker, B.M. The effects of ethyl alcohol on the heart. J.A.M.A. 228:741 (1974).
160. Regan, T.J. Ethyl alcohol and the heart. Circulation 44:957 (1971).
161. Burch, G.E. and Giles, T.D. Alcoholic cardiomyopathy. Concept of the disease and its treatment. Am. J. Med. 50:141 (1971).
162. Mitchell, J. and Cohen, L. Alcohol and the heart. Mod. Concepts Cardiovasc. Dis. 39:109 (1970).
163. Demakis, J.D. et al. The natural course of alcoholic cardiomyopathy. Ann. Int. Med. 80:293 (1974).
164. Alexander, C.S. Idiopathic heart disease. Analysis of 100 cases with special reference to chronic alcoholism. Am. J. Med. 41:213 (1966).
165. Burch, G.E. and De Pasquale, N.P. Alcoholic cardiomyopathy. Am. J. Cardiol. 23:723 (1969).
166. Fowler, N.O. et al. Primary myocardial disease. Circulation 23:498 (1961).
167. Bridgen, W. and Robinson, J. Alcoholic heart disease. Brit. Med. J. 2:1283 (1964).
168. Burch, G.E. and Walsh, J.J. Cardiac insufficiency in chronic alcoholism. Am. J. Cardiol. 6:864 (1960).
169. Gould, L. et al. Hemodynamic effects of ethanol in patients with cardiac disease. Quart. J. Stud. Alc. 33:714 (1972).
170. Wendt, V.E. et al. Acute effects of alcohol on the human myocardium. Am. J. Cardiol. 17:804 (1966).
171. Jesrani, M.U. et al. Acetaldehyde and the myocardial depressant effects of ethanol. Circulation 44:(Supplement 2) 127 (1971).
172. Walsh, M.J. and Truitt, E.B. Release of norepinephrine in plasma and urine by acetaldehyde and ethanol in cats and rabbits. Fed. Proc. 27:601 (1968).
173. De La Cruz, C. et al. Effects of ethanol on ventricular electrical stability in the chronic alcoholic animal. Clin. Res. 24:419 (1976).
174. Ahmed, S.S. et al. Depression of myocardial contractility with low doses of ethanol in normal man. Circulation 48:378 (1973).
175. Perman, E.S. Effect of ethyl alcohol on the secretion of the adrenal medulla of the cat. Acta Physiol. Scand. 48:323 (1960).
176. Laurie, W. Alcohol as a cause of sudden unexpected death. Med. J. Aust. 1:1224 (1971).
177. Evans, W. The electrocardiogram of alcoholic myocardiopathy. Brit. Heart J. 21:445 (1956).
178. Priest, R.G. et al. Electrocardiogram in alcoholism and accompanying physical disease. Brit. Med. J. 1:1453 (1966).

179. Wendkos, M.H. The influence of autonomic imbalance on the human electrocardiogram: Unstable T-waves in emotionally unstable persons. *Am. Heart J.* 28:549 (1944).
180. Wendkos, M.H. and Logue, R.B. Unstable T-waves in leads II, and III in neurocirculatory asthenia. *Am. Heart J.* 31:711 (1946).
181. Wendkos, M.H. The use of pharmacologic agents to differentiate between "functional" and "organic" T-wave abnormalities. *Triangle* 7:177 (1966).
182. Hiss, R.G. et al. Electrocardiographic findings in 67,375 asymptomatic subjects: Non-specific T-wave changes. *Am. J. Cardiol.* 6:178 (1960).
183. Brunner, D., Wendkos, M.H. and Hanne-Paparo, N. T-wave abnormalities in the electrocardiogram of top ranking athletes without demonstrable organic heart disease. *Am. Heart J.* 81:743 (1971).
184. Heyer, H.E. et al. Alterations in the form of the electrocardiogram in patients with mental disease. *Am. J. Med. Sci.* 214:23 (1947).
185. Blom, G.E. A review of electrocardiographic changes in emotional states with a clinical note on electrocardiograms of 193 psychotic patients. *J. Nerv. Ment. Dis.* 113:283 (1951).
186. Groom, D. Enigmatic T-waves. *J. South Carolina Med. Assoc.* 54:170 (1958).
187. Sjostrand, T. Experimental variations in the T-wave of the electrocardiogram. *Acta. Med. Scand.* 138:191 (1950).
188. Surawicz, B. Assessing abnormal electrocardiographic patterns in the absence of heart disease. *Cardiovasc. Med.* 2:629 (1977).
189. Wasserburger, R.H. and Lorenz, T.H. The effect of hyperventilation and Pro-Banthine on isolated RST segments and T-wave abnormalities. *Am. Heart. J.* 51:666 (1956).
190. Rotman, M. et al. Non-specific T-wave changes: A follow-up study utilizing the T-wave screen. *Arch. Int. Med.* 130:895 (1972).
191. Rosen, I.L. and Gardberg, M. The effects of non-pathologic factors on the electrocardiogram: Results of observations under controlled conditions. *Am. Heart J.* 53:494 (1957).
192. Littman, D. Abnormal electrocardiograms in the absence of demonstrable heart disease. *Am. J. Med.* 5:337 (1948).
193. Barron, G.P. et al. Histological manifestations of a magnesium deficiency in the rat and rabbit. *Proc. Soc. Exper. Biol. Med.* 70:225 (1949).
194. Schrader, C.A. et al. Symptomatology and pathology of potassium and magnesium deficiencies in the rat. *J. Nutrition* 14:85 (1937).
195. Moore, L.A. et al. Cardiovascular and other lesions in calves fed diets low in magnesium. *Arch. Path.* 26:820 (1938).
196. Hibbs, R.G. et al. Alcoholic myocardiopathy. An electron microscopic study. *Am. Heart J.* 69:766 (1965).
197. Hibbs, R.G. et al. Alcoholic myocardiopathy. A histochemical study. *Am. Heart J.* 69:748 (1965).
198. Ferrans, V.J. Isoproterenol-induced myocardial necrosis: A histochemical and electron microscopic study. *Am. Heart J.* 68:71 (1964).
199. Factor, S.M. Intramyocardial small vessel disease in chronic alcoholism. *Am. Heart J.* 92:561 (1976).
200. Pentar, K. et al. Alcoholic myocardiopathy. *Canad. M.A.J.* 93:103 (1965).
201. Myerson, R.M. Effects of alcohol on cardiac and muscular function. In: *Biological Basis for Alcoholism*, Y. Israel and J. Mardones, eds. John Wiley and Sons, New York, p. 183 (1971).
202. Seneviratne, B.I. Acute cardiomyopathy with rhabdomyolysis in chronic alcoholism. *Brit. Med. J.* 4:378 (1975).
203. Wendkos, M.H. (Unpublished observations).
204. Fisher, J. and Abrams, J. Life-threatening ventricular tachyarrhythmias in delirium tremens. *Arch. Int. Med.* 137:1238 (1977).

205. Nakano, J. and Prancan, A.V. Effects of adrenergic blockade on cardiovascular responses to ethanol and acetaldehyde. *Arch. Int. Pharmacodyn. Ther.* 196:259 (1972).
206. Sereny, G. Effects of Alcohol on the Electrocardiogram Circulation 44:558 (1971).

CHAPTER 5

Obstructive Asphyxia

For the most part, whenever sudden unexpected deaths in hospitalized psychotics have been traced to an obstructive type of asphyxia, the underlying cause has been found to be the entry of poorly masticated food into the major air passages.[1] Nevertheless, it must not be assumed that asphyxial fatalities due to alimentary strangulation have been limited to psychiatric patients alone. Even the Hebrew scholars whose observations were made a part of the Talmudic literature centuries ago had admonished that "one must not converse while eating because the windpipe might open before the gullet and thus endanger one's life."[2] In addition, historians have noted that as early as the 10th century, instruments had been devised to deal with this particular problem.[3]

"CAFE CORONARY"

More recently, this type of paraprandial death has been investigated rather intensively by Haugen[4,5] who introduced "Cafe Coronary" as a sobriquet to describe this particular type of fatality in the general population. Moreover, in the view of Haugen, an important contributory cause for such deaths was the combination of atrocious table manners and an excessive consumption of alcoholic beverages at meal time, especially when the victim was dining at some public eating facility.[4]

Similarly, with respect to asphyxial deaths from alimentary strangulation in regressed psychotics, it seems fairly evident that such fatalities were largely the result of the sort of capricious eating habits which, so often, are exhibited by patients of this genre. This particular trait, which is familiar to all hospital personnel in psychiatric institutions, has been clearly delineated by Appel, Myers, and Morris[6] in connection with their description of the behavioral characteristics of deteriorated chronic schizophrenics. As they noted, "the most striking changes in symptomatology with regard to regressed schizophrenics pertain to the eating habits of these individuals. Whereas formerly malnutrition represented a dangerous complication, these patients appear to display a voracious appetite, to the extent that they may be referred to as food grabbers. Some of these patients show a preference, for a short time, for certain types of food and a compulsion to react to stronger stimuli and eat the preferred food first. They often also eat with extreme rapidity (tachyphagia) and after licking their own plates clean will frequently attempt to finish the rations allotted to other patients. Although some may remain at the food grabbing stage, the majority progress rapidly to a more advanced stage characterized by the habit of placing into the mouth various objects without regard for edibility. These symptoms appear to be reminiscent of early infantile or disturbed infantile behavior."[6]

Case Report No. 1

Although these authors did not discuss the possible *lethal* consequences of such behavioral traits, a report which appeared in 1965[7] described a typical asphyxial death resulting from such capricious eating habits. The regressed schizophrenic, in this instance, was a veteran of World War II who died very suddenly and unexpectedly at the age of 41; sixteen years earlier he was admitted to the hospital because of seclusiveness, apathy, hallucinations, lack of insight and judgment, and characteristic catatonic behavior.

"Following treatment with phenothiazines which he received between 1956 and the time of death, there was some improvement in his psychiatric status, and eventually he was permitted to eat his meals in the main dining room of the hospital. At such times he was admonished frequently by the dieticians to eat slowly and chew his food properly because it was observed that often he gulped his food down quickly without properly masticating it, even though his teeth were adequate in number and in a state of fairly good repair. His last meal was consumed on August 9, 1960 and as was frequently his custom, he left the dining room with his mouth crammed full of food. Less than 30 minutes later, one of the nursing assistants found him lying on the hospital grounds near the dining area in an apparently moribund state. Attempts to resuscitate him were unsuccessful. Relatively large amounts of recently eaten and partly chewed liver and carrots were removed manually from his pharynx before his body was removed to the hospital morgue. An autopsy performed soon afterward disclosed that death was due to asphyxiation resulting from obstruction of the air passages by a partially masticated bolus of food containing liver and carrots. It was presumed that he left the dining area with his mouth full of food which then possibly became lodged in his larynx and trachea when he had made an involuntary sudden inspiratory effort."[7]

Case Report No. 2

A somewhat similar case was described by Von Brauchitsch and May.[1] The decedent was a chronic undifferentiated schizophrenic woman who died suddenly at the age of 52 after a prolonged hospitalization lasting 19 years. The nursing staff had observed that, customarily, prior to the time of death the decedent would "grab her food tray at mealtime, throw all its contents on the floor and wolf down her food in animal fashion. On the day of her death she suffocated suddenly when she tried to swallow an entire quarter of a grapefruit without first chewing it. Attempts to remove it were unsuccessful and within minutes she was dead."

PHENOTHIAZINES AS A DUBIOUS RISK FACTOR

Brief accounts of other fatalities due to alimentary strangulation in phenothiazine-treated hospitalized psychotics can be found in articles by Farber,[8] by Feldman,[9] by Zlotlow and Paganini,[10] by Childers,[11] by Hollister and Kosek,[12] and by Moore and Book.[13] However, it is noteworthy that in these publications the eating habits of the decedents were not discussed. Instead, it was implied by the respective authors that phenothiazine therapy was in some way involved in their asphyxial deaths.

However, only Farber[8] and Feldman[9] were more specific in inculpating these drugs with respect to such accidental deaths. Nevertheless, it is questionable whether their "explanation" necessarily was correct. If their hypothesis was interpreted properly, it seemingly was proposed by them that the unmasticated victuals which had entered the major air passages of the decedents remained there allegedly because the phenothiazine they had consumed previously had "interfered with their respiratory defenses." No further clarification of this term was provided by them and, so, it could be presumed that the intention of this autoptic notion was to indicate that the phenothiazine could be blamed for the fatalities on the basis that if it had not been employed, the patients would have succeeded in dislodging the obstructing foreign body.

Clearly, such a view is at variance with a number of clinical observations. Thus, as far as can be determined, intensive investigations up to now concerning the possible side effects of phenothiazine compounds have not disclosed that an impairment of the swallowing or other pharyngeal reflexes represents a charactterististic action of these psychoactive agents.[14] Moreover, various statements in the reports of Reinert and Herrman[15] and of Richardson et al[16] have served as a reminder that, in the years before phenothiazines became available, alimentary strangulation constituted one of the common causes of sudden death in disturbed psychotic patients. In addition, Richardson et al made the point that in their experience no differences were found when a comparison was made between the incidence of alimentary strangulation in hospitalized psychotics during the ten years after phenothiazines became available at their institutions and the incidence of the same complication in the ten years before these drugs were released for the treatment of psychiatric disorders. Finally, it should be recalled that even in nonpsychotics "atrocious eating habits" have been noted to be the major cause of sudden deaths from alimentary strangulation.[4]

Other meaningful data related to the problem of alimentary strangulation in hospitalized psychotics have been provided by the survey conducted by Von Brauchitsch and May.[1] Commendably, the "asphyxial" fatalities these authors investigated were divided by them into two separate groups: a) the pseudo-asphyxial deaths resulting from the aspiration of regurgitated gastric contents leading to death from aspiration pneumonia and b) those abrupt truly asphyxial deaths resulting from the sudden aspiration of a bolus of incompletely masticated food. The other variables they considered were the consumption of phenothiazines prior to the time of death as well as the behavioral traits and eating habits exhibited by the decedents prior to the time of death. Then, on the basis of an analysis of such data, they concluded they were "unable to establish a direct connection between psychotropic medication and death from aspiration." Moreover, when their tabulation of deaths from alimentary strangulation was examined closely, it became evident that acute asphyxial death due to alimentary strangulation occurred 50% more often in psychotics who had not received phenothiazine compounds than in those who had been receiving these psychotropic agents before the time of death. Also, in their experience, nontraumatic sudden deaths due to "choking on food" were encountered almost always in ambulatory psychotics who were regressed, difficult to manage, and prone to "wolf" down food without chewing it properly.

Moreover, on the basis of information pertaining to the doses of chlorpromazine required to manage the behavioral disturbance as well as the severity of the behavioral disturbance in the psychotics whose deaths were reported by Farber,[8] by Feldman,[9] by Zlotlow and Paganini,[10] by Childers,[11] by Hollister and Kosek,[12] and by Moore and Book,[13] it would be proper to infer that capricious eating habits constituted a conspicuous feature of their affliction. Consequently, it could be assumed that it was this particular attribute—rather than the phenothiazine therapy the decedents had received—which was chiefly responsible for the fatalities these respective authors had discussed.

Some Brief Case Reports

In the report by Feldman[9] there is actually only a brief statement that "one day following breakfast, a 28-year-old seizure-prone schizophrenic patient who required a daily dose of 2000 mg of chlorpromazine in order to control his extreme degree of agitation suddenly collapsed and at postmortem examination it was found that there was food obstructing the bronchi."

The article by Farber,[8] like that of Feldman, was an extremely brief case report. His patient was a 30-year-old female schizophrenic who had been receiving 800 mg of chlorpromazine daily to control her extremely agitated behavior. The length of her hospitalization and the duration of treatment with chlorpromazine were not mentioned. The information pertaining to the sudden unexpected death of this decedent clearly indicated that shortly after she had finished her dinner, she suddenly became very dyspneic and soon thereafter collapsed. Within minutes she was pulseless and clearly dead. The statement pertaining to the postmortem examination showed that the presence of partially masticated food within the main bronchi and bronchioles constituted the only noteworthy autopsy finding.

The patient of Zlotlow and Paganini[10] was a 23-year-old male who had been admitted to the hospital in 1939 with a diagnosis of dementia praecox of the catatonic type. Because he remained noisy, disturbed, destructive, hallucinated, and seclusive, a prefrontal lobotomy was performed in January of 1950. Despite this procedure, however, his condition remained essentially unchanged. In addition, between May of 1955 and his death on March 18, 1956, he received a daily ration of reserpine and chlorpromazine although these drugs did not materially alter his mood or behavior. On the day of his death, the patient was in the dining room where he "suddenly turned blue, fell off the chair, and died with his mouth full of food. Autopsy findings confirmed the diagnosis of asphyxia due to foreign body in the trachea."

The brief data in the paper by Childers[11] pertained to a female schizophrenic who had been hospitalized for 10 years and who had been receiving 200 mg of chlorpromazine daily for several months prior to the time of death. With regard to her demise, the author simply stated that she "swallowed a bolus of food and died of asphyxiation."

The case reported by Hollister and Kosek[12] was a man who became psychotic at the age of 45 following a head injury received in an automobile accident in 1948. His chronic brain syndrome was manifested by irritability, assaultiveness, and defective intellect requiring his continuous hospitalization since 1948. In 1956, because it was difficult to control his behavioral disturbances, treatment with thioridazine hydrochloride, 200 mg a day and chlorpromazine 900 mg a day was instituted, and he continued to receive these psychoactive preparations until the time of his death, which occurred on January 3, 1963. On that day while at dinner, he fell to the floor with his mouth still full of half-chewed food. No vital signs were apparent and resuscitative measures proved to be unsuccessful. Prior to the terminal episode, the patient had been considered to be in good general health without any recorded episodes of syncope or seizures. Postmortem examination revealed masses of partially chewed food in the pharynx and in the trachea just below the larynx. Mild pulmonary congestion and edema were present. The brain did not show any microscopic evidence of trauma."

So far as can be determined, the same entity can be held accountable for the three paraprandial deaths described by Moore and Book[13] even though the substance occluding the air passages was identified by those authors as "gastric contents" or "partially digested food." Of the three asphyxial deaths reported by Moore and Book, the first occurred in a 19-year-old man who was admitted to the hospital on January 24, 1961 with a diagnosis of "chronic undifferentiated schizophrenic reaction." His eating habits and the degree of behavioral disturbance were not mentioned but it was stated that from February 20, 1961 to February 28, 1961 he received chlorpromazine (750-1800 mg daily) and from February 28, 1961 to the day he died on July 24, 1961, he was given thioridazine hydrochloride (1950 mg daily). "Shortly after he had eaten his meal on July 24, 1961, he became weak, breathless, pale, then cyanotic and died a few minutes afterward. At autopsy occlusion of the larynx by aspirated gastric contents was found."

The second death occurred in a 52-year-old man on April 29, 1962 in the hospital where he had been confined continuously for 29 years because of a diagnosis of "mental deficiency with psychosis." Presumably, his psychotic behavior had become more pronounced about six months before the time of death because he had not received any phenothiazines until December 26, 1961. On that date, thioridazine and phenmetrazine were prescribed and he continued to receive these agents until the time of death. The daily dose of the thioridazine was 1050 mg and of phenmetrazine it was 75 mg. "At 4:35 p.m. on the day of his death, shortly after the evening meal, he convulsed, slumped forward in his chair, emptied his bladder and expired. The autopsy disclosed the following: complete occlusion of the larynx by gastric contents; congestion of the lungs; mild generalized atherosclerosis in keeping with the patient's age; slight obesity."

The third death occurred on April 9, 1966 in a 53-year-old mentally retarded female. Moderate doses of chlorpromazine were administered daily between 1961 and the time of death. The temporal relationship between the sudden unexpected death and mealtime was not mentioned. Nevertheless, the "autopsy disclosed the following: marked congestion of the lungs; partially digested food in the oral cavity and trachea; slight obesity."

Discussion

Thus, it should be evident from these case reports that the information they contained does not in any way dismiss the likelihood that the paraprandial asphyxial deaths occurred primarily because of behavioral traits rather than on the basis of phenothiazine administration. These data, then, would seem to reinforce other observations, already cited which indicate that in hospitalized psychotics, alimentary strangulation correlates positively only with capricious eating habits; accordingly, it is evident that such a behavioral trait constitutes the major risk factor with respect to paraprandial asphyxia in the mentally ill.

Moreover, it must be recognized that ultimately a diagnosis of alimentary strangulation must rest on autopsy confirmation of the presence of food in the major airways. Thus, the remarks of Messert[17] are particularly noteworthy and therefore they will be quoted without any deletions: "In cases of sudden unexplained deaths, pathologists who think of looking for the tell-tale chunk in the hypopharynx often find it, whereas those who do not, will not. One of us has had the experience of suggesting, during postmortem examinations in two cases of unexplained sudden death, that the hypopharynx be removed and examined. The pathologist reluctantly followed this advice only to find in one case a chunk of meat and in the other a large molar."

Messert also made the point that the suddenness of death in some of the reported cases of alimentary strangulation implies that pure hypoxia is not the only lethal factor. It is his thesis that because of stimulation of afferent nerve fibers in the respiratory passages, sudden occlusions of these structures can result in a reflex cardiac arrest. Thus, he recommends that even if the offending object is removed promptly, the additional need for cardiopulmonary resuscitation should not be overlooked. Support for this view is provided by the experimental observations of Coffman and Gregg[18] who noted that tracheal occlusion was followed almost immediately by the development of ventricular fibrillation. Moreover inasmuch as other data have indicated that clamping the trachea resulted in the prompt elaboration of excessive amounts of catecholamines,[19] it is conceivable that, in the presence of any degree of coronary arteriosclerosis, alimentary strangulation could favor the development of this same type of lifethreatening ventricular tachyarrhythmia.

However, ventricular fibrillation might not be the only cause for a companionate cardiac arrest in instances of obstructive asphyxia. Alternatively, the occluding foreign body could stimulate vagal receptors in the trachea which, in the presence of the associated acute hypoxic state, would result in a negative chronotropic effect and thereby favor the occurrence of complete cardiac standstill. Such an explanation would be in accord with the thesis adopted by Frankel, et al, who had invoked stimulation of vagal receptors in the trachea to account for the occurrence of a sudden cardiac arrest in artificially ventilated tetraplegic patients.[20]

EMERGENCY TREATMENT

In view of the foregoing considerations, it should be evident that the emergency treatment of acute asphyxia resulting from alimentary strangulation must include not only the procedures which will facilitate the prompt dislodgement of the alimentary obturator from the air passages but also those efforts customarily employed for the treatment of acute cardiac arrest. Therefore, an outline of the emergency measures which should be followed in such a setting has been inserted in the Appendix of this monograph.

FATAL ASTHMA

Another and less common type of sudden death in psychotics resulting from an obstructive asphyxial mechanism is the sort in which the obturator of the air passages was not derived from any external source; instead, it consisted of inspissated mucus that plugs the medium sized bronchi in adult psychiatric patients who, prior to the time of death, had not exhibited evidences of status asthmaticus. This entity was first described in 1963[21] and, as far as can be determined, no subsequent fatalities of a similar nature have been reported. However, this circumstance conceivably could be more the result of a lack of recognition of this particular fatal syndrome rather than its actual rarity. The article which was published in 1963 discussed findings of this sort in only two such decedents.

Case Report No. 1

The first was a 69-year-old white male veteran of World War I whose behavior first became noticeably bizarre at the age of 45. At that time he became withdrawn and confused. Gradually this gross change in his personality became more pronounced and, because of his inability to function satisfactorily outside of a hospital setting, he was admitted at the age of 51 to a neuropsychiatric center. At the time of his admission in 1942 he was quiet, neat, and clean, but exhibited the usual delusional and hallucinatory features of a chronic hebephrenic type of schizophrenic reaction. After approximately 17 years of hospitalization there was little evidence of improvement. The only psychotrophic drug which he received during his entire hospital stay was trifluoperazine in a dosage of 10 mg twice a day; this was administered regularly from July 12, 1960, until the day of his death on August 6, 1960.

Respiratory symptoms first appeared on May 2, 1960 at the age of 69. Physical examination at that time disclosed evidence of diffuse bronchitis. From then until his death, the patient experienced episodic attacks of mild dyspnea. A persistent moderate eosinophilia, which was unassociated with any parasitic infestation, was noted in repeated blood counts. The chest roentgenographic findings between 1955 and July 26, 1960, were considered to be compatible with a moderate degree of pulmonary emphysema and a congenital depression of the sternum. In the morning and after lunch on August 6, 1960, he appeared to be in his usual state of health and was free of any respiratory distress. Later that afternoon the ward nurse noted that he was lying in bed without showing any signs of life.

Postmortem Findings

A postmortem examination the following day disclosed extensive pleural adhesions on the right side and diffuse emphysema and congestion of both lungs. In addition, the bronchi were thickened and filled with mucus plugs through which many eosinophiles were scattered. The bronchial epithelium was edematous and contained goblet cells. The trachea also was very congested and contained large quantities of grayish mucus which almost completely filled the lumen. The heart weighed 375 gm and none of the chambers were dilated. There was no evidence of ventricular hypertrophy and there were only minimal arteriosclerotic changes of the coronary arteries. However, there were fairly extensive atheromatous changes involving the abdominal aorta. The brain weighed 1425 gm and there was no evidence of significant parenchymal or vascular disease.

Case Repoort No. 2

The other decedent was a 45-year-old Negro male veteran of World War II who already had displayed evidence of bizarre behavior before he was inducted into the Army in 1942 at the age of 26. On March 12, 1945 he was admitted to the hospital where a diagnosis of schizophrenic reaction of the paranoid type was made. In 1948 he received a course of insulin shock therapy without benefit. The clinical psychologist, in his evaluation in 1950, concluded that the test results were characteristic of a personality structure in which a psychotic process had been at work for some time. The patient received the following drugs: varying amounts of chlorpromazine between June 30, 1959 and December 18, 1959: 10 mg trifluoperazine once a day, and 1 mg benzotropine once a day between December 18, 1959 and March 20, 1961; and 100 mg thioridazine, daily between March 20, 1961, and March 25, 1961. No psychoactive drugs had been administered between March 25, 1961 and the day of his death on April 16, 1961.

The only significant nonrespiratory medical illness was an episode of hematemesis in 1947. At that time, roentgenographic studies confirmed the presence of a duodenal ulcer, which responded to medical treatment. In 1953 there was a reactivation of the duodenal ulcer, which again responded to medical management; follow-up roentgenographic studies indicated satisfactory healing of the ulcer. The first indication of any respiratory abnormality was the discovery in March, 1960, of physical findings interpreted to be due to bronchial asthma and bronchitis. However, the patient never manifested any repiratory distress until September 1960, when he developed dyspnea and an unproductive cough. In January 1961, the medical consultant noted the presence of sibilant rales over both lung fields and suspected a chronic sinus infection associated with pulmonary emphysema. Several nasal polyps were noted at the same time.

On March 25, 1961, when the patient was transferred to the Medical Service because of paroxysmal dyspnea, wheezing and coughing, the physical findings were characteristic of pulmonary emphysema and bronchial asthma. The latter completely disappeared by April 5, 1961, after he had received conventional treatment for bronchial asthma. Between April 5, 1961, and the day of his death on April 16, 1961, he did not require any epinephrine injections. Blood counts remained normal and no eosinophilia was noted. On April 16, 1961, the ward nurse noted that the patient was lying in bed in an unconscious state. Closer inspection indicated that he was lifeless. All of that day prior to his death, the patient had been ambulatory and had appeared to be entirely free of respiratory distress. His wife had visited him several hours earlier and subsequently confirmed the fact that he had been free of respiratory distress at that time.

Postmortem Findings

Postmortem examination disclosed marked congestion of the tracheal mucosa, which was covered by a thick reddish mucoid secretion. The right lung weighed 310 gm and the left lung, 305 gm. Both lungs were markedly emphysematous and congested. The larger bronchi were thickened and congested. They contained an excessive amount of obstructing reddish mucoid material which contained polymorphonuclear leukocytes and eosinophiles. The bronchial epithelium was edematous and seemingly contained many goblet cells. The heart weighed 355 gm and the myocardium, valves, and coronary arteries appeared to be normal. A few small, scattered, slightly raised atheromatous patches covered the aortic intima. The adrenal glands were grossly normal. Study of the brain and its vasculature disclosed little of significance.

Discussion

Thus, in view of the clinical and postmortem data pertaining to these two deceased schizophrenics, it must be agreed that it was appropriate to identify their terminal affliction as "lethal bronchophraxis without status asthmaticus."[21] However, it must be recognized also that when such a sobriquet was selected, the purpose was merely to designate the disparity between the extensive endogenous bronchial obstruction and the status of the decedents in terms of their respiratory symptoms prior to the time of death. Thus, there is not any adequate understanding of the underlying pathogenesis of this seemingly unique obstructive asphyxial syndrome.

Clearly, in these two instances, there was a link between an asthmatic diathesis and the subsequent development of the endogenous plugging of the bronchi but, as yet, the occurrence of bronchophrenic mucus at the time when there was little respiratory distresss cannot be explained fully. Perhaps, as has been suggested[21] the underlying cause may have been an atypical, and even an acquired, form of adult mucovisidosis. Admittedly, there is little factual data to support such a hypothesis but, on the other hand, because of the increased goblet cell activity observed in the bronchial epithelium of both decedents and the history of peptic ulceration in one of them, it is conceivable that such an entity could have been the basis for the plugging of the bronchi and its dire consequences, even though there were no concurrent symptoms of status asthmaticus (the condition most commonly associated with sudden death due to obstructing mucus plugs in the bronchi).[22] In this connection it is noteworthy that between 1960 and 1962 several publications have averred that peptic ulceration can be one of the features of mucoviscidosis[23] and numerous other reports have demonstrated that one clinical form of cystic fibrosis is the "adult" type and that, in this variety of the disease, its pulmonary component constitutes its most conspicuous feature.[24]

Moreover, because Plachta had claimed that phenothiazines can impair ciliary function in the air passages some consideration was given to the possibility that the administration of such drugs may have contributed to the fatal pulmonary complication in these two decedents. However, such an "explanation" was discarded when it was discovered that one of these two decedents had not received these particular psychotropic agents while he had been undergoing treatment for his asthmatic symptoms and that the other patient had received only small doses of trifluoperazine, a preparation which actually has been recommended as a sedative in the treatment of patients afflicted with bronchial asthma.[25]

Thus, it seems likely that sudden deaths in the psychiatric patient which are due to obstructive asphyxia can be related, primarily, to either the evolution of particular underlying medical impairments or to certain behavioral traits. Moreover, as has been indicated already, there is a sizeable body of experiential data to support the view that it is the deteriorated psychotic who is most likely to die suddenly from alimentary strangulation. Therefore, it is this group of patients who must be watched carefully at mealtime if this catastrophe is to be prevented. Correspondingly, inasmuch as recovery from alimentary strangulation must depend on the prompt use of effective measures designed to dislodge an obstructing endotracheal bolus of food, it is recommended that all health professionals responsible for the care of hospitalized psychiatric patients should become familiar with the material in the APPENDIX of this monograph which explains the procedure to be followed in order to prevent a fatality resulting from this type of complication.

REFERENCES

1. von Brauchitsch, H. and May, W. Deaths from aspiration and asphyxiation in a mental hospital. *Arch. Gen. Psychiat.* 18:129 (1968).
2. Herman, N. Asphyxiation by food. *New Eng. J. Med.* 289:757 (1973).
3. Spink, M.S. and Lewis, G.L. *Albucasis: On Surgery and Instruments.* A Definitive Edition of the Arabic Text with English Translation and Commentary. University of California Press, Berkeley and Los Angeles (1973).
4. Haugen, R.K. The cafe coronary: Sudden deaths in restaurants. *J.A.M.A.* 186:142 (1963).
5. Haugen, R.K. and Eller, W.C. Food asphyxiation—restaurant rescue. *New Eng. J. Med.* 209:81 (1973).
6. Bellak, L., ed. *Schizophrenia.* Logos Press (1958).
7. Wendkos, M.H. and Clay, B.W. Unusual causes for sudden unexpected deaths of regressed hospitalized schizophrenic patients. *J. Am. Geriatrics Soc.* 13:663 (1965).
8. Farber, I.J. Drug fatalities. *Am. J. Psych.* 114:371 (1957).
9. Feldman, P.E. An unusual death associated with tranquilizer therapy. *Am. J. Psych.* 113:1032 (1957).
10. Zlotlow, M. and Paganini, A.E. Fatalities in Patients Receiving Chlorpromazine and Reserpine During 1956-1957 at Pilgrim State Hospital. *Am. J. Psych.* 115:154 (1958).
11. Childers, R.T. Four deaths associated with chlorpromazine. *Am. J. Psych.* 119:374 (1962).
12. Hollister, L.E. and Kosek, J.C. Sudden death during treatment with phenothiazine derivatives. *J.A.M.A.* 192:1035 (1965).

13. Moore, M.T. and Book, M.H. Sudden death in phenothiazine therapy: A clinoco-pathologic study of 12 cases. *Psychiatr. Quart.* 44:389 (1970).
14. Hussar, A.E. and Bragg, D.G. The effect of chlorpromazine on the swallowing function in chronic schizophrenic patients. *Am. J. Psych.* 126:570 (1969).
15. Reinert, R.E. and Hermann, C.G. Unexplained deaths during chlorpromazine therapy. *J. Nerv. Ment. Dis.* 131:435 (1960).
16. Richardson, H.L. et al. Intramyocardial lesions in patients dying suddenly and unexpectedly. *J.A.M.A.* 195:254 (1966).
17. Messert, B. Asphyxiation by food. *New Eng. J. Med.* 289:756 (1973).
18. Coffman, J.D. and Gregg, D.E. Ventricular fibrillation during myocardial anoxia due to asphyxia. *Am. J. Physiol.* 198:955 (1960).
19. Goldfein, A. In: *Psysiology of Emotions*, A. Simon, ed. Charles C. Thomas, Springfield, Illinois (1961).
20. Frankel, H.P. et al. Mechanisms of reflex cardiac arrest in tetraplegic patients. *Lancet* 2:1183 (1975).
21. Wendkos, M.H. Lethal bronchophraxis in asthmatic schizophrenics without status asthmaticus. *Am. Rev. Resp. Dis.* 87:907 (1963).
22. Messer, J.W. et al. Causes of death and pathologic findings in 304 cases of bronchial asthma. *Dis. Chest.* 38:616 (1960).
23. Bernard, E. et al. The role of mucoviscidosis in the pathogenesis of the emphysema digestive ulcer association. *Presse Med.* 70:861 (1962).
24. Schwartz, E.E. and Holsclaw, D.S. Pulmonary involvement in Adults With Cystic Fibrosis. *Am. J. Roentg.* 122:708 (1974).
25. Wells, R.E. Physiologic Concepts in the Treatment of Bronchial Asthma. *Med. Clin. N. Amer.* 44:1279 (1960).

CHAPTER 6

Synsomnial Deaths

Inasmuch as it is now known that the majority of non-suicidal sudden deaths in hospitalized adult psychiatric patients are traceable to atherosclerotic coronary artery disease (see Chapter 3), and since coronary patients in the general population are at increased risk of dying suddenly while asleep[1] one could expect that reports concerning "naturally caused" synsomnial sudden deaths in psychiatric patients would frequently allude to sudden cardiac arrests identified with the presence of occlusive lesions in the extramural coronary arteries. However, as far as can be determined, it has been only an exceptional report that has described a synsomnial death in a psychiatric patient as being clearly due to such a cardiovascular entity.

Thus, the autopsy and clinical data presented by Reinert and Hermann in 1960[2] regarding four schizophrenic adults who had died while they were asleep, indicated that a significant degree of stenosis of the extramural coronary arteries was present in only one instance; in the remaining three decedents, the pathologist was unable to ascertain the cause of death. Accordingly, to Reinert and Hermann, these three other synsomnial fatalities represented a puzzling development.

In addition, since it was known that two of these decedents had manifested seizures while they were still alive, these authors had speculated that in these two particular instances the cardiac arrest may have occurred during an unwitnessed seizure.

However, they postulated also that the three seemingly mystifying synsomnial fatalities, collectively, were "related to spontaneous depression of autonomic regulation particularly occurring during sleep." Although, at the time, this explanation was heuristic its validity now is supported by recent studies which have been able to establish an association between REM sleep and coordinate autonomically-generated life threatening ventricular tachyarrhythmias.[1,3,4,35]

SLEEP APNEA SYNDROME

Moreover, inasmuch as the only significant postmortem finding with respect to these three decedents was "widespread visceral congestion," there is the possibility that the so-called sleep apnea syndrome could be blamed for these deaths. Characteristic features of this particular synsomnial syndrome which only recently has attracted the attention of investigators[5-7] are nocturnal asphyxial episodes with a resultant hypoxemia and respiratory acidosis as well as hemodynamic changes of a sort which would favor the occurrence of a life threatening ventricular arrhythmia.[5-7] Thus, its manifestations comprise pathophysiologic responses which correspond to those usually encountered in other types of obstructive asphyxia described elsewhere (see Chapter 5). However, the sleep apnea syndrome, unlike other asphyxial entities, is one which easily can be overlooked because a routine autopsy may not disclose the nasopharyngeal obstruction usually responsible for its occurrence. Thus, since its preeminent clinical manifestation is an exaggerated form of periodic and noisy breathing during sleep, such a history invariably should prompt the prosector to exclude this possible cause of death, particularly when the problem is one of explaining a seeemingly mystifying synsomnial cardiac arrest.

GENETIC PREDISPOSITION

Two synsomnial sudden deaths in psychiatric patients which were reported by Wilson and Reece in 1964[8] are unique inasmuch as a genetic factor would seem to be the basis for the sudden cardiac arrests in these two instances. These particular decedents were a pair of identical schizophrenic twins and their sudden deaths at the age of 32 years remained unexplained even after an autopsy had been completed. The schizophrenic illness in these two women first became apparent in 1955 but they were not admitted to a "mental hospital" until January of 1961. A behavioral trait which both manifested was the refusal to eat the food presented to them at mealtime and also the rejection through vomiting of any antipsychotic medication which they had been requested to swallow. Presumably, these acts were prompted by a delusion that both the food and the drugs were poisonous. Because of their failure to eat properly, both of these sisters had lost considerable weight and on April 10, 1962 thioridazine (400 mg daily) and an anabolic preparation were prescribed. Moreover, whenever the thioridazine was not retained, each of these women was given an injection of 100 mg of chlorpromazine.

On April 11, 1962 the decision was made to place one twin in a special section of the hospital and the other in a different section. At approximately 8 p.m. on April 11, 1962, twin A was given an intramuscular injection of 100 mg of chlorpromazine because she had vomited the oral dose of thioridazine. At approximately the same time, twin B was given 100 mg of thioridazine by mouth which was retained. That night, following a bed check, between 11 p.m. and midnight, both twins were sleeping soundly and nothing unusual was observed by the ward personnel at that time. However, at 1 a.m. on April 12, 1962, it was evident that twin A had died in her sleep. Immediately thereafter the condition of twin B was investigated and it was found that she too had died while asleep.

Autopsies of both twins were performed and the findings were identical except for the presence of endometriosis in twin A. Cholesterol gall stones were present in both twins but all other organs were normal both macroscopically and microscopically except for the presence of widespread terminal visceral congestion. Wilson and Reece concluded their paper with the following statement: "This would not be the first report where schizophrenics have died with ill-defined causes and times in perplexing circumstances. However, a rational acceptance of the death of either twin leaves unexplained the unique feature of our report, namely their simultaneous deaths. Their deaths were likely due to a combination of nutritional, toxic, and psychic factors; however, it is unlikely that these factors could have brought simultaneous death except in twins."

Thus, such a conclusion would imply that Wilson and Reece had seriously considered the possibility that the coincident and mystifying fatalities in these two identical twins were genetically-determined events. Correspondingly, then, it would seem likely that they would not have disagreed with a suggestion that an inherited susceptibility to sudden death might have been the basis for the unique experience they had described (see Chapter 14).

INHERITED DISORDER OF VENTRICULAR REPOLARIZATION

In this connection, it should be recognized that in 1976, Roy et al[9] had reported a typical synsomnial death without any proximate syncopal prodromes in a 14-year-old boy who, up until then, had been considered to be in excellent health but whose family history had indicated otherwise; his electrocardiogram and the electrocardiograms of two siblings, as well as the one of his mother were all characterized by the presence of a "lengthened Q-T interval" considered to be indicative of an inherited cardiac anomaly of a sort which could be the forerunner of a life-threatening ventricular tachyarrhythmia (see Chapter 14). Clearly, inasmuch as electrocardiograms of the two decedents reported by Wilson and Reece had not been obtained prior to the time of death, and since Wilson and Reece had not explored the family history with respect to the occurrence of seemingly unexplained sudden deaths, repolarization abnormalities, and syncopal episodes in the relatives of these homozygous twins, it would be proper to assume that the affliction which may have been responsible for the sudden and simultaneous synsomnial deaths of these schizoprenic twins was an inherited disorder of ventricular repolarization.

Furthermore, this interpretation is supported by the postmortem data which indicated that the hearts of these twins were normal both grossly and histologically. Such an observation is usual, first, when a sudden death is due to an inherited susceptibility to sudden death and, second, when cardiac tissues are examined in a routine fashion (see Chapter 14).

However, this circumstance should not be taken to mean that there is not an anatomical correlate of the inherited susceptibility to sudden death syndrome. Observations made by T.N. James[10] have demonstrated that the role of inheritance in relation to mystifying sudden deaths in persons without an overt congenital cardiac defect often can be firmly established by histologic study of the heart, provided the manner of sectioning this organ is performed in the manner he has advocated. His views in this regard are summarized clearly in one of his recent publications.[11] In this paper he explained that "during autopsy examination of cases of sudden death, failure to examine the brain is rare and most would consider such a study seriously inadequate particularly if no other suitable cause of death was found. On the other hand, the cardiac conduction system is rarely examined in just the same circumstances despite abundant evidence that its study may provide an equally convincing explanation of otherwise unexplained sudden deaths." Accordingly, it is likely that the sudden deaths of the schizophrenic twins described by Wilson and Reece[8] would have been clarified if the pathologist had examined the hearts of these respective decedents in the manner T.N. James frequently has found to be useful, in terms of establishing the basis for a seemingly inexplicable sudden death.

In 1964 Greiner and Nicolson reported the occurrence of three additional sudden unexpected unwitnessed synsomnial deaths in psychiatric patients.[12] The only noteworthy autopsy findings with respect to these three decedents included the presence of phenothiazine related pigment deposits in various viscera along with terminal visceral congestion. There was no reference to heart weights or the status of the extramural or intramural coronary arteries and there was no indication from the data presented by Greiner and Nicolson that they had connected these sudden unexpected deaths with the phenothiazines the decedents had received prior to the time of death. Thus, even though they linked the long-term consumption of phenothiazines to the pigment deposits they had observed, they did not blame either these drugs or the pigmentary changes in the heart for the fatalities they had described. However, the data they presented indicated clearly that these three decedents were known to be seizure prone prior to the time of death. In this respect, therefore, there was a resemblance between the three synsomnial sudden deaths described by Greiner and Nicolson and two of the three mystifying synsomnial deaths reported earlier by Reinert and Hermann.[2] Consequently, it is conceivable that Reinert and Hermann were correct when they suggested that the autonomic disturbances which accompany sleep may be an important risk factor, with respect to the occurrence of synsomnial sudden deaths in seizure-prone psychiatric patients.

In 1965, two synsomnial deaths of an entirely different sort were reported.[13] Undoubtedly, both were asphyxial in nature but like the other synsomnial deaths already discussed, both were entirely unexpected and, prior to the time of death, there was no indication of the presence of the condition responsible for these two fatalities. Nevertheless, the autopsy in each instance demonstrated that blockage of the air passages was clearly the cause of death. Discussed elsewhere, in more detail, are the unique features which characterized these two fatalities (see Chapter 5).

ALLEGED PHENOTHIAZINE–RELATED DEATHS

Subsequently, between 1966 and 1970, three additional papers appeared which reported instances of sudden unexpected unwitnessed synsomnial deaths in psychotics treated with phenothiazine. The respective authors of these three articles were St. Jean and Desautels,[14] Richardson et al,[15] and Moore and Book.[16]

The publication by St. Jean and Desautels[14] made merely a brief allusion to the occurrence of a single sudden unwitnessed unexpected synsomnial death in a 40-year-old phenothiazine-treated psychotic who, except for his mental illness, was seemingly healthy during his lifetime. The phenothiazine preparation he received was thioridazine (900 mg daily), but this drug was administered for only the last 4 days of his life. An autopsy was performed but this did not provide any reason for the fatality. No additional comments were made by the authors with respect to this incident which, to them, clearly represented a puzzling development. Moreover, because of the meager amount of available data pertaining to this particular fatality, no possible explanation for its occurrence can be suggested at this time. In this connection, it is noteworthy that St. Jean and Desautels made no attempt to inculpate the phenothiazine compound the decedent had received prior to the time of death.

By contrast, Richardson et al[15] and Moore and Book[16] not only reported cases of sudden unexpected unwitnessed synsomnial deaths in hospitalized psychotics treated with phenothiazines, but also seemed to blame the phenothiazines for their deaths. Otherwise, however, the data presented in their respective publications were quite dissimilar. The observations made by Moore and Book[16] were based on a retrospective neuropathologic study of the cerebral tissues of a miscellaneous group of phenothiazine-treated psychotics who had died suddenly and unexpectedly; only three of these deaths were sudden, unexpected, unwitnessed, and synsomnial as well. On the other hand, the conclusions of Richardson et al[15] were derived from a prospective study, the purpose of which was to compare the postmortem cardiac findings in two groups of autopsied psychiatric patients who had died during a single uninterrupted period of 18 months at the Little Rock Arkansas Veterans Administration Hospital.

One sample reported by Richardson et al[15] comprised four phenothiazine-treated psychiatric patients, all of whom had died suddenly; however, the deaths of only three could be clearly termed "synsomnial" in nature. Moreover, in this particular group, the hearts were decidedly overweight.

The other sample reported by Richardson et al[15] represented the "controls" which consisted of 49 psychiatric patients who, seemingly, within the same time frame, had neither died suddenly nor consumed phenothiazines prior to the time of death. This sample also included 21 psychiatric patients who had received "tranquilizers" prior to the time of death and who, presumably, had not died suddenly. Regrettably, Richardson et al had not provided any clinical or postmortem data with respect to these 70 decedents belonging to the "control group." Consequently, there was no information in their article pertaining to the heart weights or any other cardiac findings in the controls. In addition, they had not described the psychiatric or medical status of these "controls" or the causes of their respective deaths which, presumably, were due to "natural causes." Also omitted by these authors were the specific names of the tranquilizers which had been consumed by the 21 controls prior to the time of death.

Richardson et al[15] made only one reference to the postmortem findings in the "control group." This was a brief statement indicating that the focal histologic lesions in the hearts of the three tranquilized patients who had died suddenly while asleep were more extensive than those lesions in the hearts of approximately 70% of the 21 "controls" (consisting of tranquilized psychiatric patients who had not died suddenly). Moreover the authors did not provide specific information about the histologic findings in the hearts of the remaining 49 "controls" (the decedents who had not received tranquilizer drugs prior to the time of death). By contrast, these same investigators had provided detailed data pertaining to the gross and histologic features of the changes in the hearts of the three phenothiazine-treated decedents whose deaths were sudden, unexpected, and synsomnial.

Histologic Studies

It should be explained also that, in their histologic studies, Richardson et al had obtained multiple large blocks of tissue from the ventricular walls extending from the cardiac apex up to the aorta as well as from the interventricular septum and both atria. However, these areas were not excised until the heart had been weighed and then fixed en masse in 10% formalin and 2% sodium acetate. These blocks of tissue which measured 5.3 x 4.2 x 0.3 cm were then imbedded in paraplast and subsequently sliced and stained. The same technique was employed with respect to the three "targeted" decedents who had died in their sleep, and was used also when the hearts of the controls were examined histologically. The slices from each block were 6 to 8 micromillimeters in thickness and these were stained with hematoxylin and eosin, and with a group of "histochemical" stains commonly employed to demonstrate the presence of mucopolysaccharides; however, no lipophilic stains were used.

One of the members of the "targeted" group was a 77-year-old schizophrenic man who, for many years before he died, had been difficult to control despite the daily dosage of 400 mg of thioridazine and 200 mg of promazine. At autopsy, his heart weighed 475 gm and it was found to be flabby, soft, dilated, and dusky red. No gross changes were seen within the myocardial musculature. The extramural coronary arteries were remarkably free from atheromatous change; these vessels were translucent, smooth, glistening, and patent throughout.

The second "targeted" decedent was a mentally defective 45-year-old man who, despite daily intake of customary doses of various phenothiazines including thioridazine, was "very difficult to control" prior to the time of death. At autopsy, his heart weighed 500 gm and it, also, was dilated, soft, and flabby. The extramural coronary vessels were translucent and patent and no gross abnormalities were seen within the myocardial musculature. The lungs, liver, spleen, and abdominal viscera were markedly congested.

The third member of the targeted group was a 51-year-old schizophrenic man who, until the last year of his life, had received customary doses of various phenothiazines, including thioridazine, for many years. At autopsy, his heart weighed 480 gm and it, also, was dilated and flabby. On gross examination, it was otherwise normal except for an area of fibrosis in the left ventricle near its apex; this area measured approximately 0.5 x 0.5 cm. The extramural coronary arteries were patent throughout even though there was a minimal amount of atheromatous change in these vessels.

The histologic changes in these three *overweight* hearts were quite uniform. There was basophilic degeneration of muscle fibers and the formation of hydrocolloid bodies of various sizes and shapes throughout the ventricular musculature; moreover, these hydrocolloid bodies contained a PAS positive, diastase-resistant material. Thus, they represented deposits of mucinous acid mucopolysaccharides. In the areas of myofibrillary degeneration there was seldom any cellular exudate and dense fibrous tissue was not present. Similar colloid bodies were also present in the hearts of the controls. Myocardial nuclei frequently were box-like with peripheral condensation of nuclear chromatin. A lipochrome pigment was prominent in the cytoplasm of the myocytes in the hearts of these three cases and of the "controls."

The distribution of interstitial acid mucopolysaccharides about hyperplastic arterioles was found on the right and left side of the interventricular septum immediately beneath the endocardium. There was similar involvement of the inner one third of the myocardium of the right and left ventricles. Adjacent small vessels occasionally contained fibrin thrombi with complete obliteration of the lumina. There were only rare vascular or myofibrillary changes in the outer one third of the ventricular myocardium. The most severe lesions were in the small arterioles within the papillary muscles; these arterioles were extremely hyperplastic and acid mucopolysaccharide could be found in huge pools within the intima, media, adventitia, and surrounding interstitial tissue. Only focal myofibrillary changes were present in the atrial walls.

Moreover, it is clear that Richardson et al had considered the type of myocardiopathy they had described to be not only a formerly unrecognized unique phenothiazine-induced cardiac entity but also the reason for the sudden deaths which they had reported. They asserted also that "there is a similarity of the cases presented in this paper to case histories of sudden deaths of tranquilized patients that have been reported previously by Reinert and Hermann,[2] by Hollister and Kosek,[17] by Greiner and Nicolson,[12] and by Kelly et al;"[18] but, actually, there were certain important differences between their own postmortem findings and the autopsy data provided by these other authors.

Thus, with respect to their own decedents, the heart weight was uniformly increased due, presumably, to cardiac hypertrophy whereas heavy hearts were not a characteristic feature among the decedents discussed by the others. Conceivably, then, even if these other observers[2,12,17,18] had adopted the use of histochemical stains or block sectioning of the heart in the manner advocated by Richardson et al, they would not have found the deposits of acid mucopolysaccharide which Richardson et al had considered to be a fundamental change in the hearts of phenothiazine treated psychiatric patients whose sudden deaths had seemed to be somewhat mystifying, and acknowledged to be the result of a life threatening ventricular arrhythmia.

OTHER HISTOLOGIC STUDIES

In addition, it is important to note that for several years before the phenothiazines or other tranquilizers were introduced for the treatment of the mentally ill, pathologists who have used histochemical stains and block sectioning of the heart in connection with histologic studies of the myocardium have found "lesions" which conform in every respect with the changes Richardson et al had described. Particularly noteworthy in this regard, have been the observations reported by T.M. Scotti in 1955.[19]

This investigator had concluded, after a study of the hearts from 75 consecutive autopsies, that myocardial changes which formerly had been described as "basophilic degeneration of the heart muscle" actually were mucinous-like degenerative lesions resulting from depositions of acid mucopolysaccharide material. In connection with these tissue examinations, sections had been taken from the ventricles, atria, auricular appendages, and the interventricular septum. When there was gross evidence of recent or old infarcts, sections were obtained from areas away from the infarcts.

Staining Methods

The specimens were fixed in neutral 10% formalin; paraffin sections, made from each area, were then stained routinely by hematoxylin-eosin and periodic acid-Schiff (PAS) technique. In the group of cases with "basophilic degeneration," representative sections were stained by the following methods: (1) PAS with digestion using 1% solution of USP malt diastase in a buffered neutral saline solution for one hour at 37° C. on sections prior to treating them with collodion; (2) aqueous toluidine blue followed by rapid dehydration with absolute alcohol or acetone; (3) Mayer's mucicarmine; (4) crystal violet for amyloid; (5) Turnbull's blue for iron; (6) von Kossa's stain for calcium. Those sections that were not treated with collodion, and control sections exposed to buffer only, were washed thoroughly in water and stained by PAS and toluidine blue methods.

Discussion

Thereafter, Scotti made the following observations: "Of the 75 cases, there were 53 (71%) with "basophilic degeneration" of the myocardium. Areas of degeneration stained brilliantly with PAS and positive Schiff reactions were observed even after digestion with diastase. The PAS method was particularly useful in demonstrating early lesions that were overlooked in the first examination of a section stained with hematoxylin and eosin. However, the early indistinct changes were found more easily in the hematoxylin-eosin sections after such lesions were noted in sections with positive Schiff reactions. Lipochrome pigment was prominent in a large number of the sections with basophilic degeneration; inflammatory cells were not noted in relation to the affected fibers. The basophilic change was found most frequently in the left ventricle and next in the interventricular septum. It was found less frequently in the left atrium, the right atrium, the right ventricle, the left auricular appendage, and the right auricular appendage—in that order. Fibers with "basophilic degeneration" were present within or at the periphery of areas of fibrosis as well as in nonfibrotic areas.

"In this relatively small series, there was no significant difference with respect to the incidence of such lesions in men and women and there was no significant difference in incidence with respect to the race of the patient. Inasmuch as most of the autopsies were performed within a few hours after death and because the lesions were not more prominent in the few instances in which autolysis was observed in the myocardial fibers, the lesion was not attributed to postmortem change.

"In reviewing the causes of death and the main pathologic findings, it was noted that the basophilic degeneration was not related to any particular disease. It occurred in association with a variety of diseases; the association was most frequent with cardiovascular, cerebrovascular, and renal diseases, and also with malignant neoplasms. However, it should be noted that, preponderantly, 'basophilic degeneration' *was found when cardiac hypertrophy was present."*

Scotti noted also that basophilic degeneration passes through several phases of development. He continues:

"In an early lesion, the basophilic substance is very pale, separates the myofibrils and causes little if any fragmentation, but the affected fiber may be swollen. In this phase, the lesion is indistinct and may be overlooked in the section stained with hematoxylin and eosin. However, the substance is demonstrated vividly by the PAS method. As the material accumulates, it replaces the myofibrils. This phase probably is an intermediate one; only a thin rim of muscle remains at the periphery of the fiber and fragments of myofibrils are scattered throughout the basophilic light or dark blue granular material. With PAS technic the small masses also stain more intensely than the rest of the granular material. In the more advanced stages, some of the fibers are almost completely replaced by numerous homogeneous dark blue masses but this feature is not seen frequently. It is possible that the lesion progresses without development of conspicuous homogeneous masses or clumps of basophilic material. In such instances, although the granular substance is distinct owing to its abundance and its effect on the appearance of the fiber, it stains less intensely and is pale, sometimes appearing amphophilic rather than clearly basophilic. This form of degeneration is noted frequently in hearts with abundant lipochrome in the fibers and particularly if pigment is scattered throughout the basophilic substance.

"There is no level of myocardium which was particularly susceptible to 'basophilic degeneration.' The change may be found in the subepicardial and subendocardial region as well as deep in the myocardium. It has been observed also in the papillary muscles and even in the fibers of the conduction system.

"In this study of hearts from 75 consecutive autopsies, the incidence of 'basophilic degeneration' of the myocardium (71%) was higher than expected, probably because multiple areas of each heart were examined and all sections were stained both by hematoxylin-eosin and PAS methods. The PAS stain facilitated recognition of basophilic degeneration in an early phase, as well as lesions of slight degree that might have been overlooked in the first examination of the corresponding hematoxylin-eosin sections.

"Although the real significance of basophilic degeneration has not been determined, it has been established that such lesions are found principally in the hearts of persons over the age of 40 years although occasionally it is found in younger patients, and even in children ranging in age from 17 years to one year."

In Scotti's series, no relation between basophilic degeneration of the myocardium and renal disease or uremia was evident. Because the lesion has been observed frequently in hypertrophied hearts, it had been suggested by him that basophilic degeneration might be the morphologic equivalent of impaired vascular supply of the myocardial parenchyma. It is also noteworthy that Puccini and Stigniani[20] were unable to establish a relation between basophilic degeneration of the myocardium and any condition of the heart other than cardiac hypertrophy. It is interesting that there was hypertrophy of the heart in three young patients in their series; thus, the explanation of relative ischemia may be valid for these cases also. Correspondingly, it seems reasonable to suppose that basophilic degeneration of the myocardium would occur in a spotty manner when a lesser degree of ischemia is present.

Also, it should be recognized that the pathology Richardson et al had observed seems to resemble, in many respects, the changes which now are known to be compatible with a hypertrophic type of myocardiopathy.[21-29]

Thus, it would be important to know, at least, whether the three synsomnial sudden deaths which had been reported by these observers had occurred in a group of phenothiazine-treated psychiatric patients who, during their lifetimes, had also been treated for diabetes mellitus, or whether at autopsy the interventricular septum was thickened.

ELECTROCARDIOGRAPHIC ABNORMALITIES IN THE RICHARDSON SAMPLE

It also is of interest that despite the seeming uniformity of the histologic changes in the three hearts belonging to the "target" group, there was no corresponding uniformity with regard to the changes in their electrocardiograms. Clearly, then, the electrocardiographic findings in these instances do not conform with the view of Richardson[15] that, "the distinctive anatomical distribution of the myocardial lesions involving the arteriocapillary bed in the subendocardial region might well affect the conduction system and be reflected in the electrocardiographic tracings."

Case No. 1

In the first of these three cases, the electrocardiographic abnormality was expressive of abnormal depolarization of the left ventricle (a left bundle branch block). The decedent was a lobotomized seizure-prone schizophrenic who expired in 1964, when he was 77 years of age. Heart weight at time of death was 475 gm. The complete left bundle branch block was discovered for the first time, in a routine electrocardiogram made in August 1956, when he was 70 years old. Earlier electrocardiograms were considered to be normal but the dates when they were made were not given. After August 1956, the only follow-up electrocardiogram was one made in January 1963, when evidences of left bundle branch block still were present. Phenothiazines were prescribed for the first time in January 1956, beginning with 150 mg of chlorpromazine daily and 200 mg of prochlorperazine daily; thereafter, and until the time of his death on January 17, 1964, he received a variety of phenothiazine compounds, except between February 1957 and October 1958 when no such preparations were prescribed. Between October 1958 and the time of his death on January 17, 1964, he received 200 to 400 mg daily of thioridazine; and in September 1963, he received 200 mg a day of promazine hydrochloride.

Thus, the data pertaining to this 77-year-old decedent indicated that phenothiazines had not been administered until January 1956 and that a left bundle branch block was discovered for the first time in August 1956; a base line electrocardiogram had not been obtained before any phenothiazine therapy was begun. Although, the anamnestic data with respect to this decedent indicated that there were normal findings in earlier electrocardiograms made before the onset of phenothiazine therapy, the dates of these earlier electrocardiograms were not given. Thus, it is conceivable that the left bundle branch block may have been present already when the phenothiazine therapy was started.

It is well known that a left bundle branch block commonly results from various types of myocardiopathy associated with left ventricular hypertrophy[22,24-28,30] and, in the case history extract pertaining to this decedent, the heart weight was stated to be 475 gm. This circumstance would suggest long-standing left ventricular hypertrophy; consequently, it is likely that the left bundle branch block in this instance was due to both left ventricular enlargement and to the histologic changes distributed alongside the specialized conducting tissues located in the interventricular septum.

Case No. 2

By contrast, the noteworthy findings in the electrocardiograms of the second decedent were confined to an abnormality of the T-wave and "a slight prolongation of the Q-T interval." This decedent was a mental defective who, at the age of 45, was found dead during a routine bed check on December 16, 1964. Phenothiazine therapy (thioridazine) was started on March 12, 1962 and between that date and the time of death, other phenothiazines had either been added or substituted. The first electrocardiogram was obtained on January 24, 1963, approximately 10 months after thioridazine in moderate doses had been prescribed. In this electrocardiogram (a copy was not included with the text) the findings were normal except for the presence of "nonspecific T-wave changes associated with a prolonged Q-T interval." Similar changes were observed in subsequent routine electrocardiograms made in February and March of 1964; no additional electrocardiograms were obtained prior to the time of death, and no electrocardiograms had been obtained prior to the initiation of phenothiazine therapy. In this instance it is also noteworthy that whereas the administration of thioridazine was discontinued on February 4, 1964, an abnormality of the T-wave and a "lengthening of the Q-T interval" was still present in the electrocardiogram made one month later; for this reason, it is likely that the T-wave abnormality was expressive of some type of structural myocardial abnormality such as cardiac hypertrophy and that it was not the sort of electrocardiographic change which results from thioridazine therapy (see Chapter 13). Thus, although the abnormalities in the electrocardiograms of this decedent could be classified as non-specific changes indicative of some type of structural myocardiopathy, such changes were not necessarily a reflection of the "distinctive anatomical distribution of the myocardial lesions involving the arteriocapillary bed in the subendocardial region."

Case No. 3

Least expressive of the myocardiopathy or the distribution of the histologic changes noted by Richardson et al were the findings in the electrocardiograms of the third decedent. In this instance, the noteworthy electrocardiographic deviation consisted of an intermittent abnormality of the T-wave which seemingly could be correlated merely with intermittent administration of moderate doses of chlorpromazine or thioridazine.

This decedent was a 51-year-old paranoid schizophrenic who was found dead in bed on February 26, 1965. Approximately nine years before the time of death, modest doses of chlorpromazine were prescribed and this drug therapy was continued for two years (until February 1956). Then, four years before the time of death, thioridazine in modest doses was prescribed; it was discontinued three years later (March 1964). During the last year of his life (1964-1965) he was receiving only a daily ration of phenobarbital and a 75 mg daily dose of carphenazine.

The first electrocardiogram was made in November of 1953, approximately two years before phenothiazine therapy of any kind was prescribed; this electrocardiogram allegedly was normal. In two electrocardiograms made in 1956, while he was receiving modest doses of chlorpromazine, the only significant finding was a "sinus tachycardia associated with low amplitude of the T-wave in all leads;" presumably, the T-wave changes were secondary to either the tachycardia or to the chlorpromazine therapy. A subsequent electrocardiogram made in 1958, presumably after chlorpromazine therapy was discontinued, was found to be normal, whereas in February of 1964, while he was receiving moderate doses of thioridazine "nonspecific S-T and T-wave changes were again present" in an electrocardiogram made at that time. The next electrocardiogram, made on February 15, 1965, 11 days before the patient died and when he no longer was receiving any thioridazine was "interpreted to be within normal limits." Thus, all the available data in this instance would seem to show that the electrocardiographic findings were not a reflection of either the structural myocardiopathy or the histologic changes described by Richardson et al.

Although it is known that hearts damaged due to a chronic progressive myocardiopathy can suddenly, at any particular moment in time, become cardioplegic, it would nevertheless seem appropriate to consider which mechanisms could conceivably account for the occurrence of such a catastrophe. Thus, it can be supposed, for example, that a sudden life-threatening tachyarrhythmia may have followed an abrupt rheologic alteration of the coronary microcirculation when there was already an existing marginal degree of myocardial hypoxia resulting from widespread luminal narrowing of the tiny intramural coronary vessels, in conjunction with cardiac hypertrophy.

Moreover, if there was also a stenosis involving those nutrient branches supplying vital pacemaker sites in the heart, such a vasculopathy likewise could be responsible for a sudden cardiac arrest. In this connection, it is noteworthy that the investigations of T.N. James[11,29,36] have shown that occlusions or narrowing of such nutrient arterioles can, indeed, favor the occurrence of a sudden lethal tachyarrhythmia.

Equally tenable could be an explanation based on current knowledge concerning physiologic alterations during sleep.[1,31-33,35] Inasmuch as such studies emphasize an association between REM sleep and increased nocturnal traffic along neural pathways which carry adrenergic stimuli to the heart, the net effect during that phase of sleep, in certain persons, could substantially lower the ventricular fibrillation threshold.[1,33,35] It could thus be postulated that in these three patients with overweight hearts, there was a sudden burst of adrenergic augmentation during sleep which, conceivably, led to the development of a life-threatening ventricular tachyarrhythmia and a resulting cardiac arrest. This view finds further support from data which indicate that persons with a hypertrophic variety of myocardiopathy are at increased risk of dying suddenly, at any time.[34,37,38]

As far as can be determined, the major accomplishment of the study undertaken by Moore and Book[16] was their demonstration that structural changes were absent in the brains of psychiatric patients who were uniform in only two respects: all 12 patients were receiving phenothiazines prior to the time of death and all had died suddenly. In connection with their investigation, they "took sections from representative areas with special reference to the hypothalamus, reticular activating substance, and brain stem to determine if any form of tissue alteration was present as the result of phenothiazine drugs and which conceivably could explain the cause of death." Sixteen different stains were employed by them in pursuit of this objective but, in the end, they were unable to discover any changes in these various structures.

Moore and Book advanced the following hypothesis:

"It is conjectured that some patients may have a specific nervous system susceptibility producing a concatenation of cardiovascular and respiratory dysfunction resulting in sudden death. The mode of action may lie in a disturbance of enzyme systems in the synaptic cleft and interference with ionic transmembrane migrations in motoneurons of the involved nervous system. Whether this represents a genetic predisposition or a chance occurrence in this group of patients cannot be determined at present. There is an indication that the use of more than one phenothiazine in the treatment of a patient as is so commonly practiced or the combination of a phenothiazine with some other tranquilizing drug or drugs may potentiate the effect upon the susceptible portion of the nervous system and other body tissues ensuing in death. Whether this is due to a direct action of the drugs, to elaboration of a toxic metabolite, or to an autoimmune reaction has not yet been established."

Moreover, as far as can be determined from the data supplied by Moore and Book, none of the three phenothiazine-treated psychotics who died suddenly and unexpectedly in their sleep was seizure prone. It therefore seems unlikely that their deaths can be linked to an unwitnessed fatal seizure. On the other hand, there is still the possibility that the fatalities were due to the presence of coronary arterial stenosis. Data provided from many sources have shown that young or middle-aged adults in the general population can die suddenly while asleep because of occlusive coronary artery disease, even when there is no associated coronary thrombosis or myocardial infarction.[37,38] In addition, various observations have demonstrated that frequently such occlusive sites in the extramural coronary arteries can be overlooked unless the prosector undertakes a meticulous examination of the entire course of each major branch of the coronary arterial tree.[39-42,51-54] Therefore, it is regrettable that the autopsy data with respect to the three synsomnial deaths included in the report by Moore and Book omitted any detailed description of the heart and coronary vessels; the only pathology which was mentioned was the non-specific terminal visceral congestion which usually is encountered in any instance of sudden death.

Bangungut Syndrome

Even if it is conceded that Moore and Book were correct to surmise that there was a pathophysiologic rather than a pathologic basis for the sudden deaths of these three patients, the timing of these respective fatalities would imply that it was autonomic dysfunction connected with certain sleep cycles rather than any drug effect which was responsible primarily for a sudden cardiac arrest in these instances. However, this suggestion does not exclude, necessarily, mechanisms which have been invoked to explain the occurrence of "bangungut," a unique synsomnial fatal syndrome limited to orientals without any psychiatric disorder.[45]

So far, the etiology of "bangungut" still is obscure but the view has been advanced that a reflex augmentation of vagal influences reaching the heart may be involved.[45] This observation is important inasmuch as an independent study by Lenel et al[46] has established that, in intact dogs, a life-threatening ventricular tachyarrhythmia can follow reflex slowing of the heart, when this organ is exposed simultaneously to adrenergic stimulation. Thus, inasmuch as the endocrinologic accompaniments of episodic REM activity during sleep, when dreaming is at its peak, is characterized by an excessive elaboration of adrenal hormones,[1,32,35,51] it is conceivable that a dream induced coincident reflex surge of parasympathetic influences along the neural pathways to the heart in psychiatric patients who, already, are elaborating increased amounts of steroids and catecholamines[47-52] may help to explain the occurrence of a seemingly mystifying sudden symsomnial death in patients of this genre.

Clearly, such a proposition is largely heuristic in nature but inasmuch as there is currently a lack of data with respect to correlations in psychiatric patients between the various phases of sleep and changes pertaining to the electrocardiogram and neurohumoral secretions, it would seem improper to disregard the possibility that certain seemingly mystifying synsomnial sudden deaths in psychiatric patients may be, essentially, a unique feature of an "autonomic syndrome," especially when the autopsy has been unable to explain the death. Moreover, such a thesis would seem to be supported by the isolated observations already reported by Wellens et al[57] and by Lown et al[35] with regard to the occurrence of synsomnial life-threatening ventricular tachyarrhythmias.

REFERENCES

1. Williams, J.C. et al. The risk of sleep in the cardiac patient. *Circulation* (Suppl. VI) 38:206 (1968).
2. Reinert, R.E. and Hermann, C.G. Unexplained deaths during chlorpromazine therapy. *J.Nerv. Ment. Dis.* 131:435 (1960).
3. Orr,W.C. and Shappell, S.D. REM sleep and cardiac arrhythmias. *Circulation* 52:519 (1975).
4. Rosemblatt, G. et al. Cardiac irritability during sleep and dreaming. *J. Psychosomat. Res.* 17:127 (1973).
5. Tilkian, A.G. et al. Sleep-induced apnea syndrome: Reversal of serious arrhythmias after tracheostomy. *Circulation* 52: (Suppl.II):131 (1975).
6. Tilkian, A.G. et al. Hemodynamics in sleep-induced apnea: Studies during wakefulness and sleep. *Ann. Intern. Med.* 85:714 (1976).
7. Guilleminault, C. et al. The sleep apnea syndromes, *Annu. Rev. Med.* 27:465 (1976).

8. Wilson, I.C. and Reece, J.C. Simultaneous death in schizophrenic twins. *Arch. Gen. Psych.* 11:377 (1964).
9. Roy, P.R. et al. Hereditary prolongation of the Q-T interval: Genetic observations and mangement in three families with twelve affected members. *Am. J. Cardiol.* 37:237 (1976).
10. James, T.N. Q-T prolongation and sudden death. *Mod. Concepts Cardiovasc. Dis.* 38:35 (1969).
11. James, T.N. Apoplexy of the heart. *Circulation* 57:385 (1978).
12. Greiner, A.C. and Nicolson, G.A. Pigment deposition in viscera associated with prolonged chlorpromazine therapy. *Canad. M.A.J.* 91:627 (1964).
13. Wendkos, M.H. Lethal bronchophraxis in asthmatic schizophrenics without status asthmaticus. *Am. Rev. Resp. Dis.* 87:907 (1963).
14. St. Jean, A. and Desautels, S. Electrocardiographic changes with a neuroleptic, thioridazine. *Un. Med. Canada.* 95:554 (1966).
15. Richardson, H.L. et al. Intramyocardial lesions in patients dying suddenly and unexpectedly. *J.A.M.A.* 195:254 (1966).
16. Moore, M.T. and Book, M.H. Sudden death in phenothiazine therapy: A clinco pathologic study of 12 cases. *Psych. Quart.* 44:389 (1970).
17. Hollister, L.E. and Kosek, J.C. Sudden death during treatment with phenothiazine derivatives. *J.A.M.A.* 192:1035 (1965).
18. Kelly, H.G. et al. Thioridazine hydrochloride (Mellaril): Its effects on the elctrocardiogram and a report of 2 fatalities with electrocardiographic abnormalities. *Canad. M.A.J.* 89:546 (1963).
19. Scotti, T.M. Basophilic (mucinous) degeneration of the myocardium. *Amer. J. Clin. Path.* 25:994 (1955).
20. Puccini, C. and Stigliani, R. New researches concerning the cause of basophilic degeneration of the myocardium. *Arch. "de v. Ecchi" Anat. Pat.* 15:811 (1950).
21. Blumenthal, H.T. et al. A study of lesions of the intramural coronary artery branches in diabetes mellitus. *Arch. Path.* 70:13 (1960).
22. Varnauskas, E. et al. Obscure cardiomyopathies with coronary artery changes. *Am. J. Cardiol.* 19:531 (1967).
23. Rubler, S. et al. New type of cardiomyopathy associated with diabetic glomerulosclerosis. *Am. J. Cardiol.* 30:595 (1972).
24. Hamby, R.I. et al. Diabetic cardiomyopathy. *J.A.M.A.* 229:1749 (1974).
25. Ledet, T. Histological and histochemical changes in the coronary arteries of old diabetic patients. *Diabetologia* 4:268 (1968).
26. Hamby, R.I. et al. Primary myocardial disease: Clinical, hemodynamic and angiographic correlates in 50 patients. *Am. J. Cardiol.* 25:625 (1970).
27. Hamby, R.I. Primary myocardial disease: A prospective clinical and hemodynamic evaluation of 100 patients. *Medicine* 49:55 (1970).
28. Hudson, R.E.B. The cardiomyopathies: Order from chaos. *Am. J. Cardiol.* 25:70 (1970).
29. James, T.N. An etiologic concept concerning the obscure myocardiopathies. *Progr. Cardiovasc. Dis.* 7:43 (1964).
30. Goodwin, J.F. Clarification of the cardiomyopathies. *Mod. Concepts Cardiovasc. Dis.* 41:41 (1972).
31. Jouvet, M. The neurobiology of sleep and dreaming. *J.A.M.A.* 228:1437 (1974).
32. Hobson, J.A. Sleep: Physiologic aspects. *New Eng. J. Med.* 281:1343 (1969).
33. Williams, R.L. et al. *EEG of Human Sleep: Clinical Applications.* John Wiley and Sons, New York (1974).
34. Maron, B.J. et al. Sudden death in patients with hypertrophic cardiomyopathy: Characterization of 26 patients without functional limitation. *Am. J. Cardiol.* 41:803 (1978).

35. Lown, B. et al. Basis for recurring ventricular fibrillation in the absence of coronary heart disease and its management. *New Eng. J. Med.* 294:623 (1976).
36. James, T.N. Pathology of small coronary arteries. *Am. J. Cardiol.* 20:679 (1967).
37. Moritz, A.R. and Zamcheck, N. Sudden and unexpected deaths of young soldiers: Diseases responsible for sudden deaths during World War II. *Arch. Path.* 42:459 (1946).
38. French, A.J. and Dock, W. Fatal coronary arteriosclerosis in young soldiers. *J.A.M.A.* 124:1233 (1944).
39. Goodwin, J.F. and Krikler, D.M. Arrhythmia as a Cause of Sudden Death in Hypertrophic Cardiomyopathy. *Lancet* 2:937 (1976).
40. Titus, J.L. et al. Sudden Unexpected Death as the Initial Manifestation of Ischemic Heart Disease: Clinical and Pathologic Observations. *Am. J. Cardiol.* 29:294 (1972).
41. French, A.J. and Dock, W. Fatal Coronary Arteriosclerosis in Young Soldiers. *J.A.M.A.* 124:1233 (1944).
42. Mitrani, J. et al. Coronary Atherosclerosis in Cases of Traumatic Death. (Book) Physical Activity and Aging ed. by Brunner, D. and Jokl, E. Page 241. (Published by S. Karger, Basel. (1970).
43. Brunner, D. et al. Necropsy-Established Coronary Occlusions in 549 Adult Civilian Accident Victims. (Unpublished data).
44. Rodriguez, F.L. et al. Postmortem Angiographic Studies on the Coronary Arterial Circulation: Incidence and Topography of Occlusive Coronary Lesions. *Am. Heart J.* 68:490 (1964).
45. Majoska, A.V. Sudden Death in Philipino Men: An Unexplained Syndrome. *Hawaii Med. J.* 7:469 (1948).
46. Lenel, R. et al. Factors Involved in the Production of Paroxysmal Ventricular Tachycardia Induced by Epinephrine. *Am. J. Physiol.* 153:553 (1948).
47. Nelson, G.N. et al. Correlation of Behavior and Catecholamine Metabolite Excretion. *Psychosom. Med.* 28:216 (1966).
48. Sulkowitch, H. et al. Excretion of Urinary Epinephrines in Psychiatric Disorders. *Proc. Soc. Exper. Biol. Med.* 95:245 (1957).
49. Rahe, R.H. and Arthur, R.J. Biochemical Correlates of Behavior: A Digest of Selected Studies. *Dis. Nerv. Sys.* 29:114 (1968).
50. Smith, F.L. et al. Excretion of Urinary Corticoids in Mental Patients. *J. Nerv. Ment. Dis.* 124:381 (1956).
51. Weitzman, E.D. et al. REM Sleep and Plasma Corticoids. *J. Clin. Endocrin.* 26:121 (1966).
52. Ellman, J.L. and Blaker, K.H. Diurnal Patterns of 17-Hydroxycorticosteroid Excretion in Psychiatric Illness. *Dis. Nerv. Sys.* 30:683 (1969).
53. Frink, R.J. and James, T.N. Normal Blood Supply of the Human His Bundle and Proximal Bundle Branches. *Circulation* 47:8 (1973).
54. Lie, J.T. and Titus, J.L. Pathology of the Myocardium and the Conduction System in Sudden Coronary Death. *Circulation* 52: Suppl. III-53 (1975).
55. Schwartz, C.J. and Gerrity, R.G. Anatomical Pathology of Sudden Unexpected Coronary Death. *Circulation* 52: Suppl. III-18 (1975).
56. Frink, R.J. et al. Non-Obstructive Coronary Thrombosis in Sudden Cardiac Death. *Am. J. Cardiol.* 42:48 (1978).
57. Wellens, H.J.J. et al. Ventricular Fibrillation Occurring on Arousal from Sleep by Auditory Stimuli. *Circulation* 46:661 (1972).

CHAPTER 7

Postictal Fatalities

For a long time it has been known that persons with an underlying seizure diathesis are at increased risk of dying prematurely and suddenly, as well. Moreover, it has been noted that, in most instances, a sudden death in patients of this genre has been linked to the occurrence of either a witnessed or unwitnessed epileptic episode.[1-6,9-17,31,32] On the other hand, the results of epidemiologic studies have shown that status epilepticus is a relatively infrequent precursor of such fatalities.[6-11] Supposedly, this circumstance can be related to the aggressive prompt and appropriate treatment which patients with status epilepticus usually receive.[7-8]

Experiential data have indicated also that when seizure-prone patients died suddenly, such deaths often occurred while the decedent was asleep;[12-16] furthermore, with respect to psychiatric patients, it has been observed that the prospect for survival not only was diminished materially if they also were afflicted with a seizure disorder, but also that the likelihood of a sudden death was the same whether the epilepsy was the cryptogenic or the post-lobotomy variety.[17]

Generally, in connection with such fatalities, the autopsy findings have been nonspecific in nature; usually, the only meaningful finding has been the presence of a seemingly noncardiogenic variety of pulmonary edema with or without widespread visceral congestion.[18,19] However, it should be explained also that a fatal outcome is not an invariable consequence of postictal pulmonary edema;[20-21] thus, it still is uncertain whether all postictal sudden deaths can be ascribed solely to such a pulmonary complication. Nevertheless, there is, at present, sufficient circumstantial evidence to support the thesis, first, that there is, indeed, an entity such as seizure-induced pulmonary edema, and second, that it is such an adult respiratory distress syndrome which can be responsible for a sudden death in a seizure-prone individual.

PATHOGENESIS OF PULMONARY EDEMA

Still unclear is the pathogenesis of pulmonary edema in these instances, but there is both a body of experimental data and a variety of hypotheses which suggest possible mechanisms. Thus, in their paper which was published in 1966, Huff and Fred[18] postulated that the pulmonary edema was not cardiogenic in nature, and also suggested that the underlying mechanism could be a combination of increased intracranial pressure, neurogenic and humoral influences on capillary permeability, alterations in pulmonary mechanics, and the effects of attempts to exhale or inhale while the glottis was closed.

However, since the relative importance of these respective factors was not mentioned, it is conceivable that the closed glottis is paramount. This consideration, in turn, might indicate that at times the pulmonary edema was cardiogenic rather than noncardiogenic in nature. This suggestion is based largely on observations reported by Benchimol et al[22] and by Van Liere.[23] In their studies, Benchimol showed that the Valsalva maneuver produces a marked diminution in the velocity of coronary blood flow and Van Liere has demonstrated that if there is an abrupt onset of anoxia, there will be a reflex outpouring of catecholamines. Correspondingly, inspiration or exhalation against a closed glottis could favor the occurrence of two physiologic alterations which, together, could be the precursors of a life-threatening tachyarrhythmia, an abrupt cardiac arrest, and consequently, the development of acute pulmonary edema. (See Chapters 10 and 12).

However, it is equally conceivable on the basis of experiments reported by Ostwalt et al[24] that sudden closure of the glottis can precipitate a noncardiogenic form of pulmonary edema. Moreover, in view of the findings reported earlier by Visscher et al[25] and by Robin et al[26] it was acknowledged by Ostwalt et al[24] that auxiliary factors could be a combination of increased alveolar and capillary permeability along with increased negative interstitial pressure in the lung. Also, inasmuch as seizures without a companionate edenatous pulmonary complication outnumber by far the incidence of a wet lung syndrome in epileptics, it would be tendentious to suppose that "inspiration against a closed glottis" represents, in such a patient sample, the sole explanation for the occurrence of a fatal adult respiratory stress syndrome.

Clearly, then, it would be necessary to consider which other meaningful coordinate physiologic changes during a seizure (in addition to inspiration against a closed glottis) might help to explain the development of such a life-threatening entity in seizure-prone adults.

Findings which are meaningful in this regard were reported by Harrison and Liebow;[27] these investigators showed that a precipitous rise in intracranial pressure like that which might accompany a convulsive seizure can result in the development of pulmonary edema. In addition, it has been demonstrated by Bean[29] that, in rats, the inhalation of oxygen at high pressure not only produces convulsions and concurrently a lethal form of pulmonary edema; this type of experiment simultaneously increased the elaboration of catecholamines from the adrenal gland as well. Moreover, along with the use of this experimental model, Bean was able to demonstrate that the administration of adrenergic blocking agents prevented the occurrence of the pulmonary edema and, as a result, the animals survived.[28-29]

Equally meaningful were the human studies reported by Havens et al[30] who found that the occurrence of electrically-induced convulsions was accompanied by significant elevations in the blood of both epinephrine and norepinephrine. Stone and Loew[33] observed not only that the injection of large doses of epinephrine to rabbits produced a severe degree of pulmonary edema, but also that such an effect could be prevented by the administration of adrenergic blocking agents.

PHYSIOLOGIC DERANGEMENTS IN CONVULSIVE EPISODE

There are, in addition, two other investigations which have provided further insights with respect to the important physiologic derangements which accompany a convulsive episode and, by implication, might contribute, along with an exaggeration of other adverse effects, to the mortality of seizure-prone patients. One such study was described by White et al in 1961[34] and the other was the basis of reports by Meldrum and his associates which were published in 1973.[35]

Pentylene Tetrazol-Induced Seizures

The investigations undertaken by White et al[34] were designed to evaluate the encephalographic, electrocardiographic, and other cardiovascular responses to pentylene tetrazol-induced seizures in 26 known epileptics. With regard to the cardiovascular effects, it was noted that there was a positive correlation between the levels of the arterial blood pressure and the phases of the induced seizure activity. Thus, initially there was a sharp rise in the blood pressure level and then a return to normal level as seizure activity subsided.

Cardiac irregularities also developed but these did not correlate with the blood pressure level or the phase of seizure activity. Sometimes, the irregularity was most pronounced as the seizure was subsiding and as the blood pressure was falling but, in other instances, the irregularity was evident at the height of the blood pressure rise. The nature of the cardiac irregularity varied considerably; the noteworthy findings constituted of premature auricular or ventricular rhythms, elevated or depressed S-T segments and T-waves, conduction blocks, ventricular tachycardia and prolonged bradycardia with coupling. In one patient there was electrocardiographic evidence of severe myocardial ischemia but in spite of this complication, no adverse cardiac effects apparently ensued.

Moreover, the observation by these authors that seizure activity was accompanied by simultaneous increases in heart rate, vigor of cardiac contractions, cardiac output, and peripheral vascular constriction prompted them to propose not only that discharges from autonomic centers in the brain were stimulated coordinately by the seizure activity but also that such responses indicated that the autonomic effects were essentially adrenergic in type.

Correspondingly, then, although White et al[34] had not suggested a mechanism for the pentylene tetrazol-induced ventricular arrhythmias, it would be reasonable to ascribe such findings, at least in part, to a seizure-induced augmentation of adrenergic influences. Thus, fundamentally, in terms of their pathogenesis, these arrhythmias can be considered to be similar to the neurally based arrhythmias which have been observed in a variety of other experimental settings which have resulted in the production of life-threatening ventricular arrhythmias, presumably because of an augmentation of adrenergic traffic along the neural pathways leading to the heart.[36-44]

METABOLIC AND BIOCHEMICAL CORRELATES OF SEIZURE ACTIVITY

On the other hand, the meaningful experimental data which were provided by Meldrum et al[35] pertained to the metabolic and biochemical correlates of seizure activity. In connection with their studies, Meldrum et al produced seizures in 26 primates by injecting intravenously a solution of bicuculline and found that the earliest coordinate effects of the seizure included (a) a lowered arterial oxygen tension; (b) an elevated carbon dioxide tension in the arterial blood; (c) a lowered blood pH value; (d) an elevated plasma potassium level (mean peak level = 8.7 mEq). Thus, inasmuch as such a combination of findings by themselves is known to favor the development of a life-threatening ventricular tachyarrhythmia,[43] it is not surprising that six of their animals had died suddenly after they had developed seizures in this type of experimental setting. The authors ascribed both fatalities to either an acute cardiac arrest or acute respiratory failure but regrettably they did not describe the autopsy findings insofar as these pertain to the condition of the internal viscera. Four other animals also died suddenly but the fatalities in these instances were ascribed by them to "acute cardiovascular collapse resulting from a secondary irreversible hypotension." However, neither any terminal nor preterminal electrocardiograms were obtained during the hypotensive crisis and so it is uncertain whether the hypotension was secondary to an arrhythmia which prevented an effective cardiac output or whether it was due to circulatory shock.

Clearly, then, the data provided by White et al[34] and by Mildrum[35] have introduced considerations which would seem to indicate that postictal fatalities may not be the result of a noncardiogenic form of pulmonary edema, exclusively. In this connection the observations of Benchimol[22] may be relevant, provided it is agreed that the ventilatory disturbance which accompanies a grand mal seizure is a facsimile of a Valsalva maneuver. However, even then, other requirements which must be met to support such a view would be at least a pre-existing marginal degree of coronary narrowing along with the sort of metabolic accompaniments of a seizure like those described by Meldrum and Horton.[35]

Thus, because of such considerations, it is conceivable that the synsomnial sudden deaths in seizure-prone patients, might be viewed, at least in part, as a variant of the fatal sleep apnea syndrome.[45-47] However, so far as can be determined, few investigations with respect to the synsomnial feature of postictal fatalities have been undertaken and it is for this reason that the observations by Hirsch and Martin[15] would seem to be particularly pertinent.

In this connection, it is noteworthy that, at the outset, Hirsch and Martin concluded that suffocation will not explain any such fatalities. As they stated: "we believe that it is unwarranted to assume that an epileptic found dead in bed has suffocated following a seizure simply because there is no other apparent explanation for his demise. This situation seems analogous to the now exploded myth that sudden deaths in infancy (crib deaths) are a consequence of suffocation by bedding. Although the epileptic decedent is found dead in bed and examination of the scene of death does not help to reconstruct the fatality, we have encountered not one instance which was interpreted as indicative of suffocation."[15]

> "Of particular interest to us, in view of the number of patients in this study who died during sleep or were found dead in bed, is the role that sleep plays with regard to seizures. Physiologic sleep is a common provocative diagnostic technique in the electroencephalographic laboratory in the evaluation of epileptic disturbances and, accordingly, the location of either anatomical or electrical epileptogenic abnormalities in the brain may determine the occurrence of spontaneous seizures during the waking or sleeping state. It has been observed also that bilateral synchronous paraxysmal activity generally is reduced during the period of desynchronized sleep and is suppressed to the greatest degree during the period of rapid eye movements (REM) sleep. The periods of syn-

chronous sleep, with slower thalamic rhythms dominating, tend to lower the seizure threshold and are associated with greater frequency of epileptic discharges. Spontaneous all-night electro-encephalograms in patients with petit mal and grand mal epilepsy have demonstrated an increase in spike and wave discharge rate at sleep onset with a continued increase through slow wave sleep and a marked diminution in discharge rate with the onset of REM sleep. Furthermore, it was observed that there were changes with the discharges in behavioral or autonomic parameters only during Stage I sleep.

"The role played by the autonomic nervous system both in relation to a seizure discharge and as an explanation for the cause of death in these patients is most intriguing. A number of investigators have firmly established the fact that, during a seizure, a multitude of autonomically controlled functions may be altered either directly or indirectly, and, transient cardiac arrest may be the result. However, it should be noted that such alterations differ in degree from individual to individual and it may be for this reason that only an occasional epileptic will die in his sleep. In any event, such considerations make it necessary to recognize that sudden deaths of epileptics during sleep may have a pathophysiologic basis. In the final analysis, it seems to us that these deaths must relate to acute disruption of brain stem, cardiac or respiratory functions or both, secondary to seizure discharge.

"We do not know why a seizure, apparently no different from those which the patient has survived in the past should prove fatal at a particular time. The pathogenesis of the lethal mechanism may be related to a number of variables, such as an added component to the seizure discharge, nature of the circumstances which trigger the seizure, physiologic status of the patient immediately before onset of the seizure or altered physiologic response to the seizure. Hopefully, further investigation of the factors which precipitate and govern seizures will lead to therapeutic approaches which will prevent at least some of these death in the future."[15]

ADVERSE EFFECTS OF PHENOTHIAZINE THERAPY

In addition, it has been suggested by Hollister[48] by Zlotlow and Paganini,[49] and by Plachta[50] that phenothiazine therapy could be blamed sometimes for the occurrence of sudden deaths in seizure-prone psychiatric patients. This group of observers considered the underlying mechanism to be asphyxial in nature but, as far as can be determined, both Hollister[48] as well as Zlotlow and Paganini[49] posited, first, that the deaths they had described were due to a seizure-induced obstruction of the airway because of glottal spasm and, second, that the occurrence of the seizure responsible for the glottal spasm was traceable to a lowered seizure threshold induced by the phenothiazine therapy the decedents had received for their psychiatric illness.

Glottal-Esophageal Reflux

Moreover, they ascribed the glottal spasm to the lodgement of food particles in the laryngeal area when, during the seizure attack, there was a companionate regurgitation of the stomach contents. However it is noteworthy that Reinert and Hermann[13] had explained that regurgitation and aspiration of gastric contents very frequently represent a terminal or agonal development during a fatal "fit" and hence should not be viewed as the cause of a sudden death which had occurred during a fatal convulsive episode.

The paper by Plachta[50] also embodied claims that phenothiazine therapy increased the risk of asphyxial sudden death in seizure-prone psychiatric patients but he had a different view regarding the mechanisms which were involved. Thus, Plachta attributed the deaths he had reported primarily to a hypothetical undesirable effect of the phenothiazines on ciliary activity in the major air passages and on the function of the gastro-esophageal sphincter mechanism. However, since the data pertaining to these decedents also indicated that all had been receiving, concurrently with the phenothiazines, a daily ration of one of more barbiturates, it can be assumed that all were known to be seizure-prone psychiatric patients, as well.

Nevertheless, so far as can be determined, Plachta was convinced that the administration of moderate doses of chlorpromazine or prochlorperazine for a period of 5 to 10 years to seven patients with a "chronic brain syndrome" had exerted, simultaneously, an adverse effect on certain autonomic centers in the brain which control not only the ciliary movement in the lower respiratory tract but also the integrity of the gastro-esophageal sphincter. In addition, he had proposed that, as a consequence of such a supposed phenothiazine-induced effect on the gastro-esophageal sphincter, there had occurred at a particular point in time, not only a significant degree of gastro-esophageal reflux but also an inability of the cilia in the air passages to properly dispose of any aspirated gastric contents; the net result as he perceived it, was an aspirational type of asphyxia which in turn was followed sequentially and rapidly by cerebral anoxia, a convulsion, and soon thereafter, by a sudden cardiac arrest. Moreover, inasmuch as the likelihood of any gastro-esophageal reflux is enhanced by an overdistended stomach, this circumstance, in the view of Plachta, would account for the paraprandial nature of such alleged phenothiazine-related fatalities (see Chapter 6).

The ages of the decedents ranged from 36 to 62 years and during their lifetimes these patients had received a variety of ataractics; chiefly these drugs consisted of chlorpromazine, prochloperazine, and reserpine. The doses varied considerably but it is noteworthy that the dose of chlorpromazine never exceeded 800 mg daily. Moreover, "in every instance, the patient's death occurred shortly after a morning, noon, or evening meal, exhibiting respiratory difficulty characterized by marked dyspnea, apnea, cyanosis, convulsions, inability to keep from falling off the chair, or falling onto the floor while walking. There was the associated rapid pulse, clonic or tonic spasm, with instances of pupilary dilatation, petechias, and unconsciouness, terminating in unobtainable pulse and cessation of respiration."

In only three patients, the chest x-ray and electrocardiogram were normal. In the four others, such examinations confirmed the presence of coronary disease, hypertensive cardiovascular disease, or cor pulmonale. In summarizing the autopsy findings he listed the following: (a) gastric content in the esophagus, pharyngolaryngeal fossae, trachea, major bronchi and bronchioles; (b) acute bronchiolitis; (c) severe hyperemia of the tracheal and bronchila mucus membrane; (d) pleural and pericardial petechias; (e) acute pneumonitis. However, he failed to include a description of the state of the coronary vasculature or the myocardium.

Conclusions

Thus, if one accepts the validity of Plachta's thesis, it would be necessary to include in the differential diagnosis of sudden death in phenothiazine-treated psychiatric patients with an organic brain syndrome, the triad of gastro-esophageal reflux, ciliary impairment in the major air passages, and, finally an episode of fatal syncope of a convulsive type. However, it should be explained that most pathologists would consider the autopsy findings he had described as agonal manifestations and not a basic cause for the fatalities.

PHENOTHIAZINE EFFECTS ON SEIZURE THRESHOLD

It also is of interest, in view of the issues which have been discussed so far, that numerous drug trials designed to observe the effects of phenothiazines in seizure-prone psychotics have shown that such drugs do not, indeed, lower the seizure threshold.[51-55]

Anticonvulsants Combined with Chlorpromazine

One of the first to confirm such a finding was N.W. Winkelman, whose report appeared in 1954.[51] His total patient sample consisted of 142 chlorpromazine-treated psychiatric patients; but the subgroup—which is of particular interest—comprised six epileptics, each of whom continued to receive the same daily dose of anticonvulsant drugs as that prescribed before the drug trial was initiated; with respect to these patients, the daily dose of chlorpromazine did not in any instance exceed 200 mg. The duration of the drug trial was 3 months. One of the epileptics had suffered from seizures for 33 years and he had experienced recurrent biweekly convulsions before the chlorpromazine was added to the treatment program. Another seizure patient was one who had regularly experienced three attacks of psychomotor epilepsy each week before treatment with chlorpromazine was started. Moreover, these triweekly attacks of psychomotor epilepsy had persisted even though the patient had received maximal doses of dilantin and phenobarbital and, so, before the chlorpromazine had been prescribed it was planned to perform a lobotomy. However, this procedure was abandoned when it was noted that the patient remained seizure-free while his anticonvulsants were supplemented with the modest doses of chlorpromazine employed during the drug trial. With regard to the six epileptics, it was demonstrated that the daily administration of 200 mg of chlorpromazine did not increase seizure frequency; also, in two of them, there was a dramatic cessation of seizures over a 3-months period while they had received, concurrently with their anticonvulsant drug, this same modest dose of chlorpromazine.

Another equally relevant study was described in an article by Schlichter et al, which appeared in the Canadian Medical Association Journal in 1956.[52] The results of this investigation showed that in 11 of 21 hospitalized schizophrenics there were a total of 14 "seizures" while they were receiving a daily ration of chlorpromazine. Moreover, 5 of these 11 patients were known already to be seizure-prone, as well. During the entire period of the drug trial the doses of chlorpromazine consumed by the five seizure-prone patients were 20,100 mg; 7500 mg; 500 mg; 43,500 mg; and 10,500 mg, respectively, whereas the respective doses consumed by the six patients who had not manifested seizures prior to the time of the drug trial were 10,500 mg; 10,500 mg; 10,500 mg; 11,200 mg; 45,500 mg; and 11,800 mg. Thus, on average, the preseizure consumption of chlorpromazine among those known to be actually seizure-prone amounted to 16,422 mg whereas in those without a past history of seizures, the average dose was 16,666 mg, a difference which hardly is significant.

Moreover, during the drug trial there was no greater seizure frequency in the patients who already were listed as seizure-prone. Accordingly, these data can be interpreted to signify that with respect to this group of patients there was no evidence that the phenothiazines had lowered the seizure threshold. In addition, it should be explained that, with one exception, the seizures actually were considered by these investigators to be syncopal attacks, possibly secondary to the consumption of the chlorpromazine and therefore not true epileptiform episodes.

Barbiturates Combined with Chlorpromazine

Other studies can be cited also to show that it is unlikely that phenothiazines lower the seizure threshold in known seizure patients. One such investigation reported in 1955[57] was conducted by V.L. Bonafede. From a sample of 78 known epileptics, he selected a group of 67 who were not only afflicted with a seizure disorder but were also highly disturbed and therefore frequently had required large doses of sedatives and some form of restraint in order to control agitation and assaultiveness. For this reason, these were the ones chosen for inclusion in a drug trial which sought to evaluate the effectiveness of chlorpromazine as an anti-psychotic agent and to determine what harm or benefits would accrue from the use of this phenothiazine in seizure-prone psychotics. Their average length of institutionalization was 17 years and thus an ample opportunity had been provided to obtain base line data with respect to seizure frequency and the optimal dose of anticonvulsant required to limit the number of seizures. Approximately two thirds were cases of idiopathic epilepsy; the convulsive disorder in the remainder was due to birth injuries, a previous episode of meningoencephalities or postnatal brain trauma. For the most part, the phenothiazine was administered perorally and the average daily dose was 300 mg; occasionally, it was necessary to supplement this dose with an intramuscular injection of the drug when, otherwise, it would have been difficult to control such behavior as assaultiveness.

The design of Bonafede's study allowed for observation over a 60-day period in three separate groups, the distinction being based only on the amount of barbiturate consumed during the drug trial. In one group, which comprised 11 patients, the customary dose of barbiturate was not altered; this averaged 0.3 gm daily. In this group only two patients developed seizures while receiving the chlorpromazine.

The 26 patients in the second group also continued to receive a daily ration of phenobarbital while receiving the chlorpromazine, but their average daily dose of barbiturate was reduced by one third. In 18 of this number (69%) there was no clear evidence of an increase in seizure frequency while they were receiving chlorpromazine, whereas in only 8 (31%) there was a clear increase in seizure frequency. However, in these 8 patients the pre-chlorpromazine seizure pattern was restored promptly when the dose of phenobarbital was increased to the level which had been prescribed before the start of the drug trial. Thus, the findings with respect to this group could be interpreted to indicate that it was the reduction in phenobarbital dose, rather than the administration of chlorpromazine which could be blamed for the seizure frequency in these eight patients. However, the author did not indicate what proportion of these eight patients suffered from idiopathic epilepsy compared to the proportion with epilepsy resulting from some type of organic cerebral abnormality.

The third group also consisted of 26 epileptics but in this group the customary daily dose of phenobarbital was halved after treatment with chlorpromazine was begun. In this group of epileptics the result was almost identical to that encountered in the second group. In 17 (65%) there was no clear evidence of an increase in seizure frequency while they were receiving chlorpromazine, whereas in only 9 (35%) there was a clear increase in seizure frequency. Moreover, the pre-chlorpromazine seizure frequency status of eight of these nine patients was restored when the reduced dose of phenobarbital was doubled; the ninth patient, a 29-year-old mute with the mentality of an idiot, died in status epilepticus. Nevertheless, the author interpreted these results to indicate that any observed seizure increase in this sub-group was due "essentially and specifically to the reduction of phenobarbital rather than to any action of chlorpromazine." Again, from the information supplied by the author, there was no way of knowing what the relative proportion of patients with organic cerebral disorders was among the 17 patients who did not develop seizures and the 9 patients who did develop seizures while they were receiving chlorpromazine and the half-dose of barbiturate.

Lobotomy and Combined Chlorpromazine and Anticonvulsant Therapy

A somewhat different type of study was described in 1958 by Paganini and Zlotlow.[53] Their report summarized the results of an investigation in which the patient sample consisted of 50 ambulatory chronic schizophrenics who had been hospitalized for a long period because of regressive and other forms of psychotic behavior. All had undergone a lobotomy in an attempt to control their behavior disturbance and in connection with this drug trial they were assigned to two groups of 25 each. Group I included patients who occasionally manifested seizures after the lobotomy in spite of anticonvulsant therapy whereas Group II included patients who never had developed seizures after the lobotomy. The members of both groups received perorally 200-800 mg of chlorpromazine daily and the period of observation lasted 2 years. During this time none of the 25 Group II patients developed convulsions. Moreover, during the same 2-year period, 16 of the 25 Group-I patients remained seizure-free, whereas 9 patients did not. The authors also noted that in the nine patients of Group I who continued to experience seizures, the number of fits seemed to diminish the longer the chlorpromazine was continued, even though the dose of anticonvulsant remained constant. In Group II, a single patient died, but since permission for an autopsy was refused, the exact cause of death could not be definitely ascertained. However, the nature of the death suggested that the fatality was the result of coronary occlusion. In summarizing their findings, the authors concluded that they had been unable to demonstrate that customary doses of chlorpromazine possessed an epileptogenic property.

Effects of Thioridazine and Chlorpromazine on Seizure Frequency

That seizures will follow phenothiazine therapy was again disproved by the results of two separate drug trials which were reported by M.M. Frain[54] and by P.M. Panig.[55] The investigation conducted by Frain was designed to observe the effects on seizure frequency of customary doses of thioridazine and comparable doses of chlorpromazine, whereas the observations of Panig were confined to the responses which followed the administration of only thioridazine.

The subjects included in the study undertaken by Frain[54] were 70 female psychotic epileptics who exhibited marked behavioral disturbances in addition to their seizure disorder. No information was available concerning the proportion who had undergone a lobotomy. Also, the length of the period of observation was not stated and it could not be ascertained if the maintenance dose of anticonvulsant medication during the study had been reduced. The observations made by Frain indicated that following chlorpromazine administration, psychotic behavior was markedly lessened in 58 of the 70 subjects; during the time the thioridazine was administered, a similar improvement was noted in 61 of the 70 subjects. In addition, the author averred that neither the chlorpromazine nor the thioridazine had increased seizure frequency. Equally noteworthy was his assertion that there were no important side effects related to the administration of either of these phenothiazine drugs.

The purpose of the study undertaken by Panig et al[55] was to establish the influence of thioridazine on seizure frequency in 100 known epileptics who also manifested psychotic behavioral disturbance. The patient sample included men and women and each received a moderate dose of thioridazine over a period ranging from 3 to 10 months. Presumably, the daily maintenance dose of anticonvulsant medication with respect to each of these patients had not been changed during the drug trial. When the results were tabulated, it was found that during the period of observation, seizure frequency was not increased in any of the patients and seizures disappeared completely in 23. Also, the frequency remained the same in 20; and in 41 seizures were less frequent but not completely abolished.

Aside from the results of the human studies already mentioned, a meaningful set of observations in experimental animals also has demonstrated that chlorpromazine not only does not lower the seizure threshold but instead actually raises it. A paper pertaining to this sort of investigation was published in 1956 by J.W. Bean[28] who had designed an experimental model which depended upon the administration of oxygen at high pressure in order to produce convulsions. Then, having shown that such a procedure proved to be a reliable method for eliciting this type of response in rats, he administered a single dose of chorpromazine before he exposed the tests animals to this seizure evoking stimulus.

Regularly, the result of such an experiment was a "delay in the onset of either minimal or severe neuromuscular reactions and a diminution in their severity." Moreover, it was observed by Bean that 10 daily doses of chlorpromazine protected the cardiovascular and respiratory system against the adverse effects of oxygen at high pressure and also significantly reduced the high degree of mortality which ordinarily accompanied the use of this experimental procedure.

Another noteworthy study regarding the relationship between phenothiazine therapy and seizure activity was the one reported by Logothetis in 1967.[59] Its purpose was to investigate in non-epileptics, the incidence of spontaneously occurring seizures in a group of psychiatric patients who were receiving phenothiazines and to correlate the clinical observations with electroencephalographic data.

The findings derived from this study indicated that during the period of observation (1960-1965) 10 patients, while receiving phenothiazine compounds, developed a seizure episode; in 9 of the 10 patients, the episode was a grand mal seizure and in the other instance, it was described as a focal motor type. By contrast, in the remaining 849 patients who had received similar drug therapy, no spontaneously occurring seizures had been observed. It is of interest also that the electroencephalographic changes seen in the 10 patients who suffered spontaneous seizures were similar to those in other patients receiving phenothiazines who never had convulsive seizures.

In addition, the study attempted to ascertain which phenothiazine was most likely to cause a clinically observed convulsion and it was concluded that chlorpromazine more so than thioridazine or trifluoperazine was culpable in this respect. Moreover, it was observed that whereas psychiatric patients without organic brain disease had seizures irrespective of the dose of the phenothiazine which had been consumed, in those without organic brain disease, a seizure occurred only after large doses of the responsible drug had been consumed.

In this connection, Logothetis recounted the following experiences: "The first patient was 1-year post lobotomy with no previous seizures who was maintained on 400 mg of thioridazine a day. He had a major motor seizure one month after the dose was doubled. He remained hospitalized and seizure-free for 4 more years, receiving 200 mg of thioridazine daily and no anticonvulsants. The second patient, 10 years after prefrontal lobotomy, exhibited a major motor seizure for the first time when given 800 mg of promazine for three days. Over the ensuing five years of hospitalization, continuing on thioridazine daily and receiving no anticonvulsants, he remained seizure-free."

Thus, in view of such observations, it would seem proper to infer that seizure-prone psychiatric patients, following a lobotomy, can tolerate satisfactorily moderate doses of thioridazine which, even without concurrent anticonvulsant drugs, would not be likely to induce a seizure. Correspondingly, if large doses of this particular phenothiazine are required in patients of this type, the supplementary use of a small dose of a suitable anticonvulsant preparation should prevent any major seizure episode.

Furthermore, it must be recognized that, in terms of their genesis, some attacks of fatal syncope in seizure prone psychotics resemble the numerous sudden deaths which occur annually in seemingly healthy members of the general population. The cause is atherosclerotic stenosis of the extramural coronary arteries and in the literature pertaining to sudden deaths in phenothiazine-treated seizure-prone psychotics, several cases of this sort have been described. Typical examples which clearly have no connection to prior administration of phenothiazines even though such drugs were consumed prior to the time of death are the ones reported by J.B. Dynes[14] and by Roizin, Forrest and Forrest.[56]

Effects of Dilantin Therapy Combined with Chlorpromazine

In the article by J.B. Dynes[14] the author referred to a 42-year-old patient who had been receiving for a long period of time both dilantin and chlorpromazine, prior to the time of death. The chlorpromazine had been prescribed because he had been subject to recurrent seizures. Actually, the chlorpromazine therapy was interrupted one month prior to the time of death because there was so much improvement in his psychotic state; however, the dilantin therapy was never interrupted. On the day he died, he was being examined in the Dental Clinic and while he was in the dental chair he suddenly lost consciousness. However, despite the prompt institution of artificial respiration and external cardiac massage, he did not regain consciousness and therefore he was quickly rushed to the operating room where his chest was opened. The surgeon massaged the heart which was seen to be fibrillating. Therefore, an attempt was made to restore normal rhythm with an electrical defibrillator. However, these efforts were unsuccessful and he lived for only 1 hour after the onset of the syncopal episode. An autopsy was performed soon afterward and this disclosed marked congestion of the lungs and viscera and definite arteriosclerosis of the coronary vessels. There was no evidence of an acute myocardial infarction and the brain was reported as being normal. Thus, in this instance, it can be concluded that the sudden death was due not to a seizure episode but instead, to the underlying occlusive coronary artery disease (see Chapter 10).

Chlorpromazine Therapy After Lobotomy

In their paper, Roizin, Forrest and Forrest[56] described the case of a 39-year-old schizophrenic who at the age of 28 underwent a bilateral lobotomy because, in spite of repeated electroconvulsive therapy and repeated insulin coma treatments, he continued to manifest periods of withdrawal, confusion, regression, violent behavior, defective insight and judgement. Four years after the lobotomy 900 mg of chlorpromazine daily was prescribed and he continued to receive this dose of the phenothiazine until the day of his death. Following treatment with the chlorpromazine he improved to some extent from a behavioral standpoint and during the seven years he received this preparation which was continued until the day of his death, he apparently was free of symptoms referrable to the heart. On the day he died, he was found to be lying on the floor of his hospital room executing "jerking movements of the arms." Soon afterward he appeared lifeless and he could not be revived in spite of resuscitative efforts. An autopsy disclosed the following: "(1) marked coronary atherosclerosis; (2) marked bilateral diffuse pulmonary congestion and edema with agonal aspiration of the gastric content; (3) status postoperative, old bilateral frontal lobotomies." Thus, again, in this instance, it would be proper to dismiss drug therapy or a convulsive episode as the basic cause for the sudden death; unquestionably by cause was the underlying occlusive coronary artery disease (see Chapter 3).

This experience also serves to emphasize the importance of a carefully conducted postmortem examination whenever a seizure-prone psychiatric patient dies suddenly and unexpectedly. Although it is recognized that, even after an autopsy has been performed, many sudden deaths in "epileptics" remain unexplained,[16] it is known also that not every sudden death in patients of this genre is a mystifying event. The physicians of yore may have been content to ascribe both an epileptic's illness and death to a demon, but to our generation must fall the task of tirelessly searching for the cause of the malady and the reasons those so afflicted can suddenly die.

REFERENCES

1. W.G. Lennox, *Epilepsy and Related Disorders*. Little, Brown, and Co., Boston (1960).
2. Moritz, A.R. and Zamcheck, N. Sudden and unexpected deaths of young soldiers: Diseases responsible for such deaths during World War II. *Arch. Pathol. Lab. Med.* 42:459 (1946).
3. E.A. Rodin, *The Prognosis of Patients with Epilepsy*. Charles C. Thomas, Springfield, Illinois (1968).
4. Freytag, E. and Lindenburg, R. 294 Medico-legal autopsies on epileptics. *Arch. Pathol. Lab. Med.* 78:274 (1964).
5. Kuller, L. et al. Epidemiology of sudden death. *Arch. Int. Med.* 129:714 (1972).
6. W. Pryse-Phillips. *Epilepsy* John Wright and Sons, Bristol (1969).
7. Celesia, G.G. Modern concepts of status epilepticus. *J.A.M.A.* 235:1571 (1976).
8. Siris, J.H. Treatment of status epilepticus. *J.A.M.A.* 236:2174 (1976).
9. Oxbury, J.M. and Whitty, C.W.M. Causes and consequences of status epilepticus in adults. *Brain* 94:733 (1971).
11. Rowan, A.J. and Scott, D.F. Major status epilepticus: A series of 42 patients. *Acta Neuol. Scand.* 46:573 (1970).
12. Greiner, A.C. and Nicolson, G.A. Pigment deposition in viscera associated with prolonged chlorpromazine therapy. *Can. M.A.J.* 91:627 (1964).
13. Reinert, R.E. and Hermann, C.G. Unexplained deaths during chlorpromazine therapy. *J. Nerv. Ment. Dis.* 131:435 (1960).
14. Dynes, J.B. Sudden death. *Dis. Nerv. Sys.* 30:24 (1969).
15. Hirsch, C.S. and Martin, D.L. Unexpected deaths in young epileptics. *Neurology* 21:682 (1971).
16. Terrence, C.F. et al. Unexpected, unexplained death in epileptic patients. *Neurology* 25:594 (1975).
17. Malzberg, B. *Mortality Among Patients with Mental Disease*. New York State Hospitals Press. (1934).
18. Huff, R.W. and Fred, H.L. Postictal Pulmonary Edema. *Arch. Int. Med.* 117:824 (1966).
19. Ohlmacher, A.P. Acute Pulmonary Edema as a Terminal Event in Certain Forms of Epilepsy, *Am. J. Med. Sci.* 139:417 (1910).
20. Bloom, S. Pulmonary Edema Following a Grand Mal Epileptic Seizure. *Am. Rev. Resp. Dis.* 97:292 (1968).
21. Bombrest, H.C. Pulmonary Edema Following an Epileptic Seizure. *Am. Rev. Resp. Dis.* 91:97 (1965).
22. Benchimol, A. et al. The Valsalva Maneuver and Coronary Arterial Blood Flow Velocity. *Ann. Int. Med.* 77:357 (1972).
23. E.J. van Liere. *Anoxia: Its Effect on the Body*. University of Chicago Press, Chicago (1942).
24. Ostwalt, C.E. et al. Pulmonary Edema as a Complication of Acute Airway Obstruction. *J.A.M.A.* 238:1833 (1977).
25. Visscher, M.B. et al. The Physiology and Pharmacology of Lung Edema. *Pharmacol. Rev.* 8:389 (1956).

26. Robin, E.D. et al. Pulmonary Edema. *New Eng. J. Med.* 288:292 (1973).
27. Harrison, W. and Liebow, A.A. The Effect of Increased Intracranial Pressure on the Pulmonary Circulation in Relation to Pulmonary Edema. *Circulation* 5:824 (1952).
28. Bean, J.W. Reserpine, Chlorpromazine, and the Hypothalamus in Reactions to Oxygen at High Pressure (OHP). *Am. J. Physiol.* 187:389 (1956).
29. Johnson, P.C. and Bean, J.W. Effect of Sympathetic Blocking Agents on the Toxic Action of Oxygen at High Pressure (OHP). *Am. J. Physiol.* 188:593 (1957).
30. Havens, L.L. et al. Catecholamine responses to electrically induced convulsions in man. In: *Biological Psychiatry*, J.H. Masserman, ed. Grune and Stratton Inc., New York (1959).
31. Krohn, W. Causes of death among epileptics. *Epilepsia* 4:315 (1963).
32. Schwade, E.D. Mortality in epilepsy. *J.A.M.A.* 156:1526 (1954).
33. Stone C.A. and Loew, E.R. Effect of various durgs on epinephrine-induced pulmonary edema in rabbits. *Proc. Soc. Exper. Biol. Med.* 71:122 (1949).
34. White, P.T. et al. Changes in cerebal dynamics associated with seizures. *Neurology* 11:354 (1961).
35. Meldrum, B.S. and Horton, R.W. Physiology of status epilepticus in primates. *Arch. Neurol.* 28:1 (1973).
36. Hockman, C.H. et al. Electrocardiographic changes resulting from cerebral stimulation. II. A spectrum of ventricular arrhythmias ot sympathetic origin. *Am. Heart J.* 71:695 (1966).
37. Han, J. et al. Adrenergic effects on ventricular vulnerability. *Circ. Res.* 14:516 (1964).
38. Kralios, F. et al. Effects of sympathetic nerve branch stimulation on ventricular recovery properties and cardiac rhythm. *Am. J. Cardiol.* 31:142 (1973).
39. Verrier, R.L. et al. Effect of posterior hypothalamic stimulation on ventricular fibrillation threshold. *Am. J. Physiol.* 228:923 (1975).
40. Satinsky, J. et al. Ventricular fibrillation induced by hypothalamic stimulation during coronary occlusion. *Circulation* (Suppl. 2 44:60 (1971).
41. Kolman, B.S. et al. The effect of vagus nerve stimulation upon vulnerability of the canine ventricle: Role of sympathetic-parasympathetic interactions. *Circulation* 52:578 (1975).
42. Levitt, B. et al. Role of the nervous system in the genesis of cardiac rhythm disorders. *Am. J. Cardiol.* 37:1111 (1976).
43. Wolf, S. Neural mechanisms in sudden cardiac deaths. *Trans. Am. Clin. Climatolog. Assoc.* 79:158 (1967).
44. Wolf, S. Central autonomic influences on cardiac rate and rhythm. *Mod. Concepts Cardiovasc. Dis.* 38:29: (1969).
45. Tilkian, A.G. et al. Hemodynamics in sleep-induced apnea: Studies during wakefulness and sleep. *Ann. Int. Med.* 85:714 (1976).
46. Tilkian, A.G. et al. Sleep-induced apnea syndrome: Reversal of serious arrhythmias after tracheostomy. *Circulation* (Suppl. 2) 52:131 (1975).
47. Guilleminault, C. et al. The sleep apnea syndromes. *Ann. Rev. Med.* 27:465 (1976).
48. Hollister, L.E. Unexpected asphyxial death and tranquilizing drugs. *Am. J. Psychiatr.* 114:366 (1957).
49. Zlotlow, M. and Paganini, A.E. Fatalities in patients receiving chlorpromazine and reserpine during 1956-1957 at Pilgrim State Hospital. *Am. J. Psychiatr.* 115:154 (1958).
50. Plachta, A. Asphyxia relatively inherent in tranquilization: Review of the literature and report of 7 cases. *Arch. Gen. Psych.* 12:152 (1965).
51. Winkelman, N.W. Chorpromazine in the treatment of neuro-psychiatric disorders. *J.A.M.A.* 155:18 (1954).
52. Schlichter, W. et al. Seizures occurring during intensive chlorpromazine therapy. *Can. M.A.J.* 74:364 (1956).
53. Paganini, A.E. and Zlotlow, M. Two-year follow-up study of the relationship of chlorpromazine and the incidence of convulsions in 50 post-lobotomy patients. *Am. J. Psychiat.* 114:839 (1958).

54. Frain, M.M. Preliminary report on Mellaril® in epilepsy. *Am. J. Psychiat.* 117:547 (1961).
55. Panig, P.M. et al. Thioridazine hydrochloride in the treatment of behavior disorders in epileptics. *Am. J. Psychiat.* 117:832 (1961).
56. Roizin, L. et al. Combined histopathologic and biochemical studies following long-term chlorpromazine therapy. *Trans. Amer. Neurol. Assoc.* 88:258 (1963).
57. Bonafede, V.I. Chlorpromazine (Thorazine) treatment of disturbed epileptic patient. *Arch. Neurol. Psych.* 74:158 (1955).
58. Lomas, J. et al. Complications of chlorpromazine therapy in 800 mental hospital patients. *Lancet* 1:1144 (1955).
59. Logothetis, J. Spontaneous epileptic seizures and electroencephalographic changes in the course of phenothiazine therapy. *Neurology* 17:869 (1967).

CHAPTER 8

Fatal Megacolon In The Psychiatric Patient

One acquired type of chronic progressive visceropathy in psychotics which can be responsible for a sudden unexpected death is a megacolon of the sort originally reported in 1936.[1] Since then, instances of megacolon in mental patients have been reported by Lee and Bebb in 1951[2]; by Dean and Murry in 1952[3]; by Gabriel et al in 1953[4]; by Ehrentheil and Wells in 1955[5]; by Watkins, Oliver, and Rosenberg in 1961[6]; by Mc Kain in 1956[7]; by Burrell in 1957[8]; by Koback et al in 1962[9]; by Ansingh and Rideout in 1962[10]; by Watkins and Oliver in 1965[11]; by Wendkos and Clay in 1965[12]; by Kraft et al in 1966[13]; by Johnston and Gibson in 1970[14]; and by Mc Cormack in 1974.[15]

PATHOGENESIS

As the result of observations by a number of these authors, it is now generally agreed that the pathogenesis of this intestinal malady in the psychiatrically ill is related directly to the behavioral traits which accompany a regressive state. For the most part, it is believed that such progressive dilatation of the bowel is the result of indifference on the part of the patient to defecation stimuli.[5,12] It has also been suggested that the "disturbed autonomic nervous activity related to mental disease may be an etiologic factor."[6] However, in all likelihood, another important consideration could be the lack of communication between the patient and the hospital attendants. As a consequence of the latter circumstance, hospital personnel frequently are unaware of the existence of a situation which ordinarily would prompt the institution of measures to evacuate the bowel and remove any accumulated fecal impactions. Also, untrained ward personnel fail to consider fecal impaction/retention because there is no obvious reminder such as the soiled clothing of diarrhea. Thus, in accordance with the basic philosophy expressed by

Hussey in 1974,[16] the pathogenesis of "megacolon in the insane" would seem to involve two forms of neglect. One form is the neglect of the regressed psychotic to respond in the usual manner to defecation stimuli; the other form is the neglect of hospital attendants in psychiatric institutions to regularly check all regressed psychotics in order to determine whether there are any fecal accumulations which require removal.

PATHOLOGIC FEATURES

The patholigic features common to this particular type of acquired megacolon in mental patients also have been studied.[11] Consequently, three anatomical hallmarks have been established: 1) a pronounced distention of the colon (the diameter may sometimes exceed 15 cm and the circumference of the most dilated segment may exceed 50 cm); 2) a thickening of the muscular coat of that portion of the gut which is chiefly affected; 3) the persistence of ganglion cells in the myenteric plexus. Other findings which are sometimes present include thinning of the mucous membrane and intraluminal stercoraceous ulcers; the latter are due to irritation of the mucous membrances by localized inspissated fecal accumulations. Generally, too, the intestinal contents in the dilated segments of the bowel consist of a pasty mass of fecal material.

LOCALIZATION

In terms of localization, this type of acquired megacolon may be confined to the pelvic portion of the large bowel only or it may involve the entire length of this viscus. Accordingly, it has been suggested by Kraft et al[13] that the more limited variety in psychotic patients be termed the megasigmoid syndrome. However, this sort of classification is actually an arbitrary one. Furthermore, it does not seem to be particularly advantageous from the standpoint of diagnosis of this particular psychosis-related visceropathy or the treatment of its complications. As far as is known, any acquired "megacolon in the insane," regardless of its extent, can be the basis for a life-threatening intestinal obstruction by virtue of a volvulus of the sigmoid colon or a large fecal impaction.[9] In addition, it has been observed that although the megacolonic process initially may involve only the rectosigmoid portion of the bowel, it later can extend in retrograde fashion to affect longer segments of this structure.[9]

CLINICAL FEATURES

Although the clinical expressions of an acquired megacolon commonly include bouts of constipation and fecal impaction complicated by obstruction, it has been observed frequently that the obstructive symptoms associated with this entity are due, instead, to a volvulus involving the sigmoid portion of the gut.[11,14] However, even prior to the development of any acute obstructive symptoms, the presence and extent of this intestinal anomaly in the psychiatrically ill can be established by means of radiologic studies. Without the barium enema, the distended sigmoid colon usually can be seen below the left diaphragm and the meteorism may be so pronounced that the diaphragm will be displaced upward giving the illusion that the dilated gut is located in the thoracic cavity. Thus, a routine teleorentgenogram of the chest often can indicate its presence.

USE OF ENEMATA

Although, in the nonoperated patient, it is the barium enema which ultimately will confirm the diagnosis of acquired "megacolon in the insane" and demonstrate its extent, it must be recognized that the procedure sometimes may not be entirely innocuous if the amount of the barium mixture instilled into the bowel corresponds to its full capacity. In one case cited by Watkins, Oliver, and Rosenberg[6] 15 quarts of barium mixture were required to fill the rectum, sigmoid, and ascending colon. However, on average, 4 to 6 quarts of the barium solution should suffice to demonstrate the presence of an acquired "megacolon in the insane." Nevertheless, it must be recognized that the instillation of even these lesser amounts of the barium mixture can be responsible for life-threatening complications. As Koback et al[9] have mentioned the introduction of large amounts of a barium solution into an atonic bowel already filled with fecal concrements may increase the likelihood of either an obstruction or a rupture of the bowel. Moreover, it must be appreciated that even without this type of radiologic study, a stercoraceous ulcer sometimes can be the basis for a perforation of the bowel and a resulting lethal peritonitis.[13]

The authors who seem to be the ones most concerned about the possible hazards of a barium enema study in psychotics with an acquired megacolon were Ansingh and Rideout.[10] Accordingly, their paper emphasized that after the enlargement of the barium-filled colon has been delineated "frequent plates of the abdomen should be taken to satisfy onself that the colon is empty of stool." Moreover, they advocated that "after the study has been completed, saline enemas and laxatives should be given until one is satisfied that all barium has been expelled."

However, the barium enema is not the only type of enema which constitutes a hazard in psychotics with an acquired megacolon. Recently, Mc Cormack reported two cases of sudden death in psychotics with acquired megacolon[15] and in both instances the autopsy demonstrated that the fatal outcome was ascribable to cecal rupture and fecal peritonitis following the use of soap enemata administered for the relief of obstructive symptoms.

Case Report No. 1

One of the decedents reported by Mc Cormack was an 82-year-old man who had been hospitalized continuously for 42 years because of a chronic schizophrenic reaction. Four days before he died he developed evidences of intestinal obstruction thought to be secondary to fecal impaction. However, before the patient was scheduled for surgery, repeated soap enemata were prescribed. These proved to be unsuccessful in providing any relief and before a laparotomy could be performed, he died suddenly. Necropsy demonstrated a markedly distended cecum and colon but most of the sigmoid and rectum were empty. The cecum was paper thin and there was evidence of a fecal peritonitis which had resulted from a perforation of the cecum. The rupture of the cecum in this instance was attributed to increased intraluminal pressure induced by the repeated use of soap enemata.

Case Report No. 2

The other decedent reported by Mc Cormack was a 79-year-old female with a 13-year history of manic depressive illness who suddenly developed evidences of large bowel obstruction. Repeated attempts were made to evacuate the bowel by the use of soap enemata and shortly following the last of these enemata "she developed acute pulmonary edema, tachycardia, and hypotension and died soon afterward." At necropsy "the colon was found to be grossly dilated throughout its length. The cecum was especially distended and thinned and there was a slit-like anterior perforation. A fecal peritonitis was present also. The feces inside the gut were soft and foamy and there was no organic obstruction. Ganglion cells were present at all levels of the large bowel."

Moreover, in connection with the sudden deaths from cecal rupture in these two decedents with psychotogenic megacolon, Mc Cormack made the following observations which, in his view, provided an explanation for the fatal outcome: "A cecum which is already distended and thinned will tolerate a proportionately smaller increase in intraluminal pressure before splitting and it is significant that both patients had enemata with inevitable increase in intraluminal pressures immediately before a sudden physical deterioration occurred."[15]

Case Report No. 3

However, sudden deaths from the use of enemata in psychotic patients with acquired megacolon have also occurred without any rupture of the bowel. A representative case of this sort is the one which was described in 1965 by Wendkos and Clay.[12] The decedent was a 47-year-old regressed schizophrenic whose megacolon was discovered four years before he died. At that time, because of recurrent episodes of vomiting and pyrexia, various studies including a barium enema examination had been made and this radiologic study confirmed the diagnosis. Moreover, the attacks of vomiting and pyrexia were attributed to repeated fecal impactions.

Three years before he died, a resection of a dilated sigmoid colon was performed and the remaining portions of the colon were joined with an end-to-end anastamosis. At the time of operation it was noted that the sigmoid colon was redundant and almost four times its normal length and at least double its normal diameter. Moreover, it was observed then that the dilatation of the colon was limited primarily to the sigmoid portion of the bowel.

Following this surgical procedure, his postoperative course was uneventful and until the day of this death he had not presented any problems which required his transfer to the medical service. However, on that day (December 8, 1961) there was an obvious change in his physical condition. Suddenly, he began to groan a great deal and despite his mental state it became evident that he was experiencing abdominal discomfort. At 11:30 a.m. of that day when he was examined at Medical Service, the abdomen was found to be distended and there was obvious diffuse abdominal tenderness. No peristalsis could be heard but the vital signs were not in any way alarming. Also, it had been reported that he had developed some diarrhea earlier that day. The leucocyte count was not elevated and there was no disproportionate increase in the number of polymorphonuclear leucocytes. The surgical consultant considered the findings to be indicative of intestinal obstruction secondary to fecal impaction and it was recommended that attempts be made to evacuate the bowel by means of soapsud enemata. Accordingly, over a period of about 4 hours, two such enemata were administered; by this means considerable fecal material was removed. Nevertheless, the abdominal pain persisted and then approximately one half hour after the administration of the second enema, evidences of mild shock developed. The patient appeared apprehensive and became very restless. The pulse became rapid and weak and the blood pressure level could not be determined. Later, respiratory distress and cyanosis were noted and, then, very suddenly the patient became unresponsive; emergency resuscitative measures were unsuccessful.

The autopsy findings indicated that the patient had died from intestinal obstruction associated with an acquired megacolon. The cecum and colon were filled with a large quantity of pasty, yellow feculant material and the colon was enormously dilated. The dilatation extended for a distance of 60 cm proximal to the internal rectal sphincter. Below this sphincter the diameter was only 10 cm. The site of the previous colonic resection was completely healed. The coronary arteries were normal and there was no gross evidence of any myocardial abnormality. Grossly, the brain was normal except for congestion of the brain stem and cerebellum. The cerebral vasculature was normal and there was no evidence of atheromatous degeneration.

Thus, the terminal events in this case resembled those which have followed the use of enemata in children with congenital megacolon.[17] Richards and Hiatt,[18] who have attempted to explain this type of untoward reaction in such patients, have concluded that the phenomenon is the result of water intoxication resulting from the sudden absorption of relatively large amounts of water when nonisotonic solutions are instilled into an obstructed, distended bowel. Accordingly, in their view, the sudden post-enema shock-like state and subsequent death were ascribed to "altered function of essential structures particularly the central nervous system, caused by a sudden increase in intracellular water content."

Clearly, the observations of Richards and Hiatt, as well as the events pertaining to this decedent, would suggest a need to be cautious with respect to the introduction of sizeable amounts of nonisotonic solutions into the bowel of psychotics with an acquired megacolon, particularly when a complicating feature is an obstruction believed to be solely the result of fecal impactions.

SURGICAL CONSIDERATIONS

Moreover, inasmuch as a surgical approach rather than the use of enemata would be indicated when an intestinal obstruction associated with an acquired "megacolon in the insane" is secondary to a volvulus of the pelvic colon, it is important to determine when obstructive symptoms in conjunction with a psychotogenic megacolon are the result of fecal impactions alone and when they are due to a volvulus. In all likelihood, a volvulus occurs more frequently than is generally supposed and many operative successes in psychotics with acquired megacolon and a complicating volvulus already have been adequately documented.[6-11] Thus, it would be inappropriate to delay operative intervention when the interest of a psychotic with an acquired megacolon and a companionate low intestinal obstruction would seem to be served best by opting for a surgical procedure instead of an enema.

Case Report

In support of this view, an experience reported by Koback et al[9] can be cited. "The decedent was a 69-year-old white man who had been confined to mental institutions since 1923 because of a chronic schizophrenic reaction of the undifferentiated type. His last illness began on July 6, 1959 when he did not eat his supper and vomited. Because of this and a drop in blood pressure, he was transferred to the surgical service. His abdomen was rigid and a boggy mass was discovered in the pelvis. His blood pressure was 90/80 and his pulse rate was 90; his white blood count was 12,150 with 83% neurophiles. Volvulus was suspected. Despite administration of plasma, blood, and other fluids, the patient remained in shock for approximately 7 hours when his blood pressure improved but the improvement did not persist. Despite inability to maintain the blood pressure at a desirable level, surgery was deemed necessary to relieve the obstruction. As soon as the abdomen was opened, the patient again suffered severe shock which persisted despite all efforts. A massive black sigmoidal volvulus was found with megacolon extending to the hepatic flexure. Gangrene involved the colon to the upper portion of the rectum. In view of the extent of the lesion and the impossibility of performing a simple exteriorization, a resection was performed with an end-to-end anastamosis. However, despite energetic postoperative management, including immediate administration of antibiotic agents, the patient expired 22 hours after surgery."

PROBLEM OF SEMANTIC LIBERTIES

Any discussion of acquired "megacolon in the insane" also must refer to certain semantic liberties which sometimes have been encountered. Thus, there have been reported cases of sudden death in hospitalized psychotics which have been attributed to a megacolon when actually, from the available data, it was uncertain whether the distention of the colon was due to an intercurrent paralytic or mechanical ileus or to a truly acquired "megacolon in the insane." Two such cases were those reported by Greiner and Nicolson.[19]

Case Report No. 1

The first of these two decedents was a 33-year-old female psychotic mental defective who, after 14 years of hospitalization, was "found dead in bed." However, the protocol omitted any statements regarding intestinal symptoms other than a statement that "for two years prior to the time of death, she suffered from chronic constipation." According to the authors, this costiveness developed while she was receiving a daily ration of chlorpromazine. Also, although the decedent was a known seizure patient, no information was provided with respect to anticonvulsant therapy. An autopsy was performed but the authors did not include any description of the contents of the bowel or any description of the appearance of the colon and the extent of its enlargement.

A listing of the microscopic findings in this case indicated that there were "numerous pigment-laden machrophages in the mucosa of the large intestine; these were situated in the connective tissue surrounding the mucosal gland and Fontana's stain proved the pigment to be melanin." Thus, the pigment deposits in the colon of this decedent resembled those observed by Watkins, Oliver, and Rosenberg in one of their patients.[6] These authors similarly found "a heavy deposition of iron-negative granular brown pigment throughout the large bowel in macrophages in the lamina propria, a finding characteristic of melanosis coli and not infrequently found in association with chronic constipation."

Case Report No. 2

The other decedent whose sudden death was attributed by Greiner and Nicolson to a megacolon also was a seizure-prone mentally retarded woman who, because of her underlying psychosis, received a daily ration of chlorpromazine "to control her behavior." After 26 years of hospitalization, she died "unexpectedly" at the age of 52; there was no reference to intestinal symptoms prior to the time of death. An autopsy was performed and, as in the case of the other decedent, the necropsy disclosed "abdominal distention due to megacolon and pulmonary edema." There were no additional details with respect to the appearance of the colon or its contents. Microscopically, as in the case of the other decedent "macrophages containing melanin-like pigment were observed in the mucosa of the large intestine" but no other microscopic findings with respect to the colon were mentioned.

"Adynamic Ileus" Case Histories

Conversely, Warnes et al[20] reported three sudden deaths allegedly due to "adynamic ileus" when, in all likelihood, the fatalities should have been considered to be the result of intestinal obstruction associated with an acquired "megacolon in the insane." The case histories pertaining to these three decedents were very brief but, in view of the data they contained with respect to symptomatology and postmortem findings, it would seem justifiable to conclude that the intestinal malady Warnes et al had described should properly have been termed a psychotogenic megacolon of the sort described by various authors during the pre-phenothiazine era.[1-5] Thus, it would be difficult to accept the thesis of Warnes et al that the fatalities they had described should be linked to the administration of phenothiazines or kindred compounds.

STUDIES OF PHENOTHIAZINE EFFECTS

Attempts also have been made to inculpate the phenothiazines in connection with the experimental production of intestinal changes alleged to be indicative of a megacolon. The most noteworthy studies of this sort were those conducted by Zimmerman whose findings in adult rats were published in 1962.[21] However, it is doubtful that the intestinal dilatation he had observed was, actually, the analogue of the acquired type of megacolon which has been encountered in the psychiatrically ill.

There are several reasons for this conclusion. First, the existence of a megacolon in Zimmerman's animals was predicated exclusively on the finding that the combined weight of the small and large intestine was at least 13% of the animal's body weight. This ratio was adopted because intestinal weight in untreated rats were found to vary between 6.8% and 12.3% of the body weight.

Second, autopsies of the affected animals disclosed no abnormalities of the gut other than increased caliber and rare mucosal erosions"; moreover, "the character of the intestinal contents was normal at each level of the distended bowel." Third, there was a distinct sex difference; it was noted that "males developed megacolon with greater frequency and apparently more severely." The ratio of affected males to affected females was 22/8 respectively.

Fourth, this alleged megacolon in the rat followed only the intraperitoneal injection of chlorpromazine; the intestinal change occurred in only two fifths of the animals to whom the drug was administered in this manner. Moreover, uniformly, the peroral administration of doses of chlorpromazine—even double that injected intraperitoneally—did not produce similar effects in rat gut.

Fifth, a different rodent (guinea pig) never developed a similar intestinal response following one or more intraperitoneal injections of amounts of chlorpromazine comparable to the doses administered to the rats.

Sixth, there was no definite evidence that in the animals with an alleged megacolon, there was a hypertrophy of the muscular layer of the "affected" portions of the gut.

CONCLUSION

Thus, so far, no experimental data have been adduced which can challenge the implication that "megacolon in the insane" is a visceropathy which can be expected to diminish in frequency only as measures to combat regressive behaviour become more effective. There is no reliable evidence that psychotropic drugs are responsible for this potentially fatal entity.

REFERENCES

1. Schube, P.G. Colon in mental disease: Dementia praecox. *Am. J. Dig. Dis.* 3:528 (1936).
2. Lee, C.M. and Bebb, K.C. The pathogenesis and clinical management of megacolon with emphasis on the fallacy of the term "idiopathic." *Surgery* 30:1026 (1951).
3. Dean, G.O. and Murry, J.W. Volvulus of the sigmoid colon. *Ann. Surg.* 135:830 (1952).
4. Gabriel, I.T. et al. Volvulus of the sigmoid colon. *Gastroenterology* 24:378 (1953).
5. Ehrentheil, O.F. and Wells, E.P. Megacolon in psychotic patients. *Gastroenterology* 29:285 (1955).
6. Watkins, G.L. et al. Giant megacolon in the insane: Subtotal colectomy as a method of management. *Ann. Surg.* 153:409 (1961).
7. McKain, J. H. Acute cardiopulmonary embarrassment: Report of a case. *Amer. Surgeon* 25:421 (1956).
8. Burrell, Z.L. Acquired megacolon in the insane. *Gastroenterology* 33:625 (1957).
9. Koback, M.W. et al. Acquired megacolon in psychiatric patients. *Dis. Colon Rectum* 5:373 (1962).
10. Ansingh, H.R. and Rideout, E.M. Megacolon and recurrent sigmoid volvulus in psychotic patients. *Northwest Med.* 61:1032 (1962).
11. Watkins, G.L. and Oliver, G.A. Giant megacolon in the insane. *Gastroenterology* 48:718 (1965).
12. Wendkos, M.H. and Clay, B. Unusual causes for sudden unexpected death in regressed hospitalized schizophrenics. *J. Am. Geriatr. Soc.* 13:663 (1965).
13. Kraft, E. et al. The megasigmoid syndrome in psychotic patients. *J.A.M.A.* 195:1099 (1966).
14. Johnston, I.D.A. and Gibson, J.B. Megacolon and volvulus in psychotics. *Brit. J. Surg.* 47:394 (1970).

15. Mc Cormack, M. Cecal rupture in psychotic patients *Brit. Med. J.* 4:82 (1974).
16. Hussey, H.H. The cause of death. *J.A.M.A.* 229:75 (1974).

17. Hiatt, B. Pathologic physiology of congenital megacolon. *Ann. Surg.* 133:313 (1951).
18. Richards, M.R. and Hiatt, R.B. Untoward effects of enemata in congenital megacolon. *Pediatrics* 12:253 (1953).
19. Greiner, A.C. and Nicolson, G.A. Pigment deposition in viscera associated with prolonged clorpromazine therapy. *Can. M.A.J.* 91:627 (1964.
20. Warnes, H. et al. Adynamic ileus during psychoactive medication: A report of 3 fatal and 5 severe cases. *Can. M.A.J.* 96:1112 (1967.
21. Zimmerman, G.R. Megacolon from large doses of chlorpromazine. *Arch. Pathol. Lab. Med.* 74:59 (1962).
22. Giordano, J. et al. Fatal paralytic ileus complicating phenothiazine therapy. *South. Med. J.* 68:351 (1975).

CHAPTER 9

Fatal Hyperpyrexia

Although psychiatric patients have died suddenly from fatal hyperpyrexia secondary to heat stroke[1,2] and, conceivably, can die suddenly from malignant hyperpyrexia produced by the administration of an anesthetic, the majority of reported sudden deaths in psychiatric patients due to fatal hyperpyrexia have been ascribed to the consumption of remedial phrenotropic agents, with antidepressants heading the list of substances likely to produce this sort of life-threatening adverse effect.[3-11,13-18]

In general, a drug-related fatal hyperpyrexia has resulted from an overdose of a tricyclic antidepressant alone,[9] from an overdose of a monoamine oxidase inhibitor alone,[10,11,17] from a synergism between a monoamine oxidase inhibitor and a tricyclic antidepressant,[4-8,17] between a monoamine oxidase inhibitor and an amphetamine compound,[13,14] and between a monoamine oxidase inhibitor and a phenothiazine.[15,16] In addition, there is a single report of fatal hyperpyrexia due to the combined administration of lithium and haloperiodol.[18]

NOMENCLATURE

In terms of nomenclature, heat stroke is the usual term employed to describe an environment-related hyperpyrexia but some have considered it to be too prosaic. Accordingly, they have preferred to replace it with a Latin name. Correspondingly, inasmuch as Sirius, the Dog Star, regularly occupies a conspicous place in the sky during the mid-summer, they have chosen the cognomen of Siriasis to identify this particular malady.[19] Nevertheless, either designation serves to emphasize that environmental heat represents the most important, if not the sole "risk factor" with respect to the pathogenesis of this sort of fatal hyperpyrexia.

CLINICAL FEATURES OF HEAT STROKE

Repeated observations have confirmed that the fundamental clinical features of fatal hyperpyrexia associated with heat stroke include a lack of perspiration and a hot dry skin.[26-29,34] Thus, in this respect alone, fatal hyperpyrexia due to excessive doses of single psychotropic drugs or to a synergism between two antidepressants or between a monoamine oxidase inhibitor or lithium and another psychoactive preparation is unlike fatal hyperpyrexia secondary to a high ambient temperature. Moreover, inasmuch as heat stroke is a term which should be limited to an anhidrotic febrile illness, it is apparent that it would not be descriptive of either a case of heat exhaustion or a case of drug-related hyperpyrexia.

Correspondingly, for this reason, a proper taxonomic differentiation would be to classify Siriasis as a malignant thermogenic anhidrotic hyperpyrexia and, conversely, to consider a drug-related life-threatening febrile illness to be an example of malignant pharmacogenic hyperhidrotic hyperpyrexia. Essentially, aside from the hyperpyrexia, the characteristic clinical features of a malignant pharmacogenic hyperhidrotic hyperpyrexia include central nervous system effects (convulsions or delirium succeeded by coma) and evidences of peripheral cholinergic stimulation (excessive perspiration and excessive salivation), although it has been postulated that the hyperpyrexia may be the result of excessive accumulation of catecholamines in the brain.[40]

Although, in general, it is agreed that the hyperpyrexia resulting from a high ambient temperature is linked to the associated anhidrosis, the reason for the interruption of sweat gland activity still is unclear. Thus, one of the most recent and complete reviews of heat stroke has adopted the position that "the cessation in sweating in this febrile disorder is due to an intrinsic breakdown of the heat regulatory mechanism for reasons not known."[27]

It has also been postulated that "after prolonged exposure to heat, sweating decreases because the sweat glands become fatigued";[27] this conclusion, however, does not appear to be sufficiently explanatory.

On the other hand, others who have microscopically examined the sweat glands in persons who succumbed to a malignant anhidrotic thermogenic hyperpyrexia have provided some evidence that there may be an anatomical defect which can account for the sudden interruption of sudorific activity in persons who have collapsed because of heat stroke. Such an investigation has disclosed that the "sweat glands in heat stroke show marked cellular dehydration and degeneration, particularly in the basal cell layer which is responsible for water and electrolyte secretion."[42]

RISK-FACTORS

Psychotropic Drugs

Occasionally, a sudden death due to fatal hyperpyrexia can simply follow an overdose of chlorpromazine. Such a fatality was reported by Ayd in 1956.[12] In this instance, the patient was a "41-year-old white man who was hospitalized for chlorpromazine therapy for a schizoprenic reaction, unclassified. His past psychiatric history revealed the presence of overt schizophrenic symptomatology for four years. He had been treated with several courses of electroconvulsive therapy that produced a temporary amelioration of his symptoms. Several months prior to his admission, this patient had been treated with doses of chlorpromazine up to 400 mg per day with some symptomatic improvement. When chlorpromazine was discontinued, that patient relapsed. At the time of his readmission to the hospital, physical and neurologic examinations were negative. The psychiatric examination revealed an agitated schizoprenic with paranoid features. This patient was placed on increasing doses of chlorpromazine to a maximum of 2500 mg on the 18th treatment day. On the 19th and 20th treatment days he received 2500 mg daily. On the 21st treatment day, he had had 1800 mg and at 6 p.m. of that day his temperature was normal. However, 2 hours later he collapsed suddenly. At that time his rectal temperature was 108° F. Thereafter he had a few epileptiform seizures and lapsed into a coma. Intensive treatment of the hypothermia lowered the temperature to 104° F. but he expired 9 hours after his collapse. The postmortem examination was confined to the brain and the findings there included swelling of the neuron cells, capillary distention, and terminal petechial hemorrhages. Anatomic lesions of a destructive nature were not present."

In his discussion of this fatality, Ayd indicated that patients who received chlorpromazine, particularly in large doses, will perspire excessively and manifest symptoms of mild heat prostration, especially when the environmental temperature is unusually high. He also mentioned that the increased sensitivity to heat is not related to the dosage of chlorpromazine although patients on large doses apparently are more sensitive. He also explained that with regard to this particular patient, the fatal hyperpyrexia had occurred at a time when the environmental temperature was high. It was postulated by Ayd that the demise of this patient was due to "the toxic action of chlorpromazine on the hypothalamus and that the toxicity of chlorpromazine was accentuated by the environmental temperature." Apparently, he did not regard the marked overdose of chlorpromazine as an important "risk factor" with respect to this episode of fatal hyperpyrexia.

Evidently, although this episode of fatal hyperpyrexia occurred on a day when the ambient temperature was excessive, Ayd considered the sudden deaths to be primarily an adverse reaction to the chlorpromazine and not the result of heat stroke. Moreover, this view would be in accord with his observation that excessive doses of this drug will cause excessive sweating, especially when the environmental temperature is elevated, a feature which is absent in instances of true heat stroke.

Other Case Histories

Other heat stroke fatalities in phenothiazine-treated patients have been reported by Zelman and Guillan[1] and by Sarnquist and Larson.[2] However, the more detailed report is the one by Zelman and Guillan, who had provided clinical, epidemiologic, and postmortem data pertaining to three such decedents.

Prior to the time of death, one, a 50-year-old lobotomized patient, had been receiving 500 mg of chlorpromazine and 15 mg of trifluoperazine daily; the second, a 55-year-old man, had been receiving 37.5 mg of fluphenazine enanthate intramuscularly every two weeks; the third decedent had been receiving 450 mg of promazine daily.

These three fatal cases of heat stroke were encountered at the Topeka, Kansas Veterans Administration Hospital during an oppressive humid heat wave in mid-July 1969. Two of these decedents had been living outside the hospital without benefit of air conditioning and, in each instance, the sudden onset of convulsions represented the earliest clinical manifestation of their febrile illness. The third, who was being prepared to resume normal communal living, had left the hospital grounds temporarily to search for employment and then had returned without assistance to the hospital. Shortly after his arrival, he became delirious, and not long afterward he became comatose. Accordingly, he was taken promptly to the Medical Service but like the other two patients, he failed to recover.

At the time these three decedents had reached the Medical Service of the hospital, it was ascertained that, uniformly, their skins were hot and dry and the rectal temperatures exceeded 108° F. Eventually, one died because of "massive aspiration of copious vomitus"; another "died quickly of hyperpyrexia"; the third "survived his hyperthermia only to die 12 hours later in peripheral circulatory collapse." In each instance, "the postmortem examination showed intense circulatory congestion, visceral edema and punctate hemorrhages throught the heart and brain. In addition, a tubular necrosis of the kidney was present and in two instances a fatty metamorphosis of the liver also was a noteworthy finding."

However, although Zelman and Guillan[1] had observed the companionate presence of extreme hyperpyrexia and anhidrosis in these three phenothiazine-treated psychiatric patients before they had died suddenly on an unusually hot day, it was suggested by these observers that an important "risk factor" was the prior consumption of the phenothiazines consumed by the decedents before they had died. As Zelman and Guillan explained, "in addition to a suppressive effect on temperature regulation, phenothiazines exert anticholinergic effects peripherally, including suppression of sweating." In addition, they mentioned that "the importance of this peripheral action of the phenothiazines in our patients is suggested by the fact that no cases of simple heat exhaustion were encountered in our phenothiazine-treated patients during the period in which the fatal cases of heat stroke were seen."

However, it is uncertain whether simply the daily consumption of customary doses of a phenothiazine compound will, indeed, be sufficient to increase the likelihood of a malignant anhidrotic thermogenic hyperpyrexia when there also are present those environmental conditions which alone are known to favor the occurrence of such a catastrophe. Moreover, to suppose that the phenothiazines possess a powerful antisudorific action would be to endow these drugs with a property which apparently they do not possess.

Although dryness of the mouth is a fairly common side effect of the phenothiazines, it has been recognized by Ayd,[26] as well as others, that such an antisalivation action is not accompanied by a corresponding suppressive effect on the sweating mechanism.[12] In this same connection, it also is noteworthy that Shader and Di Mascio, in their monograph entitled "Psychotropic Drug Side Effects,"[36] have stated that "hyperpyrexia accompanied by profuse perspiration has been reported after chlorpromazine." In addition, Freyhan[43], in a study undertaken to evaluate the effectiveness of prochlorperazine in psychiatric disorders, found that "excessive sweating followed the administration of this particular phenothiazine compound." Equally impressive was the observation by Hanlon[37] that, despite its acknowledged anticholinergic properties, thioridazine given in customary doses, actually can increase salivation and perspiration.

Conclusions

Thus, such pharmacologic data pertaining to the phenothiazines seemed to show that these drugs actually induce sweating rather than inhibit it. Correspondingly, it is likely that both the anhidrosis and the hyperpyrexia in these three decedents reported by Zelman and Guillan were simply manifestations of a malignant thermogenic anhidrotic fatal hyperpyrexia resulting from exposure to an inordinately high ambient temperature.

Contributary effects of antiparkinsonian drugs. However, it is conceivable that concurrent consumption of antiparkinsonian drugs (because of their well-established anticholinergic properties) might in these two instances, have contributed to the occurrence of the fatal hyperpyrexia. These two decedents had received, concurrently with their phenothiazines, sizeable amounts of such preparations and, in view of the report by Litman which appeared in 1952,[38] it would be proper to give some consideration to the possibility that these drugs (which are known to possess an antisudorific property[38]) had enhanced the likelihood that these respective patients would develop a malignant thermogenic anhidrotic hyperpyrexia at a time when the ambient temperature was inordinately elevated.

Evidently, this view was also shared by Zelman and Guillan. This conclusion is based on their acknowlegement, in their publication, that anticholinergic agents such as antiparkinsonian drugs which customarily supplement the use of sizeable amounts of the phenothiazines "must bear a large share of responsibility for the susceptibility of psychiatric patients to heat stroke, because of their inhibition of sweating."

Moreover, the occurrence of only three episodes of fatal anhidrotic thermogenic hyperpyrexia during that week in 1969, when the ambient temperature in Topeka was inordinately elevated, would imply that phenothiazine therapy might not be a meaningful "risk factor" in this type of fatal malady. This interpretation is based on the fact that any large Veterans Administration Psychiatric Hospital—like the one in Topeka, Kansas—includes among its patient population during any day of the year, many hundreds of patients who are being treated with phenothiazine compounds. Moreover, such a patient sample would include chronic alcoholics, many elderly, and many persons with a variety of chronic brain syndromes as well as many with preexisting medical problems. Thus, among this number there would be many who would be disposed to develop heat stroke when the environmental temperature is unusually high.[2,27,29,30,38] Nevertheless, sudden deaths due to fatal hyperpyrexia in any broad segment of phenothiazine-treated psychiatric patients is practically an unknown event in most neuropsychiatric facilities, even during periods of extreme summertime heat.[41]

Chronic alcoholism as contributary factor. Also, in this connection, it is noteworthy that the autopsy of the three fatalities reported by Zelman and Guillan had revealed the presence of "fatty metamorphosis of the liver" in two instances. This finding is meaningful inasmuch as it suggests that two of the three decedents were chronic alcoholics and thus, supposedly, were additionally predisposed to develop a life-threatening heat-related affliction.[2,27,28,30,38]

Postmortem Data

So far, reports concerning deaths due to the pharmacogenic variety of malignant hyperpyrexia rarely have included detailed postmortem data. However, there is one article[16] in which the authors have stated that the impressive autopsy findings included renal tubular necrosis due to myoglobinuria and a disseminated intravascular coagulation disorder which was responsible for petechial hemorrhages in the brain, heart, kidney and skin. Thus, such observations are essentially comparable to the nature of the pathology which many investigators have described in connection with the nonexertional variety of malignant anhidrotic thermogenic fatal hyperpyrexia.[30] Indeed, this congruence should not be surprising inasmuch as it is the contention of several authorities[23,24] that the pathology associated with a fatal heat-related illness is primarily due to the hyperpyrexia per se.

At the present time, in contrast with the sparsity of autopsy findings related to a drug-related fatal hyperpyrexia, there is a substantial body of postmortem data pertaining to fatalities resulting from nonexertional thermogenic anhidrotic hyperpyrexia. Thus it has been established that because the hyperpyrexia has produced a widespread disseminated intravascular coagulopathy secondary to endothelial cellular damage,[20-23,25,30,32-35] petechiae or a hematoma usually will be present in the brain and in the heart.[30] In addition, a usual finding was evidence of renal tubular necrosis associated with myoglobinuria and evidence of myocardial necrosis.[23,30] Moreover, some observers have averred that a careful examination of the liver will disclose, without exception, microscopic or gross changes indicative of hepatic injury.[28,30]

Management

Moreover, inasmuch as the disseminated intravascular coagulation disorder has been recognized to be a regular feature of malignant thermogenic fatal hyperpyrexia, it has been suggested that while patients with this heart-related illness are still alive, it is imperative to exclude, by means of suitable laboratory studies, the presence of this particular intravascular abnormality; if its existence is thereby confirmed, low doses of heparin should be administered without delay.[21,33] In view of the observations already mentioned, such an approach would seem to be equally desirable even when a drug-related hyperpyrectic syndrome is encountered. However, it must be emphasized that such a recommendation does not diminish the importance of aggressive use of defervescence measures in the management of patients with fatal hyperpyrexia.

Case Report No. 1

In this connection, the observations reported by Brachfeld et al[39] are of interest. Their patient was a 41-year-old female who was admitted to the hospital on March 6, 1963 at 8:30 p.m. For the preceding three weeks tranylcypromine sulfate, 10 mg twice daily, had been prescribed by her family physician. When she failed to improve, she was referred for psychiatric evaluation and the suspicion of depression was confirmed. On the day of admission, she had become increasingly restless and at 7 p.m. she complained of excruciating headache. Her husband was advised to take her to the hospital but enroute she lost consciousness and started to convulse. At 9 p.m. she was deeply comatose and she did not respond to any stimuli except for an occasional generalized convulsive seizure. Her temperature at that time was 105° F. The neck was in severe opisthotonos and her extremities were in severe extensor rigidity and the hands showed extreme carpal spasm. The lungs were clear but because of the severe tonic spasms, little ventilatory exchange occurred.

"The cause of these neurological disturbances was uncertain at the time of her admission but accidental or suicidal poisoning by strychnine, atropine, or other products was considered to be likely. At this point, it was learned that the patient had received a prescription for imipramine on the day of her admission to the hospital and had taken one tablet in the afternoon. Since the monoamine oxidase inhibitor had been stopped 3 days previously, incompatability had not been anticipated."

"Convulsions were controlled by several injections of a barbiturate preparation which did not cause any excessive depression of respiration. The patient's temperature was reduced by the application of alcohol-ice-soaked towels. At 10:30 p.m. deep cyanosis supervened and a tracheostomy was performed. By 11 p.m. her temperature was at a normal level, convulsions and rigidity ceased, and her respiration was quiet although somewhat shallow. By the next morning the patient was conscious, rational, and her affect appeared appropriate. She was discharged from the hospital in good condition 6 days after admission."

Case Report No. 2

A less favorable outcome resulting from a synergism between a monoamine oxidiase inhibitor and a tricyclic antidepressant was reported in brief annotations by Davies[7] and by Bowen,[3] respectively. Davies described the case of a 23-year-old woman who had been hospitalized because of her addiction to preludin (phenmetrazine hydrochloride). The "addiction" was treated by substituting a daily ration of chlorpromazine (50 mg 4 times a day). She was sent home but later developed a reactive depression and, for this reason, she was advised to discontinue the chlorpromazine and to begin the use of phenelzine (15 mg 3 times a day). She was instructed, also, that if the phenelzine did not lift the depression in 21 days, she should then begin to use 25 mg of imipramine 3 times daily. Instead, she took between 200 and 300 mg of imipramine and, soon afterward, she developed hyperpyrexia, *profuse sweating*, extreme restlessness, and hyperexcitability followed by unconsciousness. She died in the hospital 4 hours after the onset of the reaction; just before her death, her temperature had reached 109° F. An autopsy was performed but the data in this case report indicated merely that "a postmortem examination revealed that the decedent had ingested about 200 mg of imipramine." No other autopsy findings were mentioned.

Case Report No. 3

The patient described by Bowen[3] was a 41-year-old woman who, before she was admitted to the hospital on August 28, 1964, had been treated for her depression with phenelzine (15 mg 3 times daily), desipramine (50 mg 3 times daily) and a nightly dose of chlorpromazine (amount was not mentioned). At the time of her admission, she was already comatose. The legs were rigid and ankle clonus was present; there was a sinus tachycardia with a rate of 150 per minute; her temperature was elevated to 104° F; the blood pressure was 130/70; her respirations were shallow and she was cyanotic; her pupils were dilated and the skin was flushed; both salivation and perspiration were markedly increased. That same day she died. The postmortem examination disclosed nothing of significance except for a dilated heart and a soft myocardium. A report from the Forensic Science Laboratory showed that chlorpromazine and desipramine had been found in the tissues, but only in therapeutic amounts. No phenelzine could be demonstrated but it was suggested that it still could have produced the reaction even if it had not been taken for a number of days.

PATHOGENESIS OF PHARMACOGENIC HYPOPREXIA

Still unsettled is the pathogenesis of the hyperpyrexia associated with this type of adverse drug-reaction. Clearly, because hyperhidrosis seems to be an essential element of this particular hyperpyrexic syndrome, it would seem unlikely that the elevated body temperature is due to interference with the mechanisms which operate to promote heat loss in the presence of either normal or excessive heat production. Moreover, it is of interest that in these instances of malignant pharmacogenic hyperpyrexia, sudorific activity was preserved even though cholinergic inhibition generally is considered to be one of the important pharmacologic hallmarks of a tricyclic antidepressant agent.[17]

Thus, it would be reasonable to suppose that the hyperpyrexic component of this particular syndrome is due to a drug-related disruption of the thermoregulatory functions of the central nervous system. Moreover, inasmuch as an important effect of both a monoamine oxidase inhibitor and a tricyclic antidepressant agent is to influence the degradation and release of catecholamines and other biogenic amines[17] it could be speculated that a malignant hyperhidrotic pharmacogenic hyperpyrexia is the result of a synergistic action by these respective compounds on amine metabolism. However, it must be acknowledged that the nature of the connection between such a synergism and the behavior of the heat-regulating center is still unclear. Thus, until more is understood concerning the role of biogenic amine metabolism in relation to the central control of body temperature, it would be a meaningless endeavor to attempt, at this time, to explain how synergistic drug effects on amine metabolism can induce a life-threatening febrile syndrome.

REFERENCES

1. Zelman, S. and Guillan, R. Heat stroke in phenothiazine treated patients: a report of 3 fatalities. Am. J. Psychiatr. 126:1787 (1970).
2. Sarnquist, F. and Larson, C.P. Drug-induced heat stroke. Anesthesiology 39:348 (1973).
3. Bowen, L.W. Fatal hyperpyrexia with antidepressant drugs. Brit. Med. J. 2:1465 (1964).
4. Stanley, B. and Pal, N.R. Fatal hyperpyrexia with phenelzine and imipramine. Brit. Med. J. 2:1011 (1964).
5. Luby, E. and Domino, E. Toxicity from large doses of imipramine and an monoamine oxidase inhibitor in suicidal intent. J.A.M.A. 177:68 (1961).
6. Lee, F.I. Imipramine overdosage. Report of a fatal case. Brit. Med. J. 1:338 (1961).
7. Davies, G. Side-effects of phenelzine. Brit. Med. J. 2:1019 (1960).
8. Babiak, W. Case fatality due to overdosage of combination of tranylcypromine (Parnate) and imipramine (Tofranil). Can. M.A.J. 85:377 (1961).

9. Masters, A.B. Delayed death in imipramine poisoning. *Brit. Med. J.* 3:866 (1967).
10. Matell, G. and Thorstrand, C. A case of fatal nialamid poisoning. *Acta Med. Scand.* 181:79 (1967).
11. Horden, A. Psychiatry and the tranquilizers. *New Eng. J. Med.* 265:584 (1961).
12. Ayd, F.J. Fatal hyperpyrexia during chlorpromazine therapy. *J. Clin. Exp. Psychopath. Q. Rev. Psych. Neurol.* 17:189 (1956).
13. Dally, P.J. Fatal reaction associated with tranylcypromine and methylamphetamine. *Lancet* 1:1235 (1962).
14. Mason, A. Fatal reaction associated with tranylcypromine and methylamphetamine. *Lancet* 1:1073 (1962).
15. Mac Caig, J.N. and Edmundson, J.S. Overdose of parstelin. *Brit. Med. J.* 1:923 (1965).
16. Plaats, M.M. et al. Phenelzine and trifluoperazine. *Lancet* 2:738 (1965).
17. Davis, J.M. et al. Overdosage of psychotropic drugs: A review. Part II. Antidepressants and other psychotropic agents. *Dis. Nerv. Sys.* 29:246 (1968).
18. Baastrup, P.C. et al. Adverse reactions in treatment with lithium carbonate and haloperidol. *J.A.M.A.* 236:2645 (1976).
19. Knochel, J.P. Dog days and siriasis. *J.A.M.A.* 233:513 (1975).
20. O Donnell, T.F. Acute heat stroke. Epidemiologic, biochemical, renal, and coagulation studies. *J.A.M.A.* 234:824 (1975).
21. Weber, M.V. and Blakely, J.A. The hemorrhagic diathesis of heat stroke. A consumption coagulopathy successfully treated with heparin. *Lancet* 1:1190 (1969).
22. Shibolet, S. et al. Fibrinolysis and hemorrhages in fatal heat stroke. *New Eng. J. Med.* 266:169 (1962).
23. Barcenas, C. et al. Obesity, football, dog days and siriasis: A deadly combination. *Am. Heart J.* 92:237 (1976).
24. Shapiro, Y. et al. Experimental heatstroke. A model in dogs. *Arch. Intern. Med.* 131:688 (1973).
25. Clowes, G.H.A. and O..Donnell, T.F. Current concepts; Heat stroke. *New Eng. J. Med.* 291:564 (1974).
26. Heat stroke (Editorial) *Lancet:* 2:31 (1968).
27. Eichler, A.C. et al. Heat stroke. *Am. J. Surg.* 118:855 (1969).
28. Austin, M.G. and Berry, J.W. Observations on 100 cases of heat stroke. *J.A.M.A.* 161:1525 (1956).
29. Ferris, E.B. et al. Heat stroke: Clinical and chemical observations in 44 cases. *J. Clin. Invest.* 17:249 (1938).
30. Knochel, J.P. et al. The renal, cardiovascular, hematologic and serum electrolyte abnormalities of heat stroke. *Am. J. Med.* 30:299 (1961).
31. Vertel, R.M. et al. Acute renal failure due to heat injury: An analysis of 10 cases associated with a high incidence of myoglobinuria. *Am. J. Med.* 43:435 (1967).
32. Sohal, R.S. et al. Heat stroke: An electronmicroscopic study of endothelial cell damage and disseminated intravascular coagulation. *Arch. Intern. Med.* 122:43 (1968).
33. Perchick, J.S. et al. Disseminated intravascular coagulation in heat stroke: Response to heparin therapy, *J.A.M.A.* 231:480 (1975).
34. Heat stroke. (Editorial) *Brit. Med. J.* 2:190 (1968).
35. Knochel, J.P. Disseminated intravascular coagulation in heat stroke, Response to heparin therapy. *J.A.M.A.* 231:496 (1975).
36. Shader, R.I. and De Mascio, A. *Psychotropic Drug Side Effects.* Williams and Wilkins, Baltimore (1970).
37. Hanlon, T.E. et al. The comparative effectiveness of 8 phenothiazines. *Psychopharmacologia* (Berlin) 7:89 (1965).

38. Litman, R.E. Heat sensitivity due to autonomic drugs. *J.A.M.A.* 149:635 (1952).
39. Brachfeld, J. et al. Imipramine-tranylcypromine incompatibility: near-fatal toxic reaction. *J.A.M.A.* 186:1172 (1963).
40. Jori, A. and Garattini, S. Interaction between imipramine-like agents and catecholamine-induced hyperthermia. *J. Pharm. Pharmacol.* 17:480 (1965).
41. Wendkos, M.H. Unpublished Data.
42. Baba, N. and Ruppert, R.D. Alteration of eccrine sweat gland in fatal heat stroke. *Arch. Pathol. Lab. Med.* 85:669 (1968).
43. Freyhan, F.A. The Neuroleptic Action and Effectiveness of Prochlorperazine in Psychiatric Disorders. *Psych. Res. Reports of Am. Psych. Ass.* 9:32-45 March (1958).

CHAPTER 10

Acute Exhaustive Mania

Ever since 1701, when Lancisi, the famous Italian physician, published his celebrated treatise entitled *De Subitaneis Mortibus*[1] much interest has been shown in the epidemiology of so-called natural sudden deaths. However, in the past, most epidemiologic studies regarding such sudden unexpected deaths have been concerned with fatalities linked to the presence of atherosclerotic coronary artery disease;[2-14] relatively little material pertaining to the epidemiology of psychosis-related sudden deaths has been published, even though such fatalities have been observed with regularity in institutions designed to care for the mentally ill.[15-18,43-44] For this reason, it is important to consider the epidemiologic aspects of an entity which was described, originally, by Bell in 1849[19] and, since then, has been discussed under a variety of rubrics.

CLINICAL PICTURE OF TYPICAL ATTACK

A vivid portrayal of a typical attack of this particular malady which, sometimes, is identified by an eponymic term such as "Bell's Mania" and, at other times, by such titles as "fatal catatonia"[21-22] or "Acute exhaustive psychosis,"[23] can be found in an article by Shulack, published in 1938.[24] The following is his version, which now will be quoted in its entirety:

"A young individual, in the second or third decade of life, suddenly becomes restless and excited. This psychomotor activity increases and is accompanied by hilarity or fearful anxiety in response to extrospective or introspective pressure of ideas. Work and duties are neglected. Sleep becomes difficult and often impossible. Impulsive or responsive aggressiveness increases. The individual breaks equipment or furniture or assaults his neighbor, apparently without reason. He is then admitted to the hospital. The excitement and restlessness continue day and night with only momentary respite. Excitement increases until it becomes a continual maniacal furor, in which the individual will tear off his clothes, tear the clothes to strips, take the bed apart, rip the mattress to pieces, bang, and pound almost rhythmically on the walls and windows, dash wildly from the room, assault anyone in reach, and run aimlessly, and without apparent objective, from one end of the room to the other. The pulse becomes rapid even in the periods of momentary rest. Food and fluids are refused and weight loss becomes apparent. Perspiration is profuse and continual. The blood pressure falls and the pulse becomes thready. Fever is then noted. Early in the furor it ranges around 100° F. rectally. When confined to a room, the patient will thrash against the wall or butt his head against it. If placed in restraints, either in a continuous tepid tub or bed, (in pack or sheet) the patient will strain ceaselessly against the restraints in an attempt to tear out and maintain his externally objectiveless activity. Fever increases, the pulse becomes more thready and rapid, blood pressure falls further, perspiration drips continually, the tongue becomes dry and furred. The skin becomes flushed and feels hot to the touch. After varying periods of excitement of from hours to days, the temperature may rise to 105° F. rectally or 107° F. rectally or even 110° F. rectally. The skin may become pale or cyanotic and suddenly all activity ceases, respiration and cardiac activity stop and the patient is dead. This end may come so suddenly that the attending psychiatrist is left with a chagrined surprise and the puzzlement is intensified after the postmortem examination because the autopsy generally fails to disclose any findings which could explain the death. Therefore, the usual final diagnosis is (1) an unclassified psychosis (2) exhaustion from overexertion in a state of acute mania."

Thus, it is evident that the syndrome he has depicted, which is generally acknowledged to be the paradigm of acute exhaustive mania in hospitalized psychotics, compromises three essential hallmarks. The first element in this triad is the persistent extremely violent psychotic behaviour which is not related to the ingestion of substances such as alcohol or other delirium-producing compounds. The second is a sudden fatal outcome which dramatically terminates the maniacal behaviour. The third is the absence of any meaningful anatomic changes at the postmortem examination.

Moreover, because it regularly was noted that the autopsy in such decedents failed to disclose a reason for the deaths, several reports which have appeared during the prephenothiazine era have undertaken to explain why patients with "Bell's Mania" so often died, whereas other maniacal psychotics survived. However, it appears that with but a single exception, none of the authors in question has provided a meaningful resolution of this epidemiologic dilemma.

HISTORICAL REVIEW

In 1919, an article was published by Ladame[25] in which he attributed deaths associated with lethal catatonia to "psychic shock" (a term he did not define). In accord with his thesis, the psychic shock led to a severe degree of excitement and subsequently to cachexia, cardiac weakness, and death. In addition he speculated that the psychic shock produced, concurrently, a series of "chemical disorders in the body, the primary one of which was a disintegration of lecithin which in turn resulted in death." However, he failed to provide any evidence to show that such a series of chemical disorders indeed could occur in conjunction with a mental illness exhibiting the characteristic features of "Bell's Mania."

Then in 1929, a report by Schiedegger appeared which was based on an experience with 43 deaths in acutely "excited" patients[26] and in this article the author concluded that, even though the autopsies of the decedents failed to reveal any positive findings, the fatalities should be ascribed to "changes in the subcortical centers." However, so far as could be determined, Schiedegger did not describe the nature of the alleged subcortical changes and he did not make it clear how, in his view, he could account for these alleged changes.

Subsequently, in 1934, after Davidson had noted that the necropsies of his patients had disclosed "nothing other than exhaustion following continuous excitement," he proposed that deaths associated with lethal catatonia resulted from cardiovascular collapse induced by the release of vasotoxic substances.[27] However, Davidson did not indicate exactly how the release of such vasotoxic substances came about; moreover, their presence was never actually demonstrated.

On the other hand, in 1938, Shulack contended that the mortality in this fatal psychiatric syndrome resulted from the tissue toxemia which, when combined with hyperthermia, was "too traumatic for a sensitized central nervous system and cardiovascular system, unable to bear the great functional load of hyperactivity."[24]

One year later, in 1939, Larson proposed a different theory in order to explain the sudden deaths associated with "Bell's Mania."[28] He postulated that as a result of the manic behaviour, the decedent prior to the time of the death developed marked dehydration and a hypochloremia, finally resulting in petechial hemorrhages in the brain. Larson also believed that when such behaviour-related petechial hemorrhages spread to the "vital centers of the brain," these lesions became primarily responsible for the sudden deaths he had observed. However, it should be pointed out that despite the attractiveness of this theory, it never has been demonstrated that hypochloremia or petechial hemorrhages in the brain are the usual findings in psychotics who die because of lethal catatonia.

An equally vague and ambiguous explanation for deaths in hospitalized psychotics was suggested by Malamud and Boyd in their paper which also appeared in 1939.[29] However, from their standpoint, the abnormal behaviour was not a lethal prodrome. Instead, they concluded that the actual pathogenesis of fatalities associated with lethal catatonia was a "functional abnormality of the vasomotor system resulting from a constitutional vasomotor instability." Thus, apparently, it was their view that the conjunction of the psychic turmoil and the death of their patient was a purely coincidental finding and, furthermore, that the explosive behaviour was not an important risk factor.

In 1944, Billig and Freeman[21] had observed that, "in many of these cases death comes suddenly and is probably of cerebral origin of either the respiratory or vasomotor type." However, they failed to supply a further clarification of the supposed mechanisms and their genesis.

In 1947, a psychoanalytically oriented explanation for the deadliness of lethal catatonia was presented by Adland.[23] In his view, "the acute exhaustive psychosis or exhaustive syndrome is a psychogenic illness originating in a need for self-anihilation as a solution to a problem." Thus, when all the circumstances identified with this fatal psychiatric syndrome are considered, it would appear that Adland's premise is sound; at least, it seems to account for the usual course of events during an episode of lethal catatonia.

Moreover, it should be appreciated that Adland's postulates do not reject the primacy of abnormal behavior in relation to the deaths which are an inherent part of this fatal malady. This point is mentioned because, in addition to the psychodynamic formulation he had subsumed, he indicated that the assaultiveness and excitement which are the external hallmarks of an attack of acute exhaustive psychosis may be an unconscious symbolic means of fulfilling the wish for escape through "self-anihilation." Nevertheless, it should be recognized that such a concept does not exclude the role of pathophysiologic equivalents with respect to the occurrence of a sudden cardiac arrest in patients of this genre.

In this connection, it is noteworthy that there are data to indicate that an excessive elaboration of medullary and cortical adrenal hormones will follow sustained physical activity[30] or psychic turmoil[30-31] and that such oversecretions can lead to a myocardial oxygen debt[32-33] and also to the occurrence of a life-threatening ventricular arrhythmia.[30,34-35,47] However it seems necessary to consider also the possible adverse effects of "restraint stress" during an epsidode of acute exhaustive mania.

ADVERSE EFFECTS OF RESTRAINT STRESS

Although it is a common nosocomial practice to utilize restraining measures in order to prevent physical injury to a patient in the throes of an episode of uncontrollable agitation and excitement it should be recognized that such a procedure may not be entirely innocuous.

This issue is raised because experimental and clinical data are now available to indicate that restraint per se, or the resistance to it, can favor the occurrence of a sudden death.[36-39,44] The exact mechanism still has not been clarified but it is suspected that such an intervention could evoke maladaptive autonomic responses which are likely to be followed by an acute cardiac arrest.[40]

Moreover, among the medical literature covering the period between 1965 and 1970, there have been located two articles which have described a sudden death following the application of restraints during an episode of acute exhaustive mania.[41-42] In these two instances, the decedent had received thioridazine in order to control the marked hyperactivity which had been present prior to the time of death and, for this reason, the respective authors had inferred that the sudden deaths of their patients could be due to an alleged cardiotoxicity of the drug. However, the anecdotal data pertaining to both of these fatalities would seem to emphasize the importance of restraint stress as a risk factor in relation to the occurrence of the sudden deaths they had reported.

In one of these two publications,[41] the case history had indicated that the decedent was a "44-year-old man who was admitted to the hospital for the third time on September 25, 1963 for continued treatment of a schizophrenic reaction. Treatment with chlorpromazine was started on October 24, 1963 because of increasing agitation and other psychotic symtoms. On November 4, 1963, the initial dose of 400 mg daily was quickly increased to 1600 mg daily. On November 12, thioridazine hydrochloride in the amount of 400 mg was added to the treatment program. On November 16, the patient became so assaultive that he had to be forcibly restrained. The patient had to be held by three nursing assistants while cuff restraints were applied. As this was being done, he suddenly stopped struggling, respirations stopped, and he was observed to become cyanotic and pulseless. Efforts at resuscitation were fruitless. Postmortem examination could not ascertain the cause of death. Some apparently agonal pulmonary edema and passive visceral congestion were noted.

In the other publication,[42] the case history had indicated that the decedent was a "24-year-old white woman who was admitted to the hospital in July of 1965 because of increasingly bizarre behaviour during the previous two weeks. She was delusional, confused, agitated, and apparently hallucinating. Physical examination and initial laboratory studies were within normal limits. A diagnosis of acute schizophrenic reaction was made and the patient was begun on 400 mg of chorpromaizine per day; this was increased to 2400 mg per day over the next five days with some improvement in behavior. One week after admission she developed a generalized skin erruption and therefore on the 10th hospital day, chlorpromazine and trifluoperazine were discontinued and 2100 mg per day of thioridazine hydrochloride was substituted. On the evening of the 10th day, the patient became severely agitated and assaultive and was restrained. During restraint, she fell to the floor unconscious and appeared cyanotic. No heart beat could be found and she was given immediate closed chest massage with success. Prior to transfer to the medical service, she vomited but did not appear to aspirate. An electrocardiogram taken about 30 minutes after her collapse revealed nonspecific T-wave and S-T segment changes and ventricular tachycardia. Her laboratory findings were interpreted as normal. Despite all supportive measures to maintain blood pressure, she died 10 hours after her collapse without regaining consciousness. An autopsy performed seven hours after death, revealed severe rigor mortis and liver mortis. The lungs were congested and edematous and no evidence of aspiration could be found. The heart weighed 250 gm and was unremarkable. Microscopically, there was a mild, very early brochopneumonia; the liver and spleen contained fine granular yellow brown pigment which reacted positively to the Fontana stain for melanin. A sample of blood obtained at autopsy was found to contain 0.5 mg per 100 cc of phenothiazines. The cause of death was listed as possible toxic reaction to phenothiazines."

At this juncture, because of the concern that circulatory collapse and sudden death in hyperexicted psychiatric patients may be linked to prior administration of phenothiazines, it would be of interest to cite an experience described by Saunders,[45] especially since, in this instance, the circulatory collapse followed the application of restraints. The data included in the case history indicated that the patient was

> "a 25-year-old white male, a known chronic schizo-affective schizophrenic who was admitted to the hospital on September 13, 1962 and placed on locked ward because of his loud, demanding behavior and vulgar speech. He was placed on thioridazine 50 mg 3 times a day and was noted to be less hyperactive. Subjectively, the patient felt "more at ease" but his behavior remained abusive and he continued to overwhelm both patients and personnel alike. Subsequently, he entered a depressed phase manifested by insomnia, ideas of reference and withdrawl. Trifluoperazine 2 mg twice a day was substituted for his previous medication. After a 2-week trial on this regimen with the dose gradually increased to 10 mg twice a day, the patient remained quite with-

drawn and aloof. Imipramine 25 mg 4 times a day was substituted and because there was no improvement after 19 days of treatment with this drug, the imipramine was discontinued and tranylcypromine 10 mg 3 times a day was prescribed. Six days after therapy with tranylcypromine, the patient became hyperexcitable, restless; this hyperactivity terminated in his destruction of the ward television set by smashing it against the floor. Accordingly, he was placed in restraints and soon afterward he became progressively more drowsy and lethargic, developed an elevated temperature, showed excessive salivation and diaphoresis and lapsed into unconsciousness. An essentially unchanged clinical picture persisted for the ensuing 12 hours. Accordingly, he was treated with chlorpromazine 25 mg intramuscularly and with another 25 mg of chorpromazine 1 hour later. Afterward, he received 25 mg every 6 hours and during the next 6 hours his blood pressure and temperature returned to normal, the sensorium cleared and excess salivation disappeared. He remained aloof and withdrawn as was his previous behavior, but spontaneity and response to conversation improved steadily."

As yet, there are insufficient reliable data pertaining to the incidence of sudden deaths in hospitalized psychotics during an episode of "acute exhaustive mania." According to Peele and von Loetzen,[15] who surveyed the English, German, French, and Italian psychiatric literature which appeared between 1949 and 1955, as well as the English language medical literature during the period from 1955 to 1970, it was possible to locate only 94 reported cases of "lethal catatonia" during those time spans. However, they suspected that over that same period, there were many more "catatonic" fatalities than those they had been able to find. In this connection, they explained that "some could have been recognized as fatalities resulting from Bell's mania but for one reason or another, they were unreported in the medical literature; this circumstance not uncommonly occurred, at least so far as such deaths in many American psychiatric institutions were concerned."

Moreover, the validity of their view in this regard is supported by the nature of the material to be found in the publications of Moritz and Zamcheck[46] and of Madow and Stauffer,[43] respectively. Both articles were published in 1946 and it is noteworthy that neither referred to the patients as persons afflicted with either "Bell's Mania," "lethal catatonia," or "acute exhaustive psychosis."

Details regarding the illness of the eight cases reported by Moritz and Zamcheck[46] were not supplied but according to the brief amount of data provided by the authors, these eight young soldiers had died abruptly and unexpectedly after an acute episode of "psychic turmoil" of undesignated duration, even though, it had not been possible, from the postmortem examination, to establish the cause of death. By contrast, the article by Madow and

Stauffer[43] provided considerably more anamnestic data with respect to the ten psychotics whose sudden deaths were classified by them as fatalities resulting solely from "acute agitation." This group included four women and six men ranging in age from 25 to 60 years; the average age was 44 years. On admission to the hospital, the provisional diagnosis was either schizophrenia (five patients), agitated depression (three patients), reactive depression (one patient), or toxic psychosis (one patient). Moreover, two of these ten "agitated" patients died "very acutely" whereas in the remaining eight agitated cases, death occurred from 12 to 56 days following their admission to the hospital.

Of the two patients who died "acutely," one was "a 25-year-old negro man who became irrational at work, heard voices, and was very agitated and noisy. On admission to the hospital, he was restless, confused, and very difficult to control. Physical examination was essentially normal. A mild sedative was administered but the agitation continued and he died approximately 6 hours after admission. A postmortem examination by the coroner revealed no specific cause of death."

The other hospitalized psychotic who died "acutely" was a 49 year old white man who became agitated while at work. This excitement continued until he was hospitalized. On the ward he was extremely restless and irrational. Past history was noncontributory. Physical examination showed a temperature of 105° F., pulse 125, respiration 36. The leucocyte count was 28,000 with 81% neutrophils and 19% lymphocytes. The agitation and restlessness continued and the patient died two days after admission. A postmortem examination was done and all organs were found to be essentially normal, including the brain which showed only acute and chronic passive congestion." Typical of the 8 agitated patients who died after longer periods of hospitalization was a "27-year-old white man who had been acting strangely for two to three weeks prior to hospitalization. He had been going about the neighborhood ringing door bells and, in addition, had been unable to sleep and was continually masturbating. He was markedly hyperactive and agitated on admission. Physical examination was essentially normal. Temperature on admission was 99° F. but this fluctuated irregularly and became as high as 106° F. The pulse was 110 on admission and rose at times to 130. Respirations were 25 on admission and fluctuated and reached 45 per minute. The leucocytes numbered 14,900 with neutrophils 94% and lymphocytes 6%. The blood urea nitrogen level was 27 mg per 100 cc. The patient's course in the hospital was progressively downhill and he died on the 12th day following admission. Postmortem examination showed only chronic passive congestion including the brain."

In addition, based on a statistical analysis of reported sudden deaths in psychiatric patients, Peele and von Loetzen[15] suggested that it was a nominal substitution alone which could account for the paucity of reports between 1949 and 1955 concerning sudden deaths due to lethal catatonia. Moreover, this thesis seems to be supported by the already cited data in the article by Moritz and Zamcheck which was published in 1946[46] and in the report by Madow and Stauffer which also appeared in 1946.[43] However, there may be an additional explanation for the infrequency of reports concerning "catatonic" sudden deaths from 1955 until 1970: Since 1955, successful control of agitated behavior among nonalcoholic psychiatric patients has been achieved largely because of the widespread use of phenothiazines.

REFERENCES

1. White, P.D. and Boursy, A.V. *De Subitaneis Mortibus (On Sudden Deaths)* (translation) St. Johns University Press, New York. (1971).
2. Kuller, L. et al. An epidemiologic study of sudden and unexpected deaths in adults. *Medicine* 46:341 (1967).
3. Burch, G.E. and De Pasquale, M.P. Sudden expected natural deaths. *Am. J. Med. Sci.* 249:86 (1965).
4. Biorck, G. et al. Studies on myocardial infarction in Malmo, 1935 to 1954: Morbidity and mortality in a hospital material. *Acta Med. Scand.* 159:253 (1957).
5. Vedin, J.A. Sudden death: Identification of high risk groups. *Am. Heart J.* 86:124 (1973).
6. Vedin, J.A. et al. Mortality trends in Sweden 1951-1968 with special reference to cardiovascular causes of death. *Acta Med. Scand.* 515:76 (1971).
7. Spain, D.M. et al. Coronary atherosclerosis as a cause of unexpected and unexplained death: An autopsy study from 1949-1959. *JAMA* 174:384 (1960).
8. Adelson, L. Sudden death from coronary disease: The cardiac conundrum. *Postgrad. Med.* 30:139 (1961).
9. (Book) Goldstein, S. *Sudden Death and Coronary Heart Disease.* Futura Publishers, Mt. Kisco, New York (1974).
10. Gordon, T. and Kannel, W.B. Premature mortality from coronary heart disease. The Framingham Study. *J.A.M.A.* 215:1617 (1971).
11. Hussar, A.E. Leading causes of death in institutionalized chronic schizophrenic patients: A study of 1275 autopsied protocols. *J. Nerv. Ment. Dis.* 142:45 (1966).
12. Jetter, W.W. and White, P.D. Rupture of the heart in patients in mental institutions. *Ann. Int. Med.* 21:783 (1944).
13. Fulton, M. et al. Sudden death and myocardial infarction *Circulation* (Suppl. 4) 40:182 (1969).
14. Wikland, B. Medically unattended fatal cases of ischemic heart disease in a defined population. *Acta Med. Scand.* 524 (Suppl.) (1971).
15. Peele, R. and von Loetzen, I.S. Phenothiazine deaths: A critical review. *Am. J. Psychiatry* 130:306 (1973).

16. Malzberg, B. *Mortality Among Patients With Mental Disease*. New York State Hospitals Press, New York (1934).
17. Brill, H. and Patton, R.E. Clinical statistical analysis of population changes in New York State mental hospitals since introduction of psychotropic drugs. *Am. J. Psychiatry* 119:20 (1962).
18. Hussar, A.E. Effect of tranquilizers on medical morbidity and mortality in a mental hospital. *J.A.M.A.* 179:682 (1962).
19. Bell, L.V. On a form of disease resembling mania and fever. *Am. J. Insan.* 6:97 (1849).
20. Kraines, S.H. Bell's Mania (acute delirium). *Am. J. Psychiatry* 91:29 (1934).
21. Billig, O. and Freeman, W.T. Fatal catatonia. *Am. J. Psychiatry* 100:633 (1944).
22. Fisher, K.J. and Greiner, A. Acute lethal catatonia treated by hypothermia. *Can. M.A.J.* 82:630 (1960).
23. Adland, M.L. Review, case studies, therapy and interpretation of the acute exhaustive psychoses. *Psych. Quart.* 21:38 (1947).
24. Shulack, N.R. Sudden exhaustive death in excited patients. *Psych. Quart.* 18:3 (1944).
25. Ladame, C.H. Psychose aigue idiopathiqueou foudrayante. *Arch. Suisse Neur. Psychiat.* 5:3 (1919).
26. Scheidegger, W. Katatone Todesfalle in der Psychiatrischen Klinik von Zurich von 1900 bis 1928. *Zchcher. Neurol. U. Psychiat.* 120:587 (1929).
27. Davidson, G.M. Concerning the cause of death in certain psychoses. *Am. J. Psychiatry* 91:41 (1934).
28. Larson, C.P. Fatal cases of acute manic-depressive psychosis. *Am. J. Psychiatry* 95:971 (1939).
29. Malamud, N. and Boyd, D.A. Sudden "brain death" in schizophrenia with extensive lesions in the central cortex. *Arch. Neurol. Psychiatry* 41:352 (1939).
30. Raab, W. Sudden death of a young athlete. *Arch. Pathol. Lab. Med.* 36:388 (1943).
31. Rubin, R.T. and Mandell, A.J. Adrenal cortical activity in pathologic emotional states: A review. *Am. J. Psychiatry* 123:387 (1966).
32. Raab. W. Catecholamine induced myocardial hypoxia in the presence of impaired coronary dilatability independent of external cardiac work. *Am. J. Cardiol.* 9:455 (1962).
33. Raab, W. *Hormonal and Neurogenic Cardiovascular Disorders*. Williams and Wilkins, Baltimore (1953).
34. Wallace, A.G. et al. Electrophysiologic effects of adrenergic stimulation and blockade in awake animals. *Circ. Res.* 18:140 (1966).
35. Han, J. et al. Adrenergic effects on ventricular vulnerability *Circ. Res.* 14:516 (1964).
36. Selye, H. *Experimental Cardiovascular Disorders*. Springer-Verlag, New York (1970).
37. Richter, C. On the phenomenon of sudden death in animals and man. *Psychosom. Med.* 19:190 (1957).
38. Dimsdale, J.E. Emotional causes of sudden death. *Am. J. Psychiatry* 134:1361 (1977).
39. Wolf S. Sudden death and the oxygen conserving reflex. *Am. Heart J.* 71:840 (1966).
40. Wright, K.E. and Mc Intosh, H.D. Syncope: Review of pathophysiological mechanisms. *Progr. Cardiovasc. Dis.* 13:580 (1971).
41. Hollister, L.E. and Kosek, J.C. Sudden death during treatment with phenothiazine derivatives. *J.A.M.A.* 192:1035 (1965).
42. Leestma, J.E. and Koenig, K.L. Sudden death and phenothiazines: A current controversy. *Arch. Gen. Psych.* 18:137 (1968).
43. Madow, L. and Stauffer, J. Analysis of incidence and causes of death in an acute psychopathic hospital. *Am. J. Med. Sci.* 212:471 (1946).
44. Derby, I.M. Manic depressive "exhaustion" deaths. *Psychiat. Quart.* 7:436 (1933).

45. Saunders, J.C. Adverse drug reaction following treatment with monoamine oxidase inhibitors and imipramine and similar drugs: Report of 2 cases—one successfully treated with chlorpromazine. *J. Kansas Med. Soc.* p. 471 (1965).
46. Moritz, A.R. and Zamcheck, N. Sudden and unexpected deaths of young soldiers: Diseases responsible for sudden deaths during World War II. *Arch. Pathol. Lab. Med.* 42:459 (1946).
47. Harris, A.S. et al. The induction of arrhythmias by sympathetic activity before and after occlusion of a coronary artery in the canine heart. *J. Electrocardiol.* 4:34 (1971).

CHAPTER 11

The Wet Lung Syndrome In Narcotic Addicts

Since the end of World War II, physicians affiliated with the office of the Medical Examiner in New York City have collected considerable meaningful data pertaining to sudden deaths among narcotic addicts residing there and have provided incontestable proof that such fatalities in that area often were due to a drug-induced episode of acute pulmonary edema.[1-9] Moreover, they found that, almost always, such a drug-related pulmonary complication followed the self injection, intravenously, of ordinary "street heroin;"[1-2] rarely it was a sequel to the intranasal application of heroin.

Thus, inasmuch as intravenous injection of heroin is likely to increase in frequency as narcotic addicts seek to obtain optimal mood-altering effects from their "habit" it can be anticipated that, in the future, heroin related pulmonary edema will become an increasingly important public health problem throughout the world.

DEFINING "WET LUNG SYNDROME"

Up to the present time, this particular potentially lethal pulmonary syndrome associated with the use of an opiate derivative has been variously named. Thus, whereas Siegel et al[1] have labeled it "acute intravenous narcotism" others have termed it "acute narcotism,"[2] "acute fatal reaction,"[13] or "heroin intoxication".[10,11,14] However, inasmuch as none of these designations refers to the precise nature of the complications which are involved, it is evident that even collectively they are insufficiently descriptive. Accordingly, it would seem advantageous to consider sudden deaths in narcotic addicts which are due to acute pulmonary edema as fatalities ascribable to a "fatal wet lung syndrome in narcotic addicts." Correspondingly, since it is known also that death is not invariably a sequel to narcotic induced edema of the lungs,[10,12,13,117,19,20,22] the prefix "reversible" instead of "fatal" could be applied to those instances when the victims had recovered from such a life threatening incident. Moreover, simply by inserting the appropriate words, the same sort of terminology could be used to indicate when a sudden death had resulted from a similar complication in persons who had consumed large doses of propoxyphene[26-28(a)] or even customary as well as excessive amounts of methadone.[3,4,9,29-38]

DEMOGRAPHIC AND EPIDEMIOLOGIA DATA

In addition, the medical examiner's office in New York City has attempted to estimate the number of narcotic addicts who are likely to become afflicted with a wet lung syndrome in any calendar year as well as the proportion of those with such a pulmonary complication who can be expected to die suddenly because of it. However, even though New York City has maintained for many years a registry of narcotic addicts residing there, the other information required to fully achieve this goal has not yet become available. Nevertheless, a variety of demographic, clinical, and postmortem observations have been made which, together, have provided certain meaningful insights with respect to the dimensions of the problem of sudden death resulting from a wet lung syndrome in narcotic addicts.

Thus, on the basis of retrospective data, it was shown by Siegel et al in 1966[1] that, up to that time, 87% of a large sample of narcotic users who had died of an intercurrent illness causally related to their addiction, had succumbed because of a drug-induced wet lung syndrome. Also, in 1966, Helpern and Rho[2] demonstrated that over a 12-year span extending from 1950 and through 1961, there were, in New York City, 1586 deaths from narcotic induced acute pulmonary edema. But in that article, they had not referred to the frequency of such fatalities in relation to the total number of New York City residents who, over the same period of time, were regular users of "hard" drugs. However, subsequently in 1972, Helpern provided data of this sort; but it pertained solely to deaths which had occurred in 1970.[7]

Essentially, Helpern's observations had indicated that whereas during 1970 approximately 100,000 herion addicts were residing in the greater New York City area, the office of the medical examiner there had confirmed the occurrence in that same year of 1070 deaths ascribable to a drug-related pulmonary complication (an incidence of 1.07%). Moreover, when Helpern had compared the number of deaths for 1970 which were due to the wet lung syndrome in narcotic addicts with the number of similar fatalities during earlier years, it was evident that in 1970 there were virtually as many as had been reported for the entire period between 1950 to 1959 (1070 during 1970 vs. 1076 during 1950-1959). However, inasmuch as data were not available regarding the total number of addicts who were residing in New York City over that same 12-year interval (1950-1961) it clearly could not be established whether, on an annual basis, the prevalence of sudden death due to this narcotic-related pulmonary syndrome had differed or remained stationary over the intervening years from 1950 to 1970. On the other hand, Helpern's data unequivocally had shown that the frequency of fatal episodes of a narcotic-related wet lung syndrome had risen dramatically between 1950 and 1970 among addicts 15 to 35 years of age. In all likelihood the explanation for this development is the rapid growth in the number of juveniles who, after 1960, have become narcotic addicts, as well as the growing preference, over the same time span, for intravenous administration of "street" heroin in order to satisfy a craving for optimal narcotic effects.

Additional meaningful epidemiologic observations reguarding deaths due to the fatal wet lung syndrome in narcotic addicts have been summarized by Cherubin et al, whose paper also appeared in 1972.[5] However, unlike Siegel et al or Helpern and his associates, these investigators had analyzed a set of observations pertaining mainly to deaths among narcotic addicts during 1967 in New York City.

Thus, with such information as their data base, they showed that in a sample of 9066 New York City residents who, in 1967, were known to be addicted to opiate derivates, 463 had died because of a fatal wet lung syndrome. Correspondingly, then, they had indicated that in 1967, 5.1% of the addict population of New York City had died because of a drug induced pulmonary complication. Clearly, then, on the basis of current available information, it would seem proper to conclude that, nowadays, between 1% and 5% of any large group of narcotic addicts can be expected to die because of a drug-induced episode of acute pulmonary edema, especially so long as persons of this genre prefer to inject the narcotic into their veins.

However, it is important to recognize also that occasionally, a similar hazard can be created by the intranasal application of a heroin containing powder as well.[2] Thus, the sudden development of a wet lung syndrome in a young person without a cardiac impairment cannot be considered unrelated to heroin use even when healed needle puncture sites on the body cannot be discovered and careful inquiry has been unable to confirm a history of addiction to narcotic drugs.

Moreover, in order to prevent any possible misunderstandings, it should be explained that such mortality statistics pertain only to the "fatal" and not to the "reversible" variety of the wet lung syndrome in narcotic addicts. As Duberstein and Kauffman have demonstrated[10] the salvage ratio can be high provided those afflicted with this pulmonary complication are brought, soon after its onset, to a proper treatment facility where appropriate and aggressive therapy can be instituted promptly.

This perspective is also shared by Cherubin et al[5] who noted that although a large number of heroin addicts in New York City had died of "acute narcotism" between 1964 and 1968, a much larger number had lived despite the occurrence of such a pulmonary complication. Moreover, these authors had concluded that fatalities resulting from "acute narcotism" could not be attributed to a "pharmacologic overdose" of the drug responsible for the pulmonary edema.

THERAPEUTIC CHOICES

They also had observed that aside from the benefits derived from the prompt injection of nalorphine, the patient with a wet lung syndrome generally responds to the administration of oxygen and usually makes an uneventful recovery from such a drug-related complication.

However, it should be explained that their reported favorable experience with this form of therapy should not be interpreted to mean that oxygen administration in such a setting is not an unhazardous procedure. It generally is agreed that whenever the condition being treated is some type of "adult respiratory distress syndrome" overzealous and prolonged administration of concentrated oxygen mixtures can induce rapid and progressive disruptive changes in the alveolar structures and interstitial tissues of the lungs. Thus, it must be recognized that the injudicious use of oxygen actually may impede rather than enhance the prospects of recovery in addicts with a drug related wet lung syndrome.

Moreover in the report by Duberstein and Kauffman[10] which was based on the experiences of these authors at only a single New York City hospital between July 1968 and December 1970, the data indicated that, following an aggressive course of treatment of 149 acutely ill stuporous and hypoxemic addicts, appropriately monitored by means of arterial blood gas determinations, only 13 of this sample failed to recover.

ALCOHOL AS A RISK FACTOR

It is also noteworthy that even though most narcotic addicts are also chronic alcoholics, it had been established by Duberstein and Kauffman that only 31 of these 149 patients had consumed sizeable amounts of alcoholic beverages shortly before the first mainfestation of the wet lung syndrome had appeared. Supposedly, then, concurrent intake of alcohol could not be considered an important "risk factor" with respect to the development of a wet lung syndrome in this particular sample of narcotic addicts. Moreover so far as Duberstein and Kauffman had been able to determine from their study, the prior consumption of alcohol had not influenced, to any significant degree, the prospects for recovery from an episode of drug induced pulmonary edema.

On the other hand, in connection with their toxicologic investigations of addicts whose deaths were ascribable to an adverse reaction to heroin, Garriott and Sturner had detected, in the bodies of such victims, not only sizeable amounts of morphine but also large quantities of alcohol as well.[39] Cherubin et al[5] who conducted epidemiologic studies with respect to the incidence of fatal pulmonary complications in heroin addicts stated that "the high proportion of deaths which had detectable alcohol levels suggest that alcohol might also have a role in narcotism deaths."

PERSISTENT HYPOXEMIA AS A RISK FACTOR

Persistent hypoxemia, despite continuous oxygen administration, also seemed to increase the likelihood that addicts with a wet lung syndrome would not recover. Such a correlation apparently was established by the data provided by Duberstein and Kauffman.[10] Thus, of their patient sample, which comprised 149 narcotic addicts with "acute narcotism", all except 13 had recovered; significantly, when the laboratory values with respect to these 13 decedents were compared to the laboratory values pertaining to the 136 who had recovered, it was found that irreversible hypoxemia and hypercapnia characterized the laboratory profile of only the decedents.

PATHOLOGIC FEATURES OF ACUTE PULMONARY EDEMA

The characteristic morphologic changes in the lungs of narcotic addicts who have died as a result of acute pulmonary edema already have been well documented and clearly defined by the medical personnel affiliated with the office of the medical examiner in New York City;[7] similar findings have been described by pathologists in Dade County, Florida, as well.[40] Thus, "grossly, as a result of the edema and

> congestion, the lungs show marked swelling and firmness and remained stiff even after removal from the thoracic cavity. The lung parenchyma may pit on pressure. As a rule, the total weight of the two lungs averages 1500 to 2000 mg or more. If the decedent lived for only a few hours after the development of the pulmonary edema, frothy edema fluid may be oozed from the cut surfaces of the bronchi; frequently, the

trachea appears congested and is filled with foamy fluid which may be slightly blood tinged. The blood in the major pulmonary vessels is dark red and liquid. The pleural sufaces may be intensely hemorrhagic in places, and when the lungs are incised, the lobular pattern may appear exaggerated. Frequently, the exaggerated lobular pattern of the lung parenchyma corresponds to the lobular pattern visible on the pleural surfaces. At times, the lungs are uniformly dark red while the adjoined lobules may appear bluish red or pinkish grey.

"Tremendous pulmonary congestion and edema causing the anterior margins of the lungs to meet in the midline and completely overlap the pericardial sac was seen when addicts were found dead with the needle still in the vein. In these cases, all the lobes of the lungs were so enlarged and stiff that the excised lungs remained upright when the base of each was placed on the smooth surface. In such cases, the deeply congested, almost hemorrhagic, gross appearance of the lungs suggested a fulminating influenzal, hemorrhagic bronchopneumonia; the microscopic findings resembled an acute exudative reaction associated with a primary bronchopneumonia. However, actually, these findings are evidence of a chemotactic reaction induced by the intravenous injection of the narcotic.

"If the decedent remains alive for more than 24 hours after the onset of the attack of pulmonary edema, bilateral patches of the pulmonary consolidation may be present and a layer of fibrinous exudate may be seen on the pleural surface. This pneumonic process can be confirmed readily by microscopic examination of the consolidated zones. However, the pneumonia is not primary as in influenza; instead it is secondary to either the fulminating shock-like pulmonary recation, or to aspiration of regurgitated gastric contents. Additional microscopic findings may consist of scattered granulomatous lesions characterized by the giant cell reaction which ordinarily occurs from entrapment of foreign bodies, such as particles of talc or other filler materials ordinarily present in heroin tablets or capsules primarily intended for oral administration but which the addicts had adapted for intravenous use."

Clearly, these pathologic features have been described only in association with the fatal variety of wet lung syndrome and therefore it cannot be assumed necessarily that similar changes characterize the reversible type, as well. Presumably, then, one of the determinants with respect to recoverability in addicts with a heroin-induced wet lung syndrome could be the extent of intra-alveolar edema and exudative reaction which accompanies such a drug-induced pulmonary reaction. Therefore, it is equally conceivable that narcotic addicts who repeatedly resort to "main line shooting" of "street heroin" may even recover spontaneously from recurrent relatively mild episodes of such a drug related variety of acute pulmonary edema.

It is to be expected, however, that even in addicts in this category, especially since so many of them generally are heavy smokers as well[8,17] there also would be some residual impairment of lung function. Support for this view has been supplied by the investigations of Frand et al[17] who found a persistent decrease in pulmonary diffusing capacity in narcotic addicts who had survived following an episode of drug induced pulmonary edema.

METHADONE-INDUCED PULMONARY EDEMA

Another acute noncardiogenic variety of pulmonary edema which has been encountered in narcotic addicts is the sort which has occurred not because of heroin use but, instead, as a result of methadone. Thus, when its presence has been recognized, it has been observed generally in those addicts who were enrolled in a methadone treatment program. Moreover, in most instances, when methadone was the culprit, this particular pulmonary complication was seen either after a customary or excessive number of methadone tablets were swallowed[3,9,16,29-36] or, more rarely, after the intravenous injection of a commercially available solution of methadone or one prepared by the addicts from the tablets.[18,34,37]

In many respects, a methadone-induced wet lung syndrome resembles the type ascribable to heroin, including the prospect that it sometimes may be responsible for a sudden death.[9] However, unlike an uncomplicated episode of pulmonary edema after heroin administration, which generally clears within 24 to 36 hours, a methadone-induced and equally uncomplicated attack of pulmonary edema generally persists until two to four days after its onset.[33] Thus, if radiologic studies demonstrate a persistence of pulmonary densities beyond 4 days after the appearance of a wet lung syndrome due to methadone, it is likely that such densities signify a superimposed infective or aspiration pneumonia.[38] Such a circumstance, then, would represent an indication for the use of additional measures including appropriate antibiotic therapy and injections of titrated amounts of adrenal cortical steroids.

As yet, there are relatively little published data regarding the respective or total frequency, in known heroin addicts, of either a fatal or reversible wet lung syndrome due to methadone. Nevertheless, precisely because of the paucity of reports concerning methadone induced pulmonary edema, it would seem proper to conclude that there is, indeed, a low incidence of this type of drug related pullmonary complication, and, correspondingly, only few fatalities due to methadone. Moreover, such an interpretation would be in accord with the results of an actual survey reported by Dole et al[4] who found that between 1965 and 1971 in New York City, with its extensive roster of narcotic addicts enrolled in methadone treatment programs, there were a proportionally small number of methadone-induced episodes of acute pulmonary edema.

There are, in addition, isolated case reports pertaining to methadone-induced pulmonary edema. Thus, Frand et al[30] have reported their experience with two patients who had been treated successfully for a methadone-induced reversible wet lung syndrome and Master,[18] in a brief annotation, made reference to two cases of acute pulmonary edema, with recovery, which, in one instance, proved to be due to peroral consumption of a large quantity of methadone and, in the other instance, to an intravenous injection of this narcotic compound. Also, one year earlier, a similar case had been reported by Kjeldgaard et al.[34]

On the other hand, Roizin et al, in 1972[9] reported 12 deaths in narcotic addicts over an unstated period and, although no details were supplied with respect to these fatalities, it could be inferred from the limited information the authors had provided that they had considered these deaths to be linked to a methadone-induced variety of wet lung syndrome. Then, one year later, Lipski et al[42] briefly described a single sudden death in a 31-year-old former heroin addict in New York City who had been receiving a daily 100 mg dose of methadone perorally up to the time of death; also "subsequent toxicological reports at the time of death were negative except for the presence of methadone."

Thus, they concluded that the death was methadone-related but because "the postmortem examination by the medical examiner's office had revealed no gross abnormalities of the heart or lungs" they excluded a methadone-induced wet lung syndrome as its cause. Instead, inasmuch as "a routine electrocardiogram made several days before the time of death had revealed marked prolongation of the Q-T interval and conspicuous U waves of greater amplitude than the T-waves," they ascribed the sudden death to a sudden cardiac arrest and perceived a connection between the abnormalities in the premortem electrocardiogram and the stoppage of the heart.

In order to link this sudden death to the prior administration of methadone, they postulated that the electrocardiographic abnormalities in this single electrocardiogram were the result of prior consumption of conventional doses of this drug.

Significance of ECG Findings

Essentially, then, it was the belief of these observers that the electrocardiographic findings, in this instance, signified that methadone had altered ventricular repolarization in a way which would favor the occurrence of a cardiac arresting ventricular tachyarrhythmia. Thus, they had considered such an interpretation to be primarily the reason they had ascribed to the drug the sudden death of their patient. Undeniably, in view of all the findings they had reported, Lipski et al could not suggest that a methadone-induced wet lung syndrome was responsible for the fatality and so it is conceivable that the explanation they have advanced is the correct one.

Evidently, inasmuch as the nature of the changes in this decedent's electrocardiogram could be seen to be an illusory lengthening of the Q-T interval along with a fusion of an inconspicuous T-wave with a prominent juxtaposed U wave, the abnormalities in this electrocardiogram could be construed to be the hallmark of a predisposition to develop an arrhythmogenic cardiac arrest, but it still is uncertain that the electrocardiographic findings, in this instance, were ascribable exclusively to the methadone this former addict had consumed prior to the time of death. So far as is known, these particular electrocardiographic features are not a characteristic sequel to methadone administration and, hence, it would have been important for Lipski et al to exclude other possible causes before they concluded that such electrocardiographic anomalies were expressive merely of a "methadone effect."

Actually, as a result of numerous observations during the past two decades, this particular electrocardiographic pattern which has been labeled by some a Q-T interval syndrome but, more accurately, by others as a U wave entity (see Chapter 13), has become identified frequently with an inherited susceptibility to sudden death (see Chapter 14). Thus, it is difficult to understand precisely how Lipski et al had become convinced that the electrocardiographic syndrome they had described was not, indeed, identical with the sort likely to be associated with sudden death in persons who have never been in contact with any type of narcotic preparation.

For the most part, the few reports which, up to now, have described the diagnostic features of a methadone-induced type of wet lung syndrome[16,30] have confirmed that, in almost every respect, such a noncardiogenic pulmonary complication is a counterpart of the more familiar sort of acute pulmonary edema resulting from an intravenous injection of heroin.[8,12]

PATHOGENESIS

In general, it is agreed that the earliest hallmarks of a wet lung syndrome due either to heroin or methadone are torpor, depressed respirations, and hypoxemia as well as clinical and/or radiologic evidences of patches of pulmonary edema. Moreover, it now is recognized that a rapidly fatal outcome often can be averted when the addict with a wet lung syndrome due to methadone receives, promptly, the same treatment as that advocated for heroin induced pulmonary edema.

However, even though there is general agreement that such procedures are effective in removing the edema primarily because they abolish the hypoxemia, many competent observers have acknowledged that the pathogenesis of such durg-related wet lung syndromes still has not been completely clarified. Presumably, this realization stems from an awareness that often, following intravenous injection of the narcotic, the triad of intra-alveolar edema, depressed respirations, and torpor, better defined as hypersomnolence, appear to be rapid torpor, simultaneous developments.[2,7]

Nevertheless, many authors have advanced the thesis that because the intra-alveolar edema cannot be resorbed until normal oxygen tension in the arterial blood is re-established, a drug-induced hypoventilatory hypoxemia must be considered to be chiefly responsible for the pulmonary edema.[12,14,16]

Hypoxemia as Etiologic Factor

In order to emphasize the role of hypoxemia with respect to the etiology of this type of pulmonary edema, some observers have drawn an analogy between the wet lung syndrome following heroin use and the frequently fatal type of noncardiogenic pulmonary edema associated with climbs to high altitudes, described so well by Houston in 1960[47] and subsequently investigated more intensively by others.[48-51,56-57]

In this connection, it is noteworthy that Gopinathin et al had reported in 1970[52] that the rise in pulmonary arterial pressure during the acute phase of the wet lung syndrome in narcotic addicts was comparable to the elevated pulmonary arterial pressure which follows, ordinarily, the type of hypoxia observed during simulated or actual ascents to areas beyond 3000 meters above sea level.[58]

Aside from hypoxemia, the other meaningful findings during their studies were a normal pulmonary capillary pressure and an elevation of both the cardiac index and the stroke volume index, along with a doubled pulmonary capillary blood volume. Thus, the pulmonary edema in these instances was attributed by Gopinathin et al to precapillary pulmonary hypertension and altered capillary permeability resulting from hypoxic stress.

Increased Permeability of Pulmonary Capillaries

It also is conceivable that increased permeability of the pulmonary cap illaries, perhaps in conjunction with an impairment of removal of lung water by the pulmonary lymphatics,[58] may represent one of the important elements with respect to the pathogenesis of drug-induced pulmonary edema. However, such a view would not discount the primacy of hypoxemia with regard to the onset of the Wet Lung Syndrome in narcotic addicts.

Presumably, it was this point which Master[18] and Frand et al[17] had intended to make. Although these respective investigators had acknowledged that their findings indicated that a lower concentration of arterial oxygen was one of the conspicuous correlates of this particular pulmonary complication, they also had interpreted their data to mean that the hypoxemia could have been the predecessor of a vasculopathy which would favor the egress of fluid from the vascular compartment of the lung.

Essentially, the purpose of the study reported by Master[18] was to correlate the relative arterial concentrations of oxygen and carbon dioxide with the clinical features in two separate samples of drug "intoxicated" addicts, differentiated only on the basis of lung wetness. In 2, the "intoxicating" drug was methadone; in the remaining 29 it was heroin. Allegedly, all 31 subjects were equally hypersomnolent and equally hypoventilatory but one sample (Group A), comprising 23 adults, had developed "overt pulmonary edema" whereas the other sample (Group B) comprised 8 addicts without "overt pulmonary edema."

Later, when the findings were reviewed by Master, he noted that in the Group-A subjects, the average value for arterial oxygen tension was 41 mm of mercury (normal level is $\pm$ 80 mm of mercury), the arterial pH value was 7.22 and the average value with respect to carbon dioxide tension was 59 mm of mercury; by comparison, in the Group-B subjects, the average oxygen tension value was 62 mm of mercury, the average carbon dioxide tension value was 45 mm of mercury and the average pH value was 7.37. Nevertheless, Master had concluded that such data signified that "the pathogenesis of this type of pulmonary edema remains an interesting mystery." In addition, he stated that a humoral, immunologic, or direct toxic effect of heroin on the alveolar-capillary membrane added to the mechanical effects of hypoxemia and hypercapnia on the pulmonary vasculature is apparently responsible."

Presumably, then, Master had considered the alternative possibility that the striking lowering of the arterial oxygen tension levels and associated respiratory acidosis in the Group-A subjects could have been primarily due to impaired diffusion of respiratory gases resulting from the presence of the pulmonary edema, and not, conversely, that the hypoxemia was the underlying cause for the escape of fluid from the pulmonary vascular compartment into the interstitial tissue and adjacent alveoli in these particular patients. However, inasmuch as several studies in experimental animals and in man have confirmed that hypoxemia can provoke reflex intrapulmonary vascular adjustments which favor the extrusion of plasma into formerly ventilated areas of the lung[53-55,65-76,79-81,95] it is evident that it would be injudicious to derogate the importance of lowered oxygen tension in the pathogenesis of a drug induced type of pulmonary edema.

Clinical Case Studies

The report by Frand et al which appeared in 1972[17] referred to studies they had conducted in 16 heroin addicts with acute pulmonary edema confirmed by chest roentgenograms and in 9 without apparent pulmonary edema. As soon as these 25 patients arrived at the hospital, chest x-rays, electrocardiograms, and complete blood counts were obtained and arterial blood samples were drawn to measure pH, oxygen tension, and carbon dioxide tension. Moreover, as soon as the patient regained consciousness following administration of oxygen and the intravenous injection of nalorphine, a detailed history of drug use and a reconstruction of the sequence of events leading to admission to the hospital were obtained from the patient, his friends, and his family. The studies included sequential chest x-rays, electrocardiograms, arterial blood gas determinations, and pulmonary function tests.

Results

On the basis of such information Frand et al were able to show that the clinical correlates in the 9-patient sample (no pulmonary edema) included hypoventilation and hypersomnolence and that the functional defects were limited to moderately severe hypoxemia and a mild reduction of vital capacity. On the other hand, the 16-patient sample (pulmonary edema present) not only exhibited hypoventilation and hypersomnolence; their pulmonary function studies demonstrated profound hypoxemia, right to left physiologic shunt, metabolic and respiratory acidosis, decreased lung volumes, decreased compliance, unchanged expiratory flow rates, and a moderate decrease in diffusing capacity. Moreover, the clinical, radiologic, and arterial blood gases determinations of the 16 patients with heroin-induced pulmonary edema improved rapidly within a few days, while the vital capacity, dynamic compliance, and diffusing capacity remained unchanged for several weeks following recovery from the episode of pulmonary edema. Thus, Frand et al speculated that the wet lung syndrome in narcotic addicts was secondary to an increased capillary permeability apparently due to a vasotoxic property of the narcotic agent.

Discussion

To some extent, the view that increased capillary permeability represents an integral component of the wet lung syndrome due to heroin use also has been supported by observations recently reported by Katz et al.[59] Primarily, the purpose of these investigators was to determine whether the edema fluid in heroin addicts with such a pulmonary complication was comparable to the transudate usually associated with left ventricular failure or if its character would suggest that, at least in part, the shift of fluid from the pulmonary capillaries into the alveoli was favored by damage to the endothelium of these vessels.

Inasmuch as their findings indicated that the average protein concentration of the edema fluid was more than double that observed in patients whose lung congestion was due to acute left ventricular failure, they interpreted such data to indicate that, in addicts with a drug induced pulmonary edema, there is, indeed, a vasculopathy of some type within the smaller tributaries of the pulmonary arterial circulation. However, the results of their study could not demonstrate conclusively whether such endothelial damage was due to a toxic effect exerted by the opiate or its metabolites on these vessels or to a local vascular response to hypoxemia.

Role of Endothelial Damage of Pulmonary Capillaries

The role of endothelial damage of the pulmonary capillaries in relation to the occurrence of extensive pulmonary edema was confirmed also by Rittenhouse and Merendino[60] albeit their patients were not narcotic addicts. Their report pertained to middle-aged adults who had succumbed allegedly because of severe cerebral damage resulting from air embolism at the time of aortic valve replacement for post rheumatic aortic valvular disease.

These authors had considered it to be especially noteworthy that their patients had experienced "fulminant pulmonary edema in the absence of a significant elevation in left atrial pressure." Actually, "at autopsy the lungs were grossly edematous and on microscopical examination the alveoli were filled with proteinaceous material, fibrin and red blood cells." Apparently arterial gas determinations were not obtained either during the pre-edematous phase of the terminal illness or while these decedents were treated for the complicating pulmonary edema. Thus, the findings were interpreted by these authors to indicate that the pulmonary edema was not due to left ventricular failure but, instead, was ascribable primarily to increased pulmonary capillary porosity resulting from the acute cerebral insult during the surgical procedure.

Immunologic Abnormalities

An attractive hypothesis with respect to the pathogenesis of the wet lung syndrome in narcotic addicts is the one based on the results of investigations pertaining to immunologic abnormalities in the sera of known heroin addicts. These studies were conducted by Smith et al[61] and the measurements were confined to the levels of the five classes of immunoglobins and two types of serum complement. An impressive finding in connection with their study was the significant reduction in the level of IgM in 22 heroin addicts with pulmonary edema whereas no such immunologic abnormality was detected in 42 addicts without this type of pulmonary complication, Thus, they advanced the view that there may be a possible immunologic basis for "heroin lung" and suggested that an induced abnormality of IgM and complement may be at least in part responsible for heroin induced pulmonary edema.

Neurohumoral Influences

Still to be clarified with respect to the pathogenesis of the hemodynamic and other features of the wet lung syndrome in narcotic addicts is the position which should be assigned to neurohumoral influences or vasoactive amines. Clearly, experiments like those performed by Aviado et al in canines[53] have demonstrated that, regularly, the pre-eminent hemodynamic effects in animals made anoxic by ventilating them with a gas mixture containing 5% to 10% of oxygen, were an increase in pulmonary artery pressure and an increase in pulmonary blood flow, the latter being a response to increased cardiac output; in this setting, the factor responsible for the inotropic effect on the heart was considered to be the reflex outpouring of medullary hormones from the adrenal gland in response to anoxia. The extent of pulmonary vasoconstriction was variable but pulmonary hypertension was not observed in anoxic animals unless the sympathetic nerve fibers surrounding the pulmonary artery remained intact. Also, it is noteworthy that pulmonary edema was not associated with the rise in pulmonary arterial pressure in these animals but this circumstance might be ascribed to the brevity of the anoxia during these experiments.

Role of Catecholamine Activity

The role of catecholamine activity in relation to pulmonary hypertension or pulmonary edema has been demonstrated in two other types of experiments. Thus, in the investigations conducted by J.L. Berk et al,[62] isoproterenol was infused intravenously in canines who were not hypoxic and, by means of cardiac catheterization studies, it was demonstrated that such a procedure was followed by pulmonary hypertension without any increase in the pulmonary vascular resistance; actually, their findings indicated a significant decrease in the pulmonary vascular resistance, and, hence, no significant change in the wedge pressure. As in Aviado's experiments,[53] the rise in pulmonary artery pressure following the infusion of isoproterenol was not accompanied by any pulmonary edema.

Conceivably, in these instances, the rise in pulmonary artery pressure was due to increased blood flow secondary to the inotropic action of the catecholamine on the heart. On the other hand, it has been observed by Stone and Loew,[63] that, shortly after the administration of epinephrine to rabbits, these animals died suddenly because of the development of pulmonary edema.

However, these investigators noted also that if the rabbits received a prior "protective" dose of an adrenergic blocking drug, similar doses of epinephrine did not produce pulmonary edema and did not cause the animals to die.

In this connection, it also is noteworthy that instances of pulmonary edema in man, following injections of epinephrine, also have been reported.[64] However, the data pertaining to these cases have not included measurements of the pulmonary artery pressure.

Hypoxia and Pulmonary Vessel Contractility

A determination of the influence of hypoxia directly on the contractility of excised pulmonary vessels and on the electrophysiologic accompaniments of this contractility was the major purpose of the experiments conducted by Bergofsky and Holtzman.[55] With the use of this type of experimental model, which excluded any possible effects produced by pulmonary blood flow, cardiac contractility, and the autonomic nervous system, these investigators were able to show that hypoxia affects the membrane potentials of the muscle layer in the pulmonary artery in a direction which would cause a reduction in its caliber but they did not indicate that the hypoxia concurrently produced any sort of endothelial damage.

Actions of Vasoactive Amines

Heuristic in nature are certain observations which pertain to the actions of vasoactive amines such as serotonin or histamine as well as the catecholamines, in relation to the development of pulmonary edema. Wilson, in his chapter on "Pulmonary Disease and the Microcirculation"[65] indicated that serotonin, histamine, prostaglandins, and other vasoactive agents might be implicated in states which produce damage to the pulmonary capillary network and increases in pulmonary vascular resistance. Moreover, serotonin has been found to possess other interesting properties as well. Thus, in addition to its various actions on the pulmonary circulation[71] which could favor the development of pulmonary edema, it is now known to be a substance which, through its competition with norepinephrine in the central nervous system, can influence the stages of sleep.[66] Thus, it is conceivable that a common denominator for the hypersomnolence and the pulmonary edema which characterize the Wet Lung Syndrome in narcotic addicts may prove to be biologic changes initiated by a sudden redistribution, quantitatively, of serotonin, or other vasoactive amines following a "loading" dose of heroin.

Also, highly provocative, have been the studies which have suggested a similarity of action of catecholamines and histamine in the lung/during hypoxia. Equally meaningful, in this connection, are the experimental findings which imply that heroin might augment rapidly the natural stores of histamine in that organ[77,78] and thereby alter pulmonary vascular permeability and facilitate the occurrence of pulmonary edema.

In addition, in view of the demonstration by Richardson et al[81] that beta-adrenergic blockade can modify, substantially, the circulatory response to hypoxia in man, it would seem improper to disregard the possible importance of excessive catecholamine activity as a contributory "risk factor" with respect to the production of the Wet Lung Syndrome in narcotic addicts. The concept of a connection between catecholamine activity and the occurrence of pulmonary edema in narcotic addicts seems to be strengthened also by the implications inherent in the observations among living narcotic addicts which were reported in 1941 by Himmelspach[82] and in 1968 by Sloan and Eisenman.[83]

Moreover, there are certain other available data to suggest that catecholamine-like substances abound in the bodies of addicts, whose deaths can be ascribed to acute pulmonary edema secondary to hypoventilatory hypoxia. In this connection, there are two elements to be considered. The first element is related to the autopsy findings reported by Cherubin[46] who noted that during 381 postmortem examinations of addicts with pulmonary edema and whose deaths were sudden, sizeable amounts of alcohol were detected in the tissues of one half of this number; he found also that in 24% of them there was a fatty liver of the sort usually associated with chronic alcoholism. The other element is a simultaneous accumulation in the body not only of aldehydes but also of serotonin during the metabolism of alcohol in the presence of faulty liver function.[100] This consideration is based on data which indicate that acetaldehydes, like catecholamines, possess sympatheticomimetic properties (see

Chapter 4), and on the demonstration that serotonin can augment the histamine content in the lungs.[100]

Effects of Nicotine

In the narcotic addict, the smoking habit is another external source of catecholamine-like substances likely to affect catecholamine-sensitive sites within the body. Generally, it is acknowledged that a major action of nicotine is sympathomimetic in nature[84,101] and, thus, it can be expected that the narcotic addict is exposed to adrenergic stimulation much of the time. Actually in persons of this genre, there may be observed a distinctive cigarette-related dermatologic lesion because of the development of hypersomnolence, possibly alcohol-induced, while injecting the heroin intravenously. This particular skin lesion has been described by Sapira[41] as a series of burn scars across the chest, resulting from the inadvertent release of an ignited cigarette from the mouth of the addict when, along with the sudden hypersomnolence produced by the drug, the pain from such an incident is blunted; thus, the incident is disregarded and the addict makes no attempt to brush away the ignited object. Conceivably, then, in instances when the hypersomnolence is sufficiently pronounced to lead to a hypoventilatory hypoxemia and its companionate pulmonary edema, the intake of sizeable amounts of tobacco smoke shortly before the injection of the drug can constitute an additional "risk factor" with respect to the occurrence of this alarming pulmonary complication.

Concurrent Liver Disease

Concurrent alcoholic liver disease, through its secondary effects on protein levels of the blood, could be another "risk factor" with respect to the Wet Lung Syndrome in certain narcotic addicts. So far as is known, measurements of the serum albumin levels in meaningful numbers of heroin users have not yet been reported; nevertheless, especially since many addicts tend to suffer also from malnutrition as well as from chronic alcoholism,[8] it would seem necessary to consider the possibility that a reduced oncotic pressure in the serum could be responsible, at least in part, for this particular pulmonary complication. Further support for such a view has been provided by the observations of Stein et al[85] who found that, frequently, hypoalbuminemia was an important factor in connection with the development of noncardiogenic pulmonary edema in critically ill patients suffering from a variety of debilitating diseases.

Another element, with respect to the pathogenesis of the wet lung syndrome in narcotic addicts, which should not be disregarded is the presence of liver pathology resulting from antecedent serum or viral hepatitis. In this connection, it is noteworthy that the original description by Siegel et al in 1966[1] of the postmortem findings in addicts whose sudden deaths were ascribable to this pulmonary complication, emphasized the frequency not only of pulmonary changes but also of a "cellular infiltrate in the portal areas of the liver."

Moreover, in an article which appeared one year earlier, Norris and Potter[86] had made similar observations. These investigators examined tissue specimens obtained from the livers of 36 adult narcotic addicts who had died suddenly because of a wet lung syndrome, sometime between 1957 and 1961. Police records had confirmed that all were known to be addicted to narcotics and in 31 of the 32 bodies in which the tests were made, an opiate was found; also, in 21 of the bodies measurable amounts of alcohol were present.

The liver tissue specimens examined by Norris and Potter were stained with hematoxylin and eosin and particular attention was paid to the architecture of the liver lobules, the extent of fibrous tissue, the distribution of various cellular infiltrates, the presence of fatty change, and the condition of the biliary canaliculi. Similar observations were made of liver tissue obtained from a control group of 50 adults whose deaths were sudden but unrelated to narcotic use. Furthermore, the majority of these "controls" were not known to be narcotic addicts and, in the majority, trauma was listed as the cause of death. This circumstance probably accounted for the presence of alcohol in the body fluids of 22 of these "controls."

The meaningful changes in the livers of the addict group consisted of increased cellular infiltrations in the periportal areas, lobular distortion, and scarring; moreover, in terms of incidence, these findings were present three times more frequently than in the "controls." These investigators were uncertain with respect to the cause of the inflammatory lesions they had observed but they suspected, despite the views reported earlier by Kaplan[87] that the changes were due to a preceding episode of viral hepatitis transmitted to the victim through the communal use of contaminated needles.

The investigation reported by Kaplan[87] was conducted at the United States Public Health Service Hospital attached to the United States Penitentiary located at Leavenworth, Kansas, and the subjects were 69 known heroin addicts who had been incarcerated there for a variety of offenses. All were studied to determine the frequency of abnormal liver function tests and, in 13, these findings were correlated with the results of a liver biopsy. Although narcotics were not accessible to these former addicts during their incarceration, the data reported by Kaplan showed that 7 of the 13 liver biopsies confirmed the presence of cellular periportal infiltrates. Nevertheless, Kaplan was reluctant, at that time, to conclude that such abnormal findings were the histologic remnants of a previous episode of viral hepatitis.

On the other hand, subsequent articles which have discussed medical complications in narcotic addicts have emphasized the prevalence of hepatitis in this sample of the population.[89-94] Moreover, it has been reported by Holmes et al[88] that liver biopsy studies in narcotic addicts have demonstrated the sort of hypertrophy of the smooth endoplasmic reticulum in the hepatocytes one might expect to find when drugs are being metabolized by hepatic microsomes. Thus, it is likely that, in some complex manner, as yet incompletely understood, the presence of post inflammatory or other changes in the liver, either alone or in conjunction with elevated levels of alcohol, may contribute to a heroin or methadone-induced maladaptive biochemical or metabolic response within the central nervous system and within the receptors and endothelial cells of the pulmonary circulation. Such a hypothesis, which remains to be tested, could explain the development of pulmonary edema which, conceivably, because of a concurrent impairment of the lymphatic tributaries located within the interstitial tissues of the lung parenchyma,[98] could not be removed effectively.

IMPERFECT CORRELATION BETWEEN TOXICOLOGIC AND POSTMORTEM FINDINGS

A puzzling feature with regard to the fatal variety of the wet lung syndrome in narcotic addicts is the occasional imperfect correlation between the toxicologic and postmortem findings.[8] Moreover, because of such a discrepancy a narcoticogenic sudden death at times may remain unrecognized as such merely because (a) the postmortem examination had not confirmed the presence of healed needle puncture sites on the body surface of the decedent; (b) the previous habits of the decedent with regard to drug abuse were unknown; (c) the toxicologic studies of the body fluids had not demonstrated sizeable amounts of morphine (the most important metabolite of heroin) in the nose, liver, or body fluids.

The most reasonable explanation for such a seemingly anomalous situation is the one which has been suggested by Garriott and Sturner.[39] These investigators measured the blood levels of morphine in 22 authenticated heroin-related fatalities and then correlated the respective concentrations of this opium alkaloid in the blood with the interval between the time the drug was injected and the time of death. In this way, it was established by them that survival time was an important factor in determining whether toxicologic investigation could help to confirm or exclude a narcoticogenic death. Thus, it must be explained, on the basis of such studies, that even when a decedent was the victim of a lethal dose of heroin, toxicological investigations may not be able to confirm the cause of death if the interval between the injection or intranasal application of the drug and the time of death had been unduly prolonged.

By contrast, an aspect of the wet lung syndrome in narcotic addicts which has not yet been clarified is the temporal relationship between the onset of the hypersomnolence and the occurrence of the pulmonary edema. Thus, Helpern and Rho, in connection with their description of "deaths from narcotism"[2] mentioned that "in many cases death or loss of consciousness has occurred so rapidly that when the body was discovered, the tourniquet was still in place on the arm and the needle of the syringe was stuck in the skin with the syringe partly filled with blood mixed with residual heroin solution" but at the same time, they added that "when death occurred in the location where the body was found it was not uncommon to discover an abundance of partly dried frothy white edema fluid oozing from the nostrils or mouth as a result of the presence of severe pulmonary edema." Clearly, then, the data provided by these investigators would indicate that there is a strong likelihood that, in terms of their respective onsets, the exudative reaction in the lungs and the hypersomnolence were simultaneously occurring phenomena.

ADDITIONAL CONSIDERATIONS

Hypersomnolence

Other observers who were concerned chiefly with the clinical aspects of the reversible type of wet lung syndrome in narcotic addicts similarly have been unable to decide whether, in their patients afflicted with this complication, hypersomnolence preceded or coincided with the onset of the pulmonary edema. Thus, according to Silber and Clerkin, whose paper appeared in 1959[14] the history with regard to four addicts with a wet lung syndrome had indicated that although "stupor" or "unconsciousness" had been the initial symptom, evidences of pulmonary edema already were discernable when these patients had been brought to the emergency room of the hospital. Therefore, it was suspected by these authors that, with respect to these four addicts, the edematous reaction had coincided with the onset of the hypersomnolence which followed the intravenous injection of the narcotic.

Hypoxemia and Respiratory Acidosis

In 1968, Steinberg and Karliner[12] reported an experience in New York

City with 16 patients who had developed an attack of pulmonary edema considered to be a complication of "heroin overdose"; of these, 14 recovered and 2 died. This publication was noteworthy because it was the first to describe laboratory evidence of hypoxemia and respiratory acidosis in a sizeable number of addicts with even a reversible wet lung syndrome. Accordingly, the presence of clinically recognizable pulmonary edema was a constant finding. However, in 14 of these 16 patients, pulmonary rales already were audible when they were seen in the emergency room where they were brought soon after they had developed their hypersomnolence, whereas in the remaining 2 patients, the diagnosis of pulmonary edema was established on the basis of radiographic findings; however, in these 2 instances, rales were found to be present on the following day.

Anoxic Brain Damage and Severe Pneumonia

The data provided by Steinberg and Karliner also indicated that of the two who died, one had several cardiac arrests, anoxic brain damage and severe pneumonia; the other decedent was found dead in bed 16 hours after admission following an initial period of clinical improvement. It also is noteworthy that only one of the 16 patients developed the Wet Lung Syndrome following the intranasal inhalation of the narcotic; the remaining 15 patients developed this pulmonary complication following intravenous injection of heroin. However, despite the completeness of the data presented by Steinberg and Karliner, their findings did not demonstrate, with any degree of certainty, whether the hypersomnolence preceded or coincided with the occurrence of the pulmonary edema in their patients.

Discussion

The paper by Duberstein and Kauffman, published in 1971[10] similarly did not provide the answer to this question. Of the 149 narcotic addicts with "heroin intoxication," whom they had studied, all, at the time of admission to the hospital, allegedly were stuporous but, inasmuch as a routine chest x-ray had not been obtained at the same time, it can be assumed on the basis of reported experiences by others[12] that Duberstein and Kauffman had underestimated the prevalence of pulmonary edema in their patient sample. Nevertheless, it was observed by these investigators that a high degree of correlation existed between laboratory evidences of hypoxia and acidosis and their own confirmation of the presence of pulmonary edema. Moreover, they did not attempt to determine whether the degree of hypersomnolence in their patients could be correlated with the level of hypoxia and acidosis or with the extent of pulmonary edema detected by clinical examination alone.

Nevertheless, on the basis of the data reviewed so far, it would seem reasonable to suppose that although the hypoxemia, which appears to be a fundamental feature of the wet lung syndrome in narcotic addicts, is, primarily, the cause of the pulmonary edema, other factors also could contribute to its occurrence. In this connection, it cannot be disregarded that the movement of fluid from the vascular compartment of the lungs into the alveoli might be facilitated, in part, by the accumulation in the lungs of vasoactive substances such as histamine and serotonin, both known to increase the permeability of the pulmonary capillary network and to alter the dynamics of the pulmonary circulation. Moreover, such a construction, as has been implied already, would be based on the following considerations: (a) the prospect of an over accumulation of serotonin in the lung structures secondary to an inefficient oxidation of an overabundance of alcohol in the tissues; (b) the presence of a coexisting liver abnormality; (c) the effects of opioids on histamine storage sites.

As yet, further details regarding the pathogenesis of the wet lung syndrome in narcotic addicts cannot be provided but it can be expected that in the years ahead, such information will become available as knowledge concerning the pathophysiology of pulmonary edema continues to advance. Nevertheless, even without this additional data, much progress has been made already toward the development of a rational treatment program in addicts afflicted with this sort of life threatening complication. Thus, there is now a substantial body of experiential evidence to show that the lives of many such patients have been saved merely by the prompt and judicious administration of narcotic antagonists such as nalorphine or naloxone coordinated with the institution, without delay, of those measures which customarily are employed for the treatment of any "adult respiratory distress syndrome,"[96,97] Therefore, a basic requirement must be the maintenance, by whatever suitable means seems to be indicated, of an adequate airway and the administration of oxygen in a manner which will avoid the hazards of oxygen toxicity.[99]

REFERENCES

1. Siegel, H. et al. The diagnosis of death from intravenous narcotism with emphasis on the pathologic aspects. *J. Forensic Sci.* 11:1 (1966).
2. Helpern, M. and Rho, Y.M. Deaths from narcotism in New York City. *N.Y. State J. Med.* 66:2391 (1966).
3. Baden, M.M. Methadone-related deaths in New York City *Int. J. Addict.* 5:489 (1970).
4. Dole, V.P. et al. Methadone poisoning. *N.Y. State J. Med.* 71:541 (1971).
5. Cherubin, C. et al. The epidemiology of death in narcotic addicts. *Am. J. Epidemiology* 96:11 (1972).
6. Siegel, H. Human pulmonary pathology associated with narcotic and other addictive drugs. *Hum. Pathol.* 3:55 (1972).

7. Helpern, M. Fatalities from narcotic addiction in New York City: Incidence, circumstances, and pathologic findings. *Hum. Pathol.* 3:13 (1972).
8. Baden, M.M. Narcotic abuse: A medical examiner's view. *N.Y. State J. Med.* 72:834 (1972).
9. Roizin, L. et al. Methadone fatalities in heroin addicts. *Psychiatr. Q.* 46:393 (1972).
10. Duberstein, J.L. and Kaufman, D.M. A clinical study of an epidemic of heroin intoxication and heroin induced pulmonary edema. *Am. J. Med.* 51:704 (1971).
11. Selzman, H.M. et al. Pulmonary edema accompanying heroin intoxication. *Cardiovasc. Res. Cent. Bull.* 6:77 (1967).
12. Steinberg, A.D. and Karliner, J.S. The clinical spectrum of heroin pulmonary edema. *Arch. Int. Med.* 122:122 (1968).
13. Stimmel, B. *Heroin Dependency: Medical, Economic, and Social Aspects.* Stratton International, New York (1975).
14. Silber, R, and Clerkin, E.P. Pulmonary edema in acute heroin poisoning: Report of 4 cases. *Am. J. Med.* 27:187 (1959).
15. Phillips, J.F. et al. Non-cardiac causes of pulmonary edema. *J.A.M.A.* 234:531 (1975).
16. Jaffe, R.B. and Koshmann, E.B. Intravenous drug abuse: Pulmonary, cardiac, and vascular complications. *Am. J. Roentgenol.* 109:107 (1970).
17. Frand, U.I. et al. Heroin-induced pulmonary edema: Sequential studies of pulmonary function. *Ann. Int. Med.* 77:29 (1972).
18. Master, K. Narcotics and pulmonary edema. *Ann. Int. Med.* 77:817 (1972).
19. Werner, A. Near fatal hyperacute reaction to intravenously administered heroin. *J.A.M.A.* 207:2277 (1969).
20. Morrison, W.J. et al. The acute pulmonary edema of heroin intoxication. *Radiology* 97:397 (1970).
21. Lynch, K. et al. Pulmonary edema in heroin overdosage. *Radiology* 94:377 (1970).
22. Karliner, J.S. et al. Lung function after pulmonary edema associated with heroin overdose. *Arch. Int. Med.* 124:350 (1969).
23. Harle, T.S. et al. Pulmonary edema without cardiomegaly. *Am. J. Roentgenol.* 103:555 (1968).
24. Saba, G.P. et al. Pulmonary complications of narcotic abuse. *Am. J. Roentgentol.* 122:733 (1974).
25. Addington, W.W. The pulmonary edema of heroin toxicity: An example of the stiff lung syndrome. *Chest* 62:199 (1972).
26. Qureshi, E.H. Propoxyphene hydrochloride poisoning. *J.A.M.A.* 188:470 (1964).
27. Karliner, J.S. Propoxyphene hydrochloride poisoning. *J.AM.A.* 199:1006 (1967).
28. Bogartz, L.J. and Miller, W.C. Pulmonary edema associated with propxyphene intoxication. *J.A.M.A.* 215:259 (1971).
28.(a) Sturner, W.Q., and Garriott, J.C. Deaths involving propoxyphene: A study of 41 cases over a 2-year period. *J.A.M.A.* 223:1125 (1973).
29. Gardener, R. Methadone misuse and deaths by overdosage. *Brit. J. Addict.* 65:113 (1970).
30. Frand, U.I. et al. Methadone-induced pulmonary edema. *Ann. Int. Med.* 76:975 (1972).
31. Presant, S. et al. Methadone-induced pulmonary edema, *Can. M.A.J.* 113:966 (1975).
32. Goldman, A.L. and Enquist, R.W. Methadone pulmonary edema. *Chest* 63:275 (1973).
33. Zyroff, J. et al. Pulmonary edema induced by oral methadone. *Radiology* 112:567 (1974).
34. Kjelgaard, J.M. et al. Methadone-induced pulmonary edema. *J.A.M.A.* 218:882 (1971).
35. Malik, S.K. et al. Pulmonary edema and oral ingestion of methadone. *J.A.M.A.* 221:915 (1972).
36. Schaaf, J.T. et al. Pulmonary edema and adult respiratory distress syndrome following methadone abuse. *Am. Rev. Respir. Dis.* 107:1047 (1973).
37. Fraser, D.W. Methadone overdose: Illicit use of pharmaceutically prepared parenteral narcotics. *J.A.M.A.* 217:1387 (1971).

38. Wilen, S.B. et al. Roentgenographic manifestations of methadone-induced pulmonary edema. *Radiology* 114:51 (1975).
39. Garriott, J.C. and Sturner, W.Q. Morphine concentrations and survival periods in acute heroin fatalities. *New Eng. J. Med.* 289:1276 (1973).
40. Wetli, C.V. et al. Narcotic addiction in Dade County, Florida: An analysis of 100 consecutive autopsies. *Arch. Pathol. Lab. Med.* 93:330 (1972).
41. Sapira, J.D. The narcotic addict as a medical patient. *Am. J. Med.* 45:554 (1968).
42. Lipski, J. et al. The effect of heroin and multiple drug abuse on the electrocardiogram. *Am. Heart J.* 86:663 (1973).
43. Smith, L.H. Medical complications of heroin addiction. *Calif. Med.* 115:42 (1971).
44. Louria, D.B. et al. The major medical complications of heroin addiction. *Ann. Int. Med.* 57:1 (1967).
45. Nelson, A.S. Medical problems associated with addiction to opioid drugs. *Int. J. Addict.* 1:50 (1966).
46. Cherubin, C.E. The medical sequelae of narcotic addiction. *Ann. Int. Med.* 67:23 (1967).
47. Houston, C.S. Acute pulmonary edema of high altitude. *New Eng. J. Med.* 263:478 (1960).
48. Hultgren, H.N. et al. Physiologic studies of pulmonary edema at high altitudes. *Circulation* 29:393 (1964).
49. Fred, H.L. et al. Acute pulmonary edema of altitude: Clinical and physiological observations. *Circulation* 25:929 (1969).
50. Penaloza, D. and Syme, F. Circulatory dynamics during high altitude pulmonary edema. *Am. J. Cardiol.* 23:369 (1969).
51. Arias-Stella, J. and Kruger, H. Pathology of high altitude pulmonary edema. *Arch. Pathol. Lab. Med.* 76:147 (1963).
52. Gopinathin, K. et al. Hemodynamic studies in heroin induced acute pulmonary edema. *Circulation* 42 (Supplement III):44 (1970).
53. Aviado, D.M. et al. Effects of anoxia on pulmonary circulation: Reflex pulmonary vasoconstriction. *Am. J. Physiol.* 189:253 (1957).
54. Whayne, T.F. and Severinghaus J.W. Experimental hypoxic pulmonary edema in the rat. *J. App. Physiol.* 25:729 (1968).
55. Bergofsky, E.H. and Holtzman, S. A study of the mechanisms involved in the pulmonary arterial pressor response to hypoxia. *Circ. Res.* 20:506 (1967).
56. Viswanathan, R. et al. Pulmonary edema of high altitude III. Pathogenesis. *Am. Rev. Respir. Dis.* 100:342 (1969).
57. Kleiner, J.P. and Nelson. W.P. High altitude pulmonary edema: A rare disease? *J.A.M.A.* 234:491 (1975).
58. Fishman, A.P. Pulmonary edema: The water-exchanging function of the lung. *Circulation* 46:390 (1972).
59. Katz, S. et al. Heroin pulmonary edema: Evidence for increased pulmonary capillary permeability. *Am. Rev. Respir. Dis.* 106:472 (1972).
60. Rittenhouse, E.A. and Merendino, K.A. Acute pulmonary edema in the absence of left ventricular failure. *Circulation* 40:823 (1969).
61. Smith, W.R. et al. High incidence of precipitins in sera of heroin addicts. *Chest* 68:651 (1975).
62. Berk, J.L. et al. Pulmonary insufficiency produced by isoproterenol. *Surg. Gynecol. Obstet.* 142:725 (1976).
63. Stone, C.A. and Loew, E.R. Effect of various drugs on epinephrine-induced pulmonary edema in rabbits. *Proc. Soc. Exper. Biol. Med.* 71:122 (1949).
64. Ersoz, N. et al. Adrenalin-induced pulmonary edema. Report of two cases. *Brit. J. Anesth.* 43:709 (1971).

65. Wilson, J.W. Pulmonary disease and the microcirculation. In: *The Microcirculation in Clinical Medicine*, R. Wells, ed. Academic Press (1973).
66. Grollman, A. and Grollman, E. *Pharmacology and Therapeutic; A Text Book for Students and Practitioners of Medicine and its Allied Professions.* 7th Ed. Lea and Febiger, Philadelphia, 1970
67. Comroe, J.H. et al. Reflex and direct cardiopulmonary effects of serotonin. *Am. J. Physiol.* 173:379 (1953).
68. Parker, B.M. et al. Serotonin-Induced pulmonary venous spasm demonstrated by selective pulmonary phlebography. *Am. Heart J.* 69:521 (1965).
69. Yoshitake, K. Pathophysiologic significances of serotonin in pulmonary circulation. *Jap. Circ. J.* 31:853 (1967).
70. Swenson, E.W. et al. Hypoxemia and edema of the lungs. In: *Experimental Pulmonary Embolism in Pulmonary Embolic Disease*, A.A. Sasahara and M. Stein, eds. Grune and Stratton, New York, 170 (1965).
71. Daicoff, G.R. et al. Serotonin-induced pulmonary venous hypertension in pulmonary embolism. *J. Thorac. Cardiovasc. Surg.* 56:810 (1968).
72. Cobb, B. and Nanson, E.M. Further studies with serotonin and experimental pulmonary embolism. *Ann. Surg.* 151:501 (1960).
73. Rudolph, A.M. and Paul, M.H. Pulmonary and systemic vascular responses to continuous infusion of serotonin in the dog. *Am. J. Physiol.* 194:263 (1958).
74. Gilbert, R.P. et al. Effects of histamine, serotonin, and epinephrine on pulmonary hemodynamics with particular reference to arterial and venous segment resistances. *Am. J. Physiol.* 194:165 (1958).
75. Aviado, D.M. and Sadavongvivad, C. Pharmacological significance of biogenic amines in the lungs: Histamine. *Br. J. Pharmacol.* 38:366 (1970).
76. Buckley, I.K. and Ryan, G.B. Increased vascular permeability. The effects of histamine and serotonin on rats mesenteric blood vessels in vivo. *Am. J. Pathol.* 55:329 (1969).
77. Feldberg, W. and Paton, W.D.M. Release of histamine from skin and muscle in the cat by opium alkaloids and other histamine liberators. *J. Physiol.* 114:490 (1951).
78. Brashear, R.E. et al. Elevated plasma histamine after heroin and morphine. *J. Lab. Clin. Med.* 83:451 (1974).
79. Pietra, G.G. et al Histamine and interstitial pulmonary edema in the dog. *Circ. Res.* 26:323 (1971).
79(a). Hendley, E.D. and Schiller, A.A. Protection against hypoxemic pulmonary edema by histaminic and adrenergic blockade. *Am. J. Physiol.* 180:378 (1955).
80. Hauge, A. Role of histamine in hypoxic pulmonary hypertension in the rat: I. Blockade or potentiation of endogenous amines, kinins, and ATP. *Circ. Res.* 22:371 (1968).
81. Richardson, D.W. et al. Modification by beta adrenergic blockade of the circulatory response to acute hypoxia in man. *J. Clin. Invest.* (1967).
82. Himmelspach, C.K. Studies on the relation of drug addiction to the autonomic nervous system. *J. Pharm. Exper. Therap.* 73:91 (1941).
83. Sloan, J.W. and Eisenman, A.J. Long persisting changes in catecholamine metabolism following addiction to and withdrawal from morphine. *Assoc. Res. Nerv. Ment. Dis.* 46:96 (1968).
84. Goodman, L.S. and Gilman, A.Z. *The Pharmacologic Basis of Therapeutics: A Text Book of Pharmacology, Toxicology and Therapeutics for Physicians and Medical Students.* MacMillan, New York, (1965).
85. Stein, L. et al. Pulmonary edema during volume infusion. *Circulation* 52:483 (1975).
86. Norris, R.F. and Potter, H.P. Hepatic inflammation in narcotic addicts: Viral hepatitis a possible cause. *Arch. Environ. Health* 11:662 (1965).

87. Kaplan, K. Chronic liver disease in narcotics addicts. *Am. J. Dig. Dis.* 8:402 (1963).
88. Holmes, A.W. et al. Addict hepatitis-toxic or viral? *J. Clin. Invest.* 48:39 (1969).
89. Marks, V. and Chapple, P.A.L. Hepatic dysfunction in heroin and cocaine users. *Brit. J. Addict.* 62:189 (1967).
90. Stimmel, B. et al. Hepatic dysfunction in heroin addicts. *J.A.M.A.* 222:811 (1972).
91. Force, E.E. et al. Liver disease in fatal narcotism. *Arch. Pathol. Lab. Med.* 97:166 (1974).
92. Steigmann, F. et al. Infectious hepatitis (homologous serum type) in drug addicts. *Gastroenterology* 15:642 (1950).
93. Alter, A. and Michael, M. Serum hepatitis in a group of drug addicts. *New Eng. J. Med.* 259:387 (1958).
94. Levine, R. and Payne, M. Homologous serum hepatitis in youthful heroin users. *Ann. Int. Med.* 53:164 (1960).
95. Barden, R.P. Pulmonary edema: Correlation of roentgenologic appearance and abnormal physiology. *Am. J. Roentgenol.* 92:495 (1964).
96. Pontoppidian, H. et al. Acute respiratory failure in the adult. *New Eng. J. Med.* (3-part article) 287:690, 743, 799 (1972).
97. Briscoe, W.A. et al. Catastrophic pulmonary failure. *Am. J. Med.* 60:248 (1976).
98. Fishman, A.P. Shock lung. A distinctive non-entity. *Circulation* 47:921 (1973).
99. Nash, G. et al. Pulmonary lesions associated with oxygen therapy and artificial ventilation. *New Eng. J. Med.* 276:368 (1967).
100. Rosenfeld, G. Inhibitory influence of ethanol on serotonin metabolism. *Proc. Soc. Exp. Biol. Med.* 103:144 (1960).
101. Grollman, A. The action of alcohol, caffeine, and tobacco on the cardiac output (and its related functions) of normal man. *J. Pharm. Exper. Therap.* 39:313 (1930).

CHAPTER 12

Myocardial Necrosis

During this century, a variety of experimental models have been devised to demonstrate that myocardial necrosis can occur even though the blood supply to the affected area remains intact. Although this has been accomplished frequently by the use of a procedure which exposes the heart to augmented adrenergic influences,[1-24] this procedure is not the only approach which has been successful in this respect.

SUMMARY OF EXPERIMENTAL METHODS

Other methods have included: 1) the administration of an adrenal cortical hormone alone[25] or in combination with a sodium phosphate buffer,[26,42] sometimes supplemented with corn oil[98] or with the adjunctive use of a stressful procedure such as physical restraint;[87] 2) the use of physical restraint alone;[31,35,71] 3) electrical stimulation of the stellate ganglion or regions in the mid-brain;[36,37,39,40,79] 4) the artificial production of intracranial bleeding;[38,56,61-63,41] 5) the removal of the parathyroid gland combined with administration of a phosphate compound;[42-44] 6) the creation of electrolyte depletion, particularly with regard to potassium or magnesium;[30,32,45-55,98] and 7) the production of hemorrhagic shock.[57,58,81-83,100]

Thus, because there is such a variety of ways in which myocardial necrosis can be induced in the experimental animal, it has been suggested by Reinchenbach and Benditt[59] and by Lehr[44] that there may be some fundamental factor, aside from myocardial hypoxia, which can account for all these experimentally produced zones of myocardial necrosis which are not linked directly or indirectly to impaired coronary flow. In this connection, it was emphasized by Reinchenbach and Benditt that the element which consistently can be found in all artificially produced myonecrotic lesions in the heart include cytologic alterations which affect the calcium pump and mitochondrial adenosine triphosphate generation.

However, in the view of Lehr,[42-44] the basic cytologic alteration which underlies the occurrence of experimentally produced myocardial necrosis—regardless of the method undertaken to produce such a lesion—is a disturbance of the kinetics of intracellular cations in the immediate vicinity of the area of myocardial damage. Moreover, within this context, Lehr has regarded as most important those electrolyte shifts which involve intracellular potassium and magnesium.[44]

Equally meaningful, in this same connection, have been the observations of Zugibe et al[112] in canines following ligation of an extramural coronary artery. The purpose of these investigations was to produce an ischemic type of myocardial necrosis and, at the same time, to study the intracellular content of potassium and sodium both after the myocardial necrosis was detectable by microscopic examination in tissues formerly supplied by the occluded vessel and also before such a myocardial lesion became visible. As a result, they were able to demonstrate that a fundamental feature of myocardial necrosis at any stage of its development was an intracellular loss of potassium and a gain of sodium.

Such findings would seem to indicate, first, that there is, indeed, a biochemical correlate of acute myocardial necrosis and, second, that its nature is the sort which would be expected to favor the occurrence of a life-threatening ventricular tachyarrhythmia.[113-116]

Additional data pertaining to a link between myocardial cytokalipenia and the occurrence of the ventricular arrhythmias are the results of separate canine experiments undertaken by Welty and Read[118] and by Brown and Mowlem.[119] Moreover, the findings of these respective investigators are noteworthy inasmuch as neither of the experimental models they employed involved a disturbance of the coronary circulation.

Thus, after Welty and Read had noted that Taurine neutralized the arrhythmogenicity of epinephrine injections in their animals, they conducted additional studies designed to establish correlations between such an effect and the content of potassium in the coronary sinus. In this way, they were able to show that whereas the induction of ventricular arrhythmias by epinephrine alone was associated with myocardial potassium loss, simultaneous effects of Taurine were not only to suppress such epinephrine-induced ventricular arrhythmias but also to prevent myocardial potassium loss. Correspondingly, they concluded that the antiarrhythmic effect of Taurine, in such a setting, was related directly to the capacity of this compound to retain potassium within the myocardium and, conversely, they interpreted their findings to indicate that the basis for the arrhythmogenic property of epinephrine was its opposite effect on this particular intramyocardial cation.

Although Brown and Mowlem[119] similarly demonstrated a link between myocardial loss of potassium and the development of ventricular arrhythmias, their observations were confined exclusively to the effects of hypercapnia. Their experiments were carried out on mongrel dogs in which the plasma potassium concentrations were measured in blood samples obtained simultaneously from the aorta and coronary sinus before, during, and following four hours of high carbon dioxide breathing. As a result, they noted that there was no significant difference between potassium concentration in aorta and coronary sinus blood before or during breathing of high carbon dioxide mixtures. However, they observed that five minutes after the animals had resumed the breathing of room air, the plasma concentration of potassium in the blood obtained from the coronary sinus was significantly higher than it was in the blood drawn from the aorta. Moreover, they demonstrated that the myocardial loss of potassium "was accompanied by severe cardiac irregularities, premature systoles, ventricular tachycardia and, sometimes, by ventricular fibrillation." Correspondingly, inasmuch as it has been shown already by Burton et al[99] that the administration to rats of a phenothiazine such as thioridazine is followed by an elevation of intramyocardial potassium and a lowering of intramyocardial sodium, the observations of Zugibe et al[112] could be interpreted to mean that the myocardial effects of such a drug would tend to diminish rather than favor the likelihood of a cardiac arresting ventricular tachyarrhythmia.

Seemingly, the association between intracellular potassium loss and myocardial necrosis has been confirmed also by the human data provided by Cruickshank et al.[60] Their investigations were confined to 40 patients with subarachnoid hemorrhage and they considered their findings to be reflective of a hypothalamic syndrome resulting from stimulation of the midbrain by the intracranial bleeding.

The changes in those patients which they perceived to be most impressive were 1) the elevated excretion of catecholamines; 2) the elevated plasma cortisol values; 3) a variety of electrocardiographic changes; and 4) a reduction in the values with respect to total body-exchangeable potassium. Thus, they postulated that, in these instances, a lowering of intracellular myocardial potassium, secondary to excessive elaboration of adrenal cortical hormones, had "rendered the heart susceptible to the necrotizing effect of catecholamines." Correspondingly, they suggested that the electrocardiographic abnormalities were ascribable to myofibrillary degeneration in the heart, induced by the hypothalamic stimulation resulting from the intracranial hemorrhage.

EFFECTS OF RESTRAINT STRESS

It would be useful at this juncture to review the animal data obtained by

Johansson et al[31] and by Guillan et al[72] with respect to the connection between myocardial necrosis and sudden death. The animal chosen by Johansson et al for their investigations was the pig. This choice was made because "evidence is accumulating that the cardiovascular system in pigs is more comparable to that in man than is that of other animals frequently used for cardiovascular research." In order to produce a suitable experimental model, they used a technique described as "restraint stress."

Method and Procedure

Basically, the method involved the use of a pharmacologic agent to prevent any form of struggle while electric shocks were applied to the animal.

In connection with these investigations, manipulations of the heart or its blood supply were avoided and the animals remained awake at all times. Moreover, the published protocol indicated that all observations were made in the same laboratory setting under carefully controlled conditions. Essentially, there were three objectives which Johansson et al had intended to achieve. First, they wished to discover a means whereby a sudden cardiac arrest would follow merely the induction of psychic turmoil. Second, they wished to establish, by means of electrocardiographic monitoring, the nature of the cardiac mechanism which immediately preceded the cardiac arrest. Third, they sought to determine, by detailed histologic study of the heart of the "treated" animals and "untreated controls," precisely which anatomical changes were associated with sudden deaths precipitated by the methods they had employed.

Throughout the procedure, cardiac activity was monitored on an electrocardiographic unit attached to the extremities and precordium of the animal. A total of 23 pigs were subjected to the restraint-stress treatment; 9 others, which were not handled in this prescribed manner, constituted the controls.

Results

Of the 23 treated animals, 3 died suddenly following the restraint-stress, 2 died during the experiment, and 1 died three hours later. The remaining 20 treated animals and the 9 untreated controls were "put to death later by bolt pistol (immediate death by brain destruction)." The cardiac arrhythmias observed throughout the period of restraint-stress in the treated animals was ventricular tachycardia (14 animals), sinus bradycardia (5 animals), sinus arrest with ventricular bradycardia (2 animals). Inexplicably, ventricular tachycardia was never followed by ventricular fibrillation and ventricular standstill. However, of the five animals with sinus bradycardia, two died suddenly from ventricular standstill, and in one of the spontaneous fatalities the ventricular standstill was preceded by a brief period of ventricular fibrillation. No cardiac arrhythmias were observed in the controls prior to the time they were killed.

Macroscopic Findings:

All animals were necropsied and the macroscopic findings were as follows: "In the three animals that died spontaneously, multiple intramural, subepicardial and subendocardial hemorrhages were seen. Coarse tigroid pale areas were observed mainly in the papillary muscles of the left ventricle." There were no abnormalities with respect to the coronary vasculature.

Histologic Findings:

Histologic examinations of multiple tissue blocks taken from various parts of the heart were also made. These tissue blocks were fixed in 10% neutral formol and in Gendre's solution for glycogen stain. Other tissue blocks were quick frozen in a cryostat for succinic dehydrogenase reaction. The fixed tissue was embedded in paraffin and cut into thin sections. These sections were stained with hematoxylin and eosin, Mallory's phosphotungstic acid hemotoxylin, Masson's trichrome which differentiated between muscle and connective tissue, and Von Kossa's stain which was used to identify calcium deposits. Sections were also stained with periodic acid-Schiff for identification of mucopolysaccharide and glycogen, Goldner's trichrome, and reticulum stain to identify elastic fibers. Moreover, in order to identify early myocardial degeneration, the acid fuschsin technique according to Poley and associates was used.

Discussion

Examination of these stained tissue sections disclosed myocardial degeneration and necrosis in all 23 hearts. This number represented the total sample of pigs subjected to restraint-stress. However, the myocardial damage was variable in extent; only a few scattered foci of fuchsinophilic degeneration and necrosis were found in some, whereas in others most of the tissue samples from the left ventricle revealed multiple necrotic foci or confluent necrosis occupying a large part of the wall.

The damaged muscle cells were found anywhere in the wall of the left ventricle but were most prominent in the inner third of the wall, particularly in the papillary muscles. The myocardial cell cytoplasm in the degenerated myocardium showed loss of cross-striation, segmentation, and fine or coarse granular disintegration. There was marked reduction of succinic dehydrogenase in the degenerated myocardium. The foci of necrosis often contained, in addition to the muscular debris, accumulations of a homogenous material positive to PAS (mucopolysaccharide deposits). By contrast, microscopic examination of heart muscle samples taken from control animals did not reveal any pathologic changes. No vascular changes were found in either experimental or control animals.

Thus, the data derived from Johansson et al have confirmed that a simple stress-producing procedure (prevention of escape by temporary restraint) can be followed by a severe cardiopathy and by a sudden death (13% of these stressed animals). Also, the electrocardiographic data in these studies had confirmed that there was a positive correlation between the presence of a sinus bradycardia and the sudden death. This finding would suggest that when restraint stress is the forerunner of a sudden cardiac arrest in pigs, the emotional correlate in such instances is the "giving-up syndrome" which has been described elsewhere in man[64-69] and in animals.[71] Moreover, the data derived from Johansson et al seems to demonstrate clearly that, even in animals, a sudden cardiac arrest can sometimes result from the combination of psychic turmoil and a noncoronary-related myocardial necrosis.

It is also noteworthy that Johansson et al were impressed by the similarity between the pathologic changes they had observed during the course of their experiments and the structural alterations in the myocardium which, generally, have been identified with the necrotic myocardiopathy resulting from the administration of catecholamine compounds.[2] Accordingly, in evaluating their findings, these investigators commented, "recent preliminary observations have shown that surgical destruction of certain regions in the central nervous system causing a reshape of animal behavior, can prevent this type of cardiac lesion." They also indicated that it would be proper "to undertake further investigations of the role played by the central nervous mechanism in the cardiac lesions" which they had described.

Another important observation in the course of their investigation pertained to the size of the degenerative lesions they had found. Frequently, these lesions were minute and, in some instances, they measured no more than 1 mm in diameter. However, Johansson et al had noted that the size of the necrotic area did not determine whether the stress-afflicted animal had died suddenly after a relatively short period of restraint stress or whether death had occurred from a different cause. Thus, because of such data, it is conceivable that some reported sudden deaths in highly agitated psychiatric patients which seemed to be unexplained even after a conventional autopsy had been performed, actually may have been due to an easily overlooked minute psychogenic area of myocardial necrosis.

EFFECTS OF CHLORPROMAZINE ADMINISTRATION

The animals chosen by Guillan et al[72] for their experiments were rabbits. Three of them belonged to the treated group and one served as a control. In this experiment, the "treatment," was the intramuscular administration of a single large dose of chlorpromazine. Each animal weighed 2 kg and the daily dose, on average, was 77 mg, 56 mg, and 65 mg per kg of body weight, respectively. Hence, simple extrapolation of such data would indicate that the three "treated" rabbits had received daily doses of chlorpromazine which corresponded to a daily intramuscular chlorpromazine injection of 5400 mg, 3900 mg, and 4500 mg to a man or woman weighing 70 kg.

All three treated rabbits died suddenly; one survived for 10 days, another survived for 8 days, and the third survived for 9 days, respectively. The animal which had survived for 10 days had received, in toto, 1550 mg of chlorpromazine; the animal which had survived for 8 days had received a total of 900 mg of the drug; the third, "treated" rabbit, which had survived for 9 days, had received a total of 1175 mg of the drug.

The treated animals had been monitored with an electrocardiograph throughout the time they had remained alive. In this way, it was demonstrated that 1) only the "treated" animals died suddenly and 2) in conjunction with the sudden cardiac arrest, there was a brief period of slow idioventricular rhythm which preceded a complete cardiac standstill.

Without any delay, the hearts of the three rabbits which had died suddenly were processed in the conventional manner prior to electron microscopic examination of the cardiac tissue. Such histologic studies demonstrated, uniformly, the presence of a nonspecific type of zonal necrotic myocardiopathy and, as Guillan et al had explained, the findings were similar to those described by Ferrans et al[11] in connection with their electron microscopic study of isoproterenol-induced myocardial necrosis in rodents. The ultrastructural changes they had noted consisted of swelling of the endoplasmic reticulum and mitochondrial damage. Thus, the data derived from the investigations by Guillan et al[72] and by Ferrans et al,[11] respectively, indicated that a similar type of myocardial necrosis could result from either *massive* doses of chlorpromazine or an anoxia-producing amount of a catecholamine preparation. On the basis of such observations, it also is conceivable that the inordinately large doses of chlorpromazine may have been responsible for a reflex elaboration of catecholamines. On the other hand, the data obtained in experiments performed by Morpurgo[74] should not be overlooked. Morpurgo had demonstrated with anesthetized rats that, whereas hypothalmic stimulation was followed by increased locomotor activity culminating in a flight reaction, an elevation of the blood pressure, and eyelid contractions before modest doses of chlorpromazine had been administered, the same procedure after chlorpromazine had been administered did not produce any of these responses. Thus, such data could signify that chlorpromazine, in doses which are not not excessive, can actually inhibit adrenergic responses resulting from hypothalamic stimulation.

EFFECTS OF INTRACRANIAL DISEASE

Autopsy data in man, which have shown a connection between intracranial pathology and noncoronary-related myocardial necrosis, would seem to be equally meaningful with respect to the pathogenesis of sudden deaths in emotionally disturbed patients. Thus, Connor,[75-78] on the basis of postmortem findings, had advanced the view that the deaths of 21 of 169 patients with intracranial disease could be ascribed to a noncoronary-related concurrent necrotic cardiac lesion which had remained undetected until the time of the postmortem examination.

Method

In connection with his studies of the hearts of these 169 patients, slices of ventricular myocardium were stained with cresyl violet and acid fuchsin, as well as with hematoxylin and eosin, before the histologic examination of these tissues was undertaken.

Findings

In this way, Connor discovered, in the hearts of 21 of the overall sample, the presence of a necrotic cardiopathy which he termed "fuchsinophilic degeneration of the myocardium." Moreover, this finding was associated with a miscellaneous group of neurologic abnormalities: intracranial hemorrhage or infarction was present in 13 patients; a brain tumor was present in 2 patients; 2 patients were under treatment for head injury; there was 1 case each of obstructive hydrocephalus, encephalitis, and postoperative complications following a thalatomy.

Conclusions

With regard to the pathogenesis of this myocardial lesion, it was concluded by Connor that "it was unlikely that coronary artery disease or hypertension played a major part in its causation." Instead, he suggested that it may have resulted from "a sudden increase in intracranial tension which, in turn, produced a rise in the level of circulating catecholamines," and in order to validate this view, he cited the observation of Shkhvatsabaia[79] that "the sudden injection of air into the lateral cerebral ventricles of rabbits will cause heart lesions."

MYOFIBRILLARY DEGENERATION

Reichenbach and Benditt[59] described comparable noncoronary-related myonecrotic lesions in the hearts of patients "dying after subarachnoid hemorrhage or with pheochromocytoma" (a tumor which characteristically floods the circulation with excessive amounts of catecholamines). In addition, these investigators explained that the myocardial lesions in these decedents resembled the sort which regularly can be produced in animals by electrical stimulation of circumscribed zones of the mid-brain.[37,39,40] Inasmuch as such an experimentally produced myonecrotic lesion has been ascribed to an augmentation of catecholamine activity resulting from such an intervention in experimental animals, Reichenbach and Benditt postulated that the genesis of the cardiac lesions they have labeled "myofibrillary degeneration" could be related, as part of a stress reaction, to "local release of increased amounts of endogenous norepinephrine from cardiac sympathetic nerve endings."

Pathologic Features

In their view, the pathologic features of myofibrillary degeneration can be distinguished readily from the "coagulation necrosis" identified with myocardial infarction exclusively due to occlusive coronary artery disease. As they explained, the salient features of myofibrillary degeneration are the following: early there is clumping and disorganization of the cardiac myofibrillae. Later, degenerative changes in cell cytoplasm and mineralization of mitochondria are manifest. Cells may either be repaired or die. In the repair of cells, evidence of new protein synthesis is found in the form of nuclear, nucleolar, and ribosomal changes. There is little evidence of inflammation. In the later stages, stromal condensation and fibrosis may become evident.

OBSERVATIONS OF COMBINATION ETIOLOGIES

Equally noteworthy are the observations by Duren and Becker[80] who reported two fatalities ascribable to the triad of sudden death, intracranial pathology, and fatal noncoronary-related "myofibrillary degeneration." One of these two decedents had been treated for a cerebral infarct and the other for an astrocytoma of the brain. However, Duren and Becker were somewhat ambivalent with respect to the relationship between the cardiac lesion and an elaboration of catecholamines secondary to the intracranial pathology.

With respect to these two fatalities, they speculated that a contributory factor may have been the associated atherosclerotic lesions of the coronary circulation but, on the other hand, they were also supportive of the view that an equally important cause could have been a rise in intramyocardial catecholamine concentrations produced by hypothalamic stimulation of catecholamine storage sites in the adrenal glands and sympathetic nerve endings located in the heart.

They observed that the necrotic lesions differed, in certain important respects, from the changes identified with a myocardial infarction resulting from occlusive coronary artery disease. For this reason, they were reluctant to consider the etiology of the necrotic lesions in the heart to be exclusively the atherosclerotic narrowing of the extramural coronary arteries, which also was present in both instances. They described the nature of the myocardial necrosis as "focal myocytolysis," a term which had been introduced by several earlier observers[84,85] to identify this particular myonecrotic lesion.

Case Study No. 1

The first of the two patients studied by Duren and Becker[80] was a 61-year-old white woman who was admitted to the neurologic department because of a right-sided hemiplegia, probably attributable to cerebral thrombosis. She was semiconscious at the time of admission, but 5 days later she suddenly became completely unconscious and coincident with that episode the electrocardiogram showed changes compatible with an acute transmural anteroseptal and lateral myocardial infarction. The patient died on the 6th day—one day after the electrocardiogram had revealed the infarct pattern.

Autopsy Findings

An autopsy was performed and confirmed the clinical diagnosis of cerebral infarction. In addition, there was massive cerebral edema with signs of cerebral compression. The heart weighed 325 gm and the coronary arteries were normal except for two sites with 75% stenosis. One such area of coronary stenosis was located in the right coronary artery and one in the anterior descending branch. The extent of the stenosis was 5 mm in the right coronary artery and 7 mm in the left coronary artery. Nowhere was there total occlusion of the lumen. The myocardium was sectioned in parallel slices from the apex to the base of the heart, but there was no gross evidence of a myocardial infarction. The ventricular wall had a fleshy reddish brown appearance throughout its entire circumference.

Histologic Findings

Histologic testing showed foci of necrotic muscle fibers and a cellular infiltrate. The affected fibers were swollen and the cytologic architecture was distorted. Contraction bands were present and loss of myofibril became apparent. The degenerating fibers showed encroachment by mononuclear cells, some of which contained phagocytosed lipofuchsin pigment and nuclear debris. There was no polymorphonuclear leucocytic infiltration and the myocardial cells surrounding the foci of degeneration were all viable without any recognizable sign of degradation.

Conclusions

The lesion was considered comparable to the focal myocytolysis described by Schlesinger and Reiner[84] as well as by others[85,86,96] who had employed a slightly different designation for such changes. Nowhere in the many sections of the heart of this particular decedent was a classical myocardial infarction present.

Case Study No. 2

The second of the two patients studied by Duren and Becker[80] was a 51-year-old man who had been admitted to the department of neurosurgery where it was established that his basic disability was related to a tumor in the region of the right temporo-occipital lobe.

Description of Deterioration

Portions of the tumor were removed surgically; postoperatively, the patient developed evidences of an elevated intracranial pressure which was ultimately treated with an appropriate drainage procedure. Seven days after the operation, an electrocardiogram disclosed signs of an acute transmural anteroseptal infarction with extention toward the lateral wall of the left ventricle. Despite these electrocardiographic findings, the results of multiple enzyme studies were within normal limits. At the same time, there was no laboratory evidence of any electrolyte disorder. The patient gradually deteriorated and 4 months after the operation died from elevated intracranial pressures.

Autopsy Findings

The autopsy did not reveal any gross abnormalities apart from those in the brain, where there was extensive growth of tumor with destruction of both left and right frontal lobes and arachnoidal extension around the brain stem. In the heart, there were no gross signs of any acute or healed myocardial infarction. The total cardiac weight was 360 gm. A postmortem coronary angiogram confirmed the presence of mild atherosclerosis restricted to the left anterior descending coronary artery. In this branch there was a localized narrowing of approximately 75%, 9 mm after its origin from the main stem. There was no thrombosis and no total occlusion in any part of the coronary arterial stem.

Histologic Findings

In sections obtained from the anteroseptal, apical, and inferior regions of the left ventricle, there were multiple lesions which were quite variable in a structural sense. Occasionally, minute foci existed where cells exhibited swollen cytoplasm, a slightly granular appearance, a loss of myofibrils, and an encroachment by mononuclear cells. However, the majority of lesions consisted of small foci of intact sarcolemmal sheets and almost a total disappearance of myofibrils. No polymorphonuclear leucocytes were present but there was a scant mononuclear cellular infiltrate. In other foci, there was a fine fibrillar meshwork of connective tissue fibers which apparently had replaced lost myocardial cells. In these foci, lymphocytes and macrophages occasionally could be seen. Definite signs of a classical myocardial infarction were not seen in any of the sections studied.

Discussion

The pathogenesis of these foci of "focal myocytolysis" was perceived by Duren and Becker to be, basically, a disturbance of hypothalamic function which, in turn, led to sympathetic overstimulation and adrenocortical stimulation. Within this context, they considered the adrenocortical stimulation to be responsible for a shift of potassium ions from within the myocardial cell toward the extracellular space, a phenomenon known to make the myocardial cell extra sensitive to norepinephrine stimulation.[87] In addition, Duren and Becker were impressed by the localization of the "focal myocytolysis" to regions of the left ventricular myocardium supplied by the stenosed extramural coronary arteries. Therefore, they concluded that the luminal narrowing may be of some significance with respect to the etiology of these myonecrotic lesions but, at the same time, they recognized that some adjunctive risk factor was responsible for their development. Within this formulation, they seemed ready to accept the proposition that a rise in intracranial pressure which led to an excessive release of catecholamines might be inculpated.

EFFECTS of PHENOTHIAZINES: PSYCHIATRIC CASE STUDIES

Besides the reports already discussed, the medical literature includes three articles concerning sudden deaths that occur in conjunction with a nonspecific and noncoronary-related myocardial necrosis in highly disturbed psychiatric patients who, prior to the time of death, had been receiving phenothiazines to control their agitation. The first of these publications by Kelly et al[88] appeared in 1963; the second paper by Hollister and Kosek,[89] appeared in 1965; the third, by Guillan et al[73] appeared in 1970.

Case Study No. 1

Although the 46-year-old patient discussed by Kelly et al[88] had been confined to the hospital continuously for 18 years prior to the time of death, the authors had not mentioned the nature of the treatment she had received during that entire period. However, they did indicate that she had been suffering from a severe behavioral disturbance due to a prior attack of postvaccinal encephalitis. The information which was provided indicated that on December 19, 1959, after it had been established that the findings in a preliminary electrocardiogram were normal, usual amounts of thioridazine were prescribed. The starting dose was 600 mg daily but because of her highly disturbed behavior, this amount proved to be inadequate. Accordingly, the daily dose was increased gradually and by February 9, 1960 she was receiving 3600 mg of thioridazine daily.

Suddenly and unexpectedly, on February 22, 1960, while she was still receiving 3600 mg of thioridazine daily she developed cardiovascular collapse and died the following day. In serial electrocardiograms made on February 23, 1960 the significant findings included periods of complete A-V heart block with the ventricular pacemaker located below the bifurcation of the A-V bundle, runs of ventricular tachycardia, or bizzare combinations of heart block and ectopic beats.

Autopsy Findings

An autopsy was performed and this disclosed the following; the heart was found to be normal in size and its weight was 300 gm. The only gross abnormality of the heart was a brownish, hyperemic, somewhat softened area in the septum, measuring 3.5 cm in diameter lying posteriorly and extending into the wall of the left ventricle. The ventricular walls were 1.1 and 0.3 cm respectively. The heart valves were normal and the coronary arteries were remarkably healthy and almost free of atheroma. There was no vascular disease demonstrable near the discolored area in the septum.

Histologic Findings

Microscopic examination of this area revealed the muscle fibers to be remarkably atrophic with narrow, often fragmented cytoplasmic bodies which occasionally lacked nuclei. The fibers were widely separated by loose and edematous connective tissue, particularly around the vascular channels of smaller caliber which were dilated and filled with red blood cells. The interstitial connective tissue contained acid mucopolysaccharide brown substance and in some areas young fibers were present. In this instance, the pathologist also added that "the myocardial changes which have been described were not those of any known cardiomyopathy," and he speculated that the myocardial lesion may have been the result of the extremely large doses of thioridazine which the patient had received prior to the time of death.

Discussion

Thus, in view of such data, and because of the findings derived from the animal studies reported by Johannson et al,[31] it is conceivable in this instance, that it would be proper to make the following assumptions: (1) the cardiac lesion was a stress-induced myonecrosis of the heart; (2) the stress was related to the evidently severe emotional disorder exhibited by the decedent prior to the time of death; (3) the emotionally-induced stress factor could have resulted in the release of large amounts of catecholamines[90-95]: (4) the development of myocardial necrosis, as in experimental animals,[1-22] was linked to the impact of high concentrations of catecholamines on the heart; (5) because of the presence of this zonal myocardial necrosis, the heart became electrically unstable[97]; (6) subsequently, the electrical instability provided the basis for an eventual abrupt cardiac arrest.[107-109]

Data are also extant which would make it likely that even large doses of thioridazine would not produce the type of nonspecific myocardial necrosis described by the pathologist in this instance. This view is based on the contrasting findings in the articles by Solymos et al[98] and by Burton et al,[99] respectively. In the paper by Solymos et al which pertained to the production and prevention of myocardial necrosis in experimental animals, it is emphasized that the noteworthy change with respect to the distribution of electrolytes within the necrotic myocardial cells was a marked increase in the concentration of the sodium ion. Moreover, these observers had interpreted such a finding to indicate that the development of the myocardial necrosis was to a large degree dependent not only on a surplus of intracellular sodium but also on an intracellular potassium loss. Observations by Lehr[44] with regard to the experimental production of myocardial necrosis are also in accord with this finding.

On the other hand, experiments by Burton et al,[99] which sought to determine the electrolyte content in the ventricular myocardium of rats following repeated intraperitoneal administrations of thioridazine, confirmed that this phenothiazine actually decreased the sodium concentration in the myocardial cells and at the same time increased their potassium content. Correspondingly, in view of the observations of Zugibe[112] regarding sodium concentration in necrotic lesions, the myonecrosis in this instance should not be considered a thioridazine-effect.

Conclusions

The results of studies of this sort would, therefore, seem to exclude thioridazine as a "risk factor" with respect to the myocardial necrosis observed by Kelly et al in their highly agitated psychiatric patient who had died suddenly due to the combined life-threatening ventricular arrhythmias and advanced degrees of A-V heart block. On the other hand, it is conceivable, inasmuch as the massive doses of thioridazine were used because the patient was highly agitated, that the patient had an excessive outpouring of catecholamines. It is therefore likely that the agitation itself was actually the underlying cause for the myocardial necrosis and the subsequent cardiac arrest.

Case Study No. 2

In the article by Hollister and Kosek,[89] the authors discuss the fatal illness of a 40-year-old chronic schizophrenic woman who had always been in good physical health. Although she was not known to have seizures, on the 46th day of her hospitalization she developed a sudden episode of syncope and died approximately 17 hours later.

Prior to the first syncopal episode, she had received unusually large doses of phenothiazine drugs in order to control her psychotic behavior. The nature of the behavioral distrubance was not described but, in view of the large doses of the phenothiazines which were prescribed, it can be presumed that she was very hyperactive and assaultive. The first phenothiazine agent she received was chlorpromazine: the maximim daily dose was 2400 mg. Six days before she died, the chlorpromazine was withdrawn abruptly, and a daily dose of 1600 mg thioridazine combined with 20 mg trifluoperazine were substituted. Six days after the chlorpromazine had been stopped, she experienced the first of many attacks of cardiac syncope that resulted in death 17 hours later.

Apparently, no one had any knowledge of anything unusual just before the time of her first syncopal episode. However, it was stated by the authors that prior to that incident, she had never lost consciousness. Also lacking was any information regarding the respiratory rate, audibility of the heart sounds or the level of the blood pressure during that first syncopal episode. In any event, "resuscitation was accomplished, followed by gastric lavage." Thirty minutes later, her vital signs were normal but she had not regained consciousness. Accordingly, she was transferred immediately to the medical ward and was attached to a cardiac monitor. Soon after her transfer to the Medical Service, she vomited and aspirated some of the vomitus. At this time, neither pulse, heart sounds, nor respirations were perceptible. Although these vital signs were restored promptly by mouth-to-mouth respiration and external cardiac massage, the patient remained unconscious until her death 17 hours after the occurrence of the original syncopal attack.

While on the Medical Service, 45 episodes of ventricular fibrillation were allegedly recorded; however, no electrocardiographic strips were included with the case report in order to indicate whether, indeed, the episodes were linked to an episode of ventricular fibrillation. In connection with these episodes of cardiac syncope, she received various drugs including digitalis, procaineamide, dilantin, molar lactate, levarterenol, and several antibiotics. Frequently, but not always, countershock therapy was required to restore a viable cardiac rhythm; however, when this procedure was used during the 45th episode of cardiac arrest, cardiac resuscitation could not be accomplished. The only comments pertaining to the autopsy were the following: "postmortem examination revealed a severe aspiration bronchopneumonia, left ventricular dilatation, and some histological myocardial changes secondary to electrode defibrillation." Thus, it is evident that the pathologist had not considered the possibility that the microscopic areas of myocardial necrosis might have antedated and actually might have created zones of electrical instability which. in turn, could have initiated the recurrent episodes of ventricular tachyarrhythmia and their companionate seizure episodes.

However, without more definitive data, it is uncertain whether the pathologist was correct to claim that the myocardial necrosis represented a tissue change produced by repeated transthoracic cardioversion interventions and that the phenothiazines the decedent had received were primarily responsible for the recurrent arrhythmias treated with repeated countershocks prior to the time this patient had succumbed. It was stated, merely, that "in 45 instances over a 14-hour period, normal cardiac rhythm was restored by *either* cardiac massage *or* external defibrillation," but there was no statement regarding the frequency of either procedure or the magnitude of the voltages which were employed. Correspondingly, it would be reasonable to suppose that electrical cardioversion was employed approximately half the time during that 14-hour period. On this basis, it could be conjectured that cardioversion was employed approximately 25 times and that the heart had been exposed to a total of 5000 watt-seconds, in divided doses, over a 14-hour span. Then, since the average electrical charge is 200 watt-seconds, a simple calculation would demonstrate that over each one-hour time span, the patient would have received a charge of 356 watt-seconds (in divided doses).

The results of such a calculation are highly significant because in a recent article by Pugh et al[101] entitled "Cardioversion and False Positive Technetium Stannous Pyrophosphate Myocardial Scintigrams," data were presented to indicate that in dogs (whose chest wall musculature is much thinner than that of man) myocardial necrosis ascribable to external countershocks occurred only in 2 of 10 dogs exposed to such treatment when the doses were repeated every 5 minutes. Moreover, in these two animals, the doses (total amounts) which were able to induce myocardial necrosis by such means was 1000 watt-seconds over a period of one half hour and 4000 watt-seconds over a period of one hour, respectively.

Thus, so long as specific information is unavailable with respect to the doses and frequency of the electrical countershocks which the patient of Hollister and Kosek had received prior to the time of death, it seems doubtful that it was the phenothiazines that the decedent had received and not the myocardial necrosis which was responsible for the recurrent episodes of cardioplegic ventricular fibrillation, one of which ultimately proved to be irreversible. Moreover, within the same context, it would seem reasonable to attribute the death of this patient to a stress-induced patchy microscopic myonecrosis secondary to a severe psychotic episode and, coordinately, to recurrent life-threatening ventricular tachyarrhythmias resulting from the microscopic myonecrotic lesions. Moreover, in this same connection, it would be important to know where in the heart of this decedent the "histologic myocardial changes" were located. Surely, if they were close to the subendocardium and not near the epicardium, it can be deduced from the observations of Di Cola et al[102,111] that the customary-sized transthoracic shocks the decedent had received intermittently were not primarily responsible for the occurrence of these particular myocardial lesions.

Case Study No. 3

Unlike the postmortem studies reported by Kelly, Fay, and Laverty[88] on the one hand, and by Hollister and Kosek[89] on the other hand, those described by Guillan et al[73] consisted of electron microscopic data. Thus, their findings pertained to the ultrastructure of the hearts which had belonged to two psychiatric patients who had been highly disturbed and who died suddenly, even though, grossly, their hearts appeared to be normal. It should be noted also that because of their psychiatric problem, both of these decedents had received varying doses of phenothiazines prior to the time of death.

One of these two hearts had been removed from a 53-year-old patient who had been "hospitalized because of irritability, hallucinations, and bizzare behavior"; the other had belonged to a 45-year-old man who, during his hospitalization for bronchial asthma, had manifested, at various times, "agitation, bizarre behavior, sleeplessness, hallucinations, and restlessness."

The noteworthy ultrastructural changes in these two hearts consisted of "foci of mitochondrial swelling with diffuse clumping of cristae into osmiophilic masses; myofibril degeneration and increased electron dense material within mitochondria." By contrast, evidence of a focal myocardial necrosis had not been detected by conventional light microscopy. Correspondingly, then, such data could imply that Madow and Stauffer, whose article was published in 1940[103] and others who also have reported their observations in the first half of the 20th century with respect to sudden deaths associated with acute exhaustive mania (see Chapter 10) may have overlooked a myonecrotic lesion in the hearts of the "catatonic fatalities" they had discussed in their respective publications.

Thus, an undoubtedly meaningful observation was the detection by Guillan et al of such ultrastructural changes in the hearts of these two "excited" psychiatric patients who had died suddenly. However, another aspect of the myonecrotic lesions they had found which needs to be considered is their pathogenesis.

In this connection, it is noteworthy that although Guillan et al conjectured that the myocardial lesions might be a phenothiazine-related phenomenon, they also acknowledged that the histologic features of these lesions resembled the cardiac changes which had been produced in animals by the administration of isoproterenol.[11] For this reason, and also because isoproterenol-induced myonecrotic lesions in animals have been shown to be histologically comparable to the myocardial necrosis observed in patients whose deaths were linked to a pheochromocytoma of the adrenal glands,[104-106] it would seem appropriate to consider the possibility that catecholamine excess was, fundamentally, the "risk factor" responsible for the patchy myocardial necrosis detected by Guillan et al in the hearts of their patients. Inasmuch as there is a substantial body of data to indicate that manic behavior in psychiatric patients is accompanied by an outpouring of catecholamines,[90-95] it would seem to be equally appropriate to connect the myocardial necrosis described by Guillan et al with the emotional disturbance exhibited by the decedents prior to the time of death, and not with premortem phenothiazine therapy.

MYOCARDIAL NECROSIS IN HEROIN ABUSER

In addition, inasmuch as it is customary at present for psychiatric-care facilities to assume the responsibility for the care of narcotic addicts, it would seem improper to disregard, in a monograph of this sort, the occurrence of a type of myocardial necrosis which can be associated with sudden death in habitual heroin users. However, so far, only one fatality associated with a distinctive myocardial necrotic lesion in patients of this genre has been reported. Such a case was described in a paper by Schwartzfarb et al which appeared in 1977[117] and, in this instance, the myocardial necrosis was associated with a rhabdomyolysis of the soleus muscle.

Case Study

This decedent, a 23-year-old heroin abuser, had been admitted to the hospital because of edema of the right leg and oliguria. Admission diagnoses were right iliofemoral thrombo—phlebitis, acute renal failure, and heroin addiction. Urinalysis was strongly positive for "blood" in the absence of hemolysis or marked hematocyturia; consequently, the attending physicians made a diagnosis of rhabdomyolysis associated with myoglobinuria. Peritoneal dialysis succeeded in lowering blood urea nitrogen and serum potassium levels but the patient died suddenly on the fourth hospital day as a result of cardiogenic shock.

In the view of Schwartzfarb et al, the rhabdomyolysis and the myocardial necrosis had a common pathogenesis and, for this reason, they surmised that some type of ill-defined systemic mechanism was involved.

Histologic Findings

Histologically, there was a striking similarity between the necrotic lesion in the skeletal and the cardiac muscles. With respect to the affected soleus muscle, the findings consisted of "marked proliferation of sarcolemmal nuclei with giant cell formation in some fields. Scattered macrophages, a mononuclear cell infiltrate, and a few plasma cells were present between muscle fibers. Although the intrinsic blood vessels were congested, no thrombi were seen. Electron microscopy of the discoid areas of soleus muscle showed fragmentation of the myofibrils with dissolution of Z lines and I bands. In other areas, regenerating fibers contained scanty, poorly organized myofibrils."

Correspondingly, "representative sections of the left ventricular free wall likewise contained foci of myocardial necrosis with sarcolemmal proliferation. A macrophage, mononuclear, and plasma cell infiltrate was seen in these areas and focal dystrophic calcification was seen in some of the necrotic fibers."

Conclusions

Thus, in view of such findings, it can be anticipated that an aggressive search for evidences of myocardial necrosis in future instances of rhabdomyolysis in heroin addicts, may detect the presence of myocardial involvement associated with this particular myopathic syndrome. However, if such investigations are undertaken, it would seem advisable to include estimations of the potassium and sodium contents of myocardial tissue, employing the method described by Zugibe et al[112] especially since Schwartzfarb et al had cited a case of narcotic-induced rhabdomyolysis associated with normal histologic findings on light microscopy despite evidences of serious muscle fiber damage disclosed during electron microscopy of the same tissues.

REFERENCES

1. Szakacs, J.E. and Cannon, A. 1-Norepinephrine myocarditis. *Amer. J. Clin. Path.* 30:425 (1958).
2. Ferrans, V.J. et al. Isoproterenol-induced myocardial necrosis. *Am. Heart J.* 68:71 (1964).
3. Ostadal, B. et al. Isoproterenol-induced acute experimental cardiac necrosis in the turtle. *Am. Heart J.* 76:645 (1968).
4. Wexler, B.C. et al. Myocardial necrosis induced by isoproterenol in rats. *Angiology* 19:665 (1968).
5. Bloom, S. and Cancilla, P.A. Myocytolysis and mitochondrial calcification in rat myocardium after low doses of isoproterenal. *Amer. J. Path.* 54:373 (1969).
6. Moss, A.J. et al. Cardiovascular effects of sustained norepinephrine infusions. *Circ. Res.* 18:596 (1966).
7. Haft, J.I. et al. Protection against epinephrine-induced myocardial necrosis by drugs that inhibit platelet aggregation. *Am. J. Cardiol.* 30:838 (1972).
8. Szakacs, J.E. and Mehlman, B. Pathologic changes induced by 1-norephinephrine. *Am. J. Cardiol.* 5:619 (1960).
9. Schenk, E.A. and Mos, A.J. Cardiovascular effects of sustained norephinephrine infusions. II Morphology. *Circ. Res.* 18:605 (1966).
10. Csapo, Z. et al. Early alterations of the cardiac muscle cell in isoproterenol-induced necroses. *Arch. Path.* 93:356 (1972).
11. Ferrans, V.J. et al. Histochemical and electron microscopical studies on the cardiac necroses produced by sympathomimetic agents. *Ann. N.Y. Acad. Sci.* 156:309 (1969).
12. Bajusz, E. and Jasmin, G. Influence of variations in electrolyte intake upon the development of cardiac necrosis produced by vasopressor amines. *Lab. Invest.* 13:756 (1964).
13. Rona, G. et al. Myocardial lesions, circulatory and electrocardiographic changes produced by isoproterenol in the dog. *Rev. Canad. de Biol.* 18:83 (1959).
14. Selye, H. and Bahusz, E. Conditioning by corticoids for the production of cardiac lesions with noradrenaline. *Acta Endocrinol.* 30:183 (1959).
15. Rona, G. et al. The significance of factors modifying the development of isoproterenol-induced myocardial necrosis. *Am. Heart J.* 66:389 (1963).
16. Rona, G. et al. An infarct-like myocardial lesion and other toxic manifestations produced by isoproterenol in the rat. *Arch. Path.* 67:443 (1959).
17. Beznak, M. Hemodynamics during the acute phase of myocardial damage caused by isoproterenol. *Canad. J. Biochem. Physiol.* 40:25 (1962).
18. Rona, G. et al. The effect of breed, age and sex on myocardial necrosis produced by isoproterenol in the rat. *J. Gerontol.* 14:169 (1959).
19. Rona, G. et al. Effect of dietary sodium and potassium content on myocardial necrosis elicited by isoproterenol. *Lab. Invest.* 10:892 (1961).
20. Chappel, C.I. et al. Comparison of cardiotoxic actions of certain sympathomimetic amines. *Canad. J. Biochem. Physiol.* 37:35 (1959).
21. Maling, H.M. et al. Some similar effects after large doses of catecholamines and myocardial infarction in dogs. *Am. J. Cardiol.* 5:628 (1960).
22. Rosenblum, I. et al. Studies of cardiac necrosis. I. Production of cardiac lesions with sympathomimetic amines. *Toxicol. Appl. Pharmacol.* 7:1 (1965).
23. Stanton, H.C. et al. Studies on isoproterenol-induced cardiomegaly in rats. *Am. Heart J.* 77:72 (1969).
24. Judd, J.T. and Wexler, B.C. Myocardial connective tissue metabolism in response to injury: Histological and chemical studies of mucopolysaccharide and collagen in rat hearts after isoproterenol-induced infarction. *Circ. Res.* 25:201 (1969).

25. Darrow, D.C. and Miller, H.C. The production of cardiac lesions by repeated injections of desoxycorticosterone acetate. *J. Clin. Invest.* 21:601 (1942).
26. D'Agostino, A.N. An electron microscopic study of cardiac necrosis produced by fluorocortisol and sodium phosphate. *Amer. J. Path.* 45:633 (1964).
27. Bajusz, E. and Selye, H. Adaptation to the cardiac necrosis-eliciting effect of stress. *Am. J. Physiol.* 199:453 (1960).
28. Selye, H. The humoral production of cardiac infarcts. *Brit. Med. J.* 1:599 (1958).
29. Nickerson, M. and Karr, G.W. Pathogenesis of electrolyte-steroid-cardiopathy. *Circ. Res.* 9:209 (1961).
30. Prioreschi, P. Role of potassium in the pathogenesis of the electrolyte-steroid-cardiopathy with necrosis. *Circ. Res.* 10:782 (1962).
31. Johansson, G. et al. Severe stress-cardiopathy in pigs. *Am. Heart J.* 87:451 (1974).
32. Selye, H. *The Pluricausal Cardiopathies.* Charles C. Thomas, Springfield, Ill. (1961).
33. Selye, H. *Experimental Cardiovascular Diseases.* Springer-Verlag, Heidelberg (1970).
34. Raab, W. et al. Sympathogenic and antiadrenergic prevention of stress-induced myocardial lesions. *Am. J. Cardiol.* 8:203 (1961).
35. Raab, W. et al. Myocardial necroses produced in domesticated rats and in wild rats by sensory and emotional stresses. *Proc. Soc. Exp. Biol. Med.* 116:665 (1964).
36. Klouda, M.A. and Brynjolffson, G. Cardiotoxic effects of electrical stimulation of stellate ganglia. *Ann. N.Y. Acad. Sci.* 156:271 (1969).
37. Chen, H.I. et al. Encephalogenic cardiomyopathy after stimulation of the brain stem in monkeys. *Am. J. Cardiol.* 33:845 (1974).
38. Greenhoot, J.H. and Reichenbach, D.D. Cardiac injury and subarachnoid hemorrhage. A clinical, pathological, and physiological correlation. *J. Neurosurg.* 30:521 (1969).
39. Melville, K.I. et al. Central nervous system stimulation and cardiac ischemic changes in monkeys. *Ann. N.Y. Acad. Sci.* 156:241 (1969).
40. Melville, K.I. et al. Cardiac ischemic changes and arrhythmias induced by hypothalamic stimulation. *Am. J. Cardiol.* 12:781 (1963).
41. Burch, G.E. et al. Acute myocardial lesions following experimentally-induced intracranial hemorrhage in mice: A histological and histochemical study. *Arch. Path.* 84:517 (1967).
42. Lehr, D. and Krukowski, M. About the mechanism of myocardial necrosis induced by sodium phosphate and adrenal corticoid overdosage. *Ann. N.Y. Acad. Sci.* 105:135 (1963).
43. Lehr, D. et al. Correlation of myocardial and renal necrosis with tissue electrolyte changes. *J.A.M.A.* 197:105 (1966).
44. Lehr, D. Tissue electrolyte alteration in disseminated myocardial necrosis. *Ann. N.Y. Acad. Sci.* 51:344 (1969).
45. Heggtveit, H.A. et al. Cardiac necrosis and calcification in experimental magnesium deficiency. A light and electron microscopic study. *Amer. J. Path.* 45:757 (1964).
46. Lowenhaupt, E. et al. Basic histologic lesions of magnesium deficiency in the rat. *Arch. Path.* 49:427 (1950).
47. Mc Allen, P.M. Myocardial changes occurring in potassium deficiency. *Brit. Heart J.* 17:5 (1955).
48. Mac Pherson, C.R. Myocardial necrosis in the potassium-depleted rat: A reassessment. *Brit. J. Exp. Path.* 37:279 (1956).
49. French, J.E. A histological study of the heart lesions in potassium-deficient rats. *Arch. Path.* 53:485 (1952).
50. Molnar, Z. et al. Cardiac changes in the potassium-depleted rat. *Arch. Path.* 74:339 (1962).
51. Emberson, J.W. and Muir, A.R. Changes in ultrastructure of rat myocardium induced by hypokalemia. *Quart. J. Exp. Physiol.* 54:36 (1969).
52. Priorischi, P. Chlorides, potassium, and experimental cardiac necrosis. *Circ. Res.* 12:55 (1963).

53. Selye, H. and Bajusz, E. Sensitization by potassium deficiency for the production of myocardial necrosis by stress. *Amer. J. Path.* 35:525 (1959).
54. Tucker, V.L. et al. Cardiac necrosis accompanying potassium deficiency and administration of corticosteroids. *Circ. Res.* 13:420 (1963).
55. Priorischi, P. Experimental cardiac necrosis and potassium: A review. *Canad. M.A.J.* 96:1221 (1967).
56. Jacob, W.A. et al. Myocardial ultrastructure and hemodynamic reactions during experimental subarachnoid hemorrhage. *J. Mol. Cell Cardiol.* 4:287 (1972).
57. Hackel, D.B. and Catchpole, B.V. Pathologic and electrocardiographic effects of hemorrhagic shock in dogs treated with 1-norephinephrine. *Lab. Invest.* 7:358 (1958).
58. Martin, A.M. and Hackel, D.B. The myocardium of the dog in hemorrhagic shock. *Lab. Invest.* 12:77 (1963).
59. Reichenbach, D.D. and Benditt, E.P. Catecholamines and cardiomyopathy: The pathogenesis and potential importance of myofibrillar degeneration. *Human Path.* 1:125 (1970).
60. Cruickshank, J.M. et al. A possible role of catecholamines, corticosteroids, and potassium in production of electrocardiographic abnormalities associated with subarachnoid hemorrhage. *Brit. Heart J.* 36:697 (1974).
61. Hawkins, W.E. and Clower, B.R. Myocardial damage after head trauma and simulated intracranial hemorrhage in mice: The role of the autonomic nervous system. *Cardiovasc. Res.* 5:524 (1971).
62. Hunt, D. and Gore, I. Myocardial lesions following experimental intracranial hemorrhage: Prevention with propranolol. *Am. Heart J.* 83:232 (1972).
63. Offerhaus, L. and van Gool, J. ECG changes and tissue catecholamines in experimental subarachnoid hemorrhage. *Cardiovasc. Res.* 3:433 (1969).
64. Alexander, G.H. An unexplained death coexistent with death wishes. *Psychosom. Med.* 5:188 (1943).
65. Coolidge, J.C. Unexpected Death in patient who wished to die. *J. Am. Psychoanal. Ass.* 17:413 (1969).
66. Engel, G.L. A life setting conducive to illness: The Giving UP-Given Up complex. *Bull. Menn. Clin.* 32:355 (1968).
67. Engel, G.L. Sudden and rapid death during psychological stress. Folklore or Folkwisdom? *Ann. Intern. Med.* 74:771 (1971).
68. Goodfriend, M. and Wolpert, E.A. Death from fright: Report of a case and literature review. *Psychosom. Med.* 38:348 (1976).
69. Harvey, W.P. and Levine, S.A. Paroxysmal ventricular tachycardia due to emotion: Possible mechanism of death from fright. *J.A.M.A.* 150:479 (1952).
70. Brow, G.R. et al. Irregularities of the heart under chloroform; their dependence on sympathetic nervous system. *JAMA* 95:715 (1930).
71. Richter, C.P. On the phenomenon of sudden death in animals and man. *Psychosom. Med.* 19:191 (1957).
72. Guillan, R.A. et al. Electrocardiographic and ultrastructural cardiac effects of phenothiazine in rabbits: A preliminary report. *Chest* 62:62 (1972).
73. Guillan, R.A. et al. Electron microscopy; sudden death in patients under phenothiazine therapy: Study of 3 cases. *J. Kansas Med. Soc.* 71:213 (1970).
74. Morpurgo, C. Pharmacological modifications of sympathetic responses elicited by hypothalamic stimulation in the rat. *Br. J. Pharmac.* 34:532 (1968).
75. Connor, R.C.R. Myocardial damage secondary to brain lesions. *Am. Heart J.* 78:145 (1969).
76. Connor, R.C.R. Focal myocytolysis and fuchsinophilic degeneration of the myocardium of patients dying with various brain lesions. *Ann. N.Y. Acad. Sci.* 156:261 (1969).

77. Connor, R.C.R. Heart damage associated with intracranial lesions. *Brit. Med. J.* 3:29 (1968).
78. Connor, R.C.R. Fuchsinophilic degeneration of myocardium in patients with intracranial lesions. *Brit. Heart J.* 32:81 (1970).
79. Shkhvatsabaia, I.K. Attempt at experimental reproduction of cardiac lesions through action on the nervous system. *Kardiologiya* 3:18 (1961).
80. Duran, D.R. and Becker, A.E. Focal myocytolysis mimicking the electrocardiographic pattern of transmural anteroseptal myocardial infarction. *Chest* 69:506 (1976).
81. Martin, A.M. and Hackel, E.B. An electron microscopic study of the progression of myocardial lesions in the dog after hemorrhagic shock. *Lab. Invest.* 15:243 (1966).
82. Martin, A.M. et al. The ultrastructure of zonal lesions of the myocardium in hemorrhagic shock. *Amer. J. Path.* 44:124 (1964).
83. Martin, A.M. et al. Mechanisms in the development of myocardial lesions in hemorrhagic shock. *Ann. N.Y. Acad. Sci.* 156:79 (1969).
84. Schlesinger, M.J. and Reiner, L. Focal myocytolysis of the heart. *Amer. J. Path.* 31:443 (1955).
85. Morales, A.R. et al. Cardiac surgery and myocardial necrosis. *Arch. Path.* 83:71 (1967).
86. Baroldi, G. Different types of myocardial necrosis in coronary heart disease: A pathophysiologic review of their functional significance. *Am. Heart J.* 89:742 (1975).
87. Selye, H. The evolution of the stress concept. *Am. J. Cardiol.* 26:289 (1970).
88. Kelly, G. et al. Thioridazine hydrochloride: Its effects on the electrocardiogram and a report of 2 fatalities with electrocardiographic abnormalities. *Canad. M.A.J.* 89:546 (1963).
89. Hollister, L.E. and Kosek, J.C. Sudden death during treatment with phenothiazine derivatives. *JAMA* 192:1035 (1965).
90. Sulkowitch, H. et al. Excretion of urinary epinephrines in psychiatric disorders. *Proc. Soc. Exper. Biol. Med.* 95:245 (1957).
91. Rahe, R.H. and Arthur, R.J. Biochemical correlates of behavior: A digest of selected studies. *Dis. Nerv. Sys.* 29:114 (1968).
92. Bunney, W.E. et al. Study of a patient with 48-hour manic-depressive cycles. II. Strong positive correlations between endocrine factors and manic defense patterns. *Arch. Gen. Psych.* 12:619 (1965).
93. Bergsman, A. The urinary excretion of adrenaline and noradrenaline in some mental diseases: A clinical and experimental study. *Acta Psychiat. Neurologica Scand.* Suppl. 133 34:11 (1959).
94. Strom-Olsen, R. and Weil-Malherbe, H. Humoral changes in manic-depressive psychosis with particular reference to the excretion of catecholamines in urine. *J. Ment. Sci.* 104:696 (1958).
95. Funkenstein, D.H. et al. Norepinephrine-like and epinephrine-like substances in psychotic and psychoneurotic patients. *Am. J. Psychiat.* 108:652 (1951-52).
96. Haerem, J.W. Myocardial lesions in sudden unexpected coronary deaths. *Am. Heart J.* 90:562 (1975).
97. James, T.N. Apoplexy of the heart. *Circulation* 57:358 (1978).
98. Solymos, B. et al. The role of electrolyte disturbances and extracellular alkalosis in metabolic cardiac necrosis and the preventive effect of amiloride. *Am. J. Cardiol.* 26:46 (1970).
99. Burton, R. et al. Water and electrolyte content of rat heart after thioridazine administration. *J. Clin. Pharmacol.* 7:271 (1967).
100. Ratliff, N.B. et al. Myocardial zonal lesions. *Circ. Shock.* 3:77 (1976).
101. Pugh, B.R. et al. Cardioversion and "false positive" technetium-99m stannous pyrophosphate myocardial scintigrams. *Circulation* 54:399 (1976).
102. Di Cola, V.C. et al. Effect of direct current countershock upon myocardial technetium-99m stannous pyrophosphate uptake. *Am. J. Cardiol.* 37:131 (1976).

103. Madow, L. and Stauffer, J. Analysis of incidence and causes of death in an acute psychopathic hospital. *Am. J. Med. Sci.* 212:471 (1946).
104. Van Vliet, P.D. et al. Focal myocarditis associated with pheochromocytoma. *New Eng. J. Med.* 274:1102 (1966).
105. Kline, I.K. Myocardial alterations associated with pheochromocytomas. *Am. J. Pathol.* 38:539 (1961).
106. Alpert, L.I. et al. Cardiomyopathy associated with a pheochromocytoma: Report of a case with ultrastructural examination of the myocardial lesions. *Arch. Path.* 93:544 (1972).
107. Verrier, R.L. et al. Ventricular vulnerability during sympathetic stimulation: Role of heart rate and blood pressure. *Cardiovasc. Res.* 8:602 (1974).
108. Schamroth, L. Genesis and evolution of ectopic ventricular rhythms. *Brit. Heart J.* 28:244 (1966).
109. Waldo, A.L. and Kaiser, G.A. A study of ventricular arrhythmias associated with acute myocardial infarctions in the canine heart. *Circulation* 47:1222 (1973).
110. Nelson, G. et al. Correlation of behavior and metabolite excretion. *Psychosom. Med.* 28:216 (1966).
111. Di Cola, V.C. et al. Myocardial uptake of technetium-99m stannous pyrophosphate following direct current transthoracic countershock. *Circulation* 54:980 (1976).
112. Zugibe, F.T. et al. Determination of myocardial alterations at autopsy in the absence of gross and microscopic changes. *Arch. Path.* 81:409 (1966).
113. Burke, W.M. et al. Effects of glucose and non-glucose infusion on myocardial potassium ion transfers and arrhythmias during ischemia. *Am. J. Cardiol.* 24:713 (1969).
114. Harris, A.S. Excitatory factors in ventricular tachycardia resulting from myocardial ischemia: Potassium a major excitant. *Science* 119:200 (1954).
115. Cherbakoff, A. et al. Relation between coronary sinus potassium and cardiac arrhythmia. *Circ. Res.* 5:517 (1957).
116. Regan, T.J. et al. Ventricular arrhythmias and potassium transfer during myocardial ischemia and intervention with procaine amide, insulin, or glucose solution. *J. Clin. Investig.* 46:1657 (1967).
117. Schwartzfarb, L. et al. Heroin-associated rhabdomyolysis with cardiac involvement. *Arch. Int. Med.* 137:1255 (1977).
118. Welty, J.D. and Read, W.O. Studies on Some Cardiac Effects of Taurine. *J. Pharm. Exper. Therap.* 144:110 (1964).
119. Brown, E.B. and Mowlem, A. Potassium Loss from the Heart During the Immediate Posthypercapnic Period. *Am. J. Physiol.* 198:962 (1960).

Chapter 13

Electrocardiographic Considerations

Inasmuch as it now is recognized that atherosclerotic coronary artery disease is the leading cause of sudden death in westernized societies[1] numerous investigators have sought to determine which features in the electrocardiogram of a known "coronary patient" would be the most likely precursors of such a catastrophe. As a result, it has been observed that the most significant of such electrocardiographic "risk factors" proved to be non-drug related S-T segment deviations[2,3] and/or repeated ventricular premature contractions[4,5-9]. With regard to the latter, those which were "fired" during the so-called vulnerable period of the ventricle have been considered to be the ones most likely to initiate a cardiac-arresting ventricular tachyarrhythmia.[8,10-11,57-59]

ECG CHANGES THAT FORECAST SUDDEN CARDIAC ARREST

In persons without ischemic heart disease, a miscellaneous and different group of changes have come to be recognized as electrocardiographic forerunners of a sudden cardiac arrest. These include the following: (a) the deep T-wave inversions which sometimes are associated with various types of intracranial pathology or neurosurgical procedures confined to the central nervous system[12-14] (b) the widened QRS complexes which can be the precursors of an asystolic cardiac arrest in persons who have developed an episode of tricyclic antidepressant intoxication (see Chapter 15); (c) the conspicuous U-wave which is identified with quinidine administration,[15,17] hypokalemia,[16,18-21] intracranial lesions,[12] or the Inherited Susceptibility to Sudden Death syndrome (see Chapter 14).

However, the combination of a subordinate T-wave and an enlargement of the juxtaposed U wave often has been described as a "prolonged Q-T interval".[12,17] As a result, many reports indicate that a "lengthening of the Q-T interval" rather than an exaggerated U wave is the electrocardiographic counterpart of the sort of ventricular repolarization abnormality likely to favor the occurrence of an arrhythmogenic cardiac arrest.[22-33,87,65] Moreover, others have claimed that the electrocardiographic change usually produced by customary doses of chlorpromazine or thioridazine can be termed a "hypokalemia-like" effect;[50] a "quinidine-like effect;[34,35] or a "cardiotoxic effect."[36] However, it should be explained that the data derived from organized investigations are not in accord with any of these interpretations with respect to such a drug induced electrocardiographic effect.

DRUG-INDUCED T-WAVE ABNORMALITIES

Actually, many well-planned surveys have shown that the only meaningful electrocardiographic abnormality produced by customary doses of chlorpromazine, thioridazine, or mesoridazine, is merely a benign alteration of the T-wave.[37-49,51-53] Morphologically, three varieties can be recognized.[38-43] Thus, a Grade I abnormality has been described as a T-wave which was not reduced in amplitude but was broadened, truncated, or bifid; flattening and broadening of the T-wave was considered a Grade II abnormality; and a T-wave inversion, infrequent in occurrence, and less than 1 mm in depth, was classified as a Grade III abnormality.

Phenothiazines

Occasionally, it has been observed that any grade of a phenothiazine-induced electrocardiographic abnormality can follow the administration of 100 mg of such drugs with an aliphatic or piperidine moiety; much more often, one of these varieties of T-wave change was seen when the daily dose ranged between 400 and 800 mg a day.[42,43,45]

In addition, it was not unusual to find that in serial electrocardiograms obtained over a fixed period while the patient continued to receive the same dose of the phenothiazine, there was a spontaneous variation in the degree of T-wave abnormality induced by the drug.[38-41] Thus, inasmuch as variations in the morphology of the T-wave similarly have been observed in serial electrocardiograms of emotionally disturbed individuals who never had received phenothiazine compounds,[54,55,56] it was suspected that such spontaneous mutations of phenothiazine-induced T-wave abnormalities might have been due, at least in part, to variable levels of emotional upheaval in the patients who were receiving these phrenotropic substances. However, it cannot be discounted that such spontaneous fluctuations in the degree of T-wave change might be related solely to the pharmacokinetics of these particular psychotropic agents.

Another meaningful feature of the T-wave change produced by the phenothiazines was the relationship of its occurrence to the daily doses of these drugs. In this connection, it is noteworthy that the findings in a large sample of thioridazine treated patients have shown that whereas there was a positive correlation between the magnitude of the mean daily dose and the incidence of T-wave malformation, there was no correlation between the amount of drug consumed and the grade of T-wave abnormality which followed the administration of doses ranging between 100 to 800 mg daily.[41,42,45] This observation would seem to indicate that although the drug altered the morphology of the T-wave, such an electrocardiographic effect should not be construed as an evidence that it is cardiotoxic. Correspondingly, the T-wave malformation produced by customary doses of thioridazine should be viewed as an entirely benign effect.

Thioridazine

Generally, a phonocardiographic study can be employed to delineate more precisely the morphologic features of a T-wave abnormality which commonly follows the administration of customary doses of thioridazine. In this connection, it can be a particularly useful means of showing the temporal relationship between the second hump of a bifid T-wave and the onset of the second heart sound. Correspondingly, it can determine whether the two components of the deflection should be considered a part of the T-wave or whether the second hump is a U wave. The latter is a deflection which is not only diastolic in time; according to competent investigators[61] its apex is inscribed between 0.04 sec. and 0.14 sec. after the onset of the second heart sound.

Moreover, it is of interest that such a study, performed by Kalbian[62] demonstrated clearly that, in the electrocardiogram of a normokalemic thioridazine-treated patient, the apex of the second hump of a bifid T-wave was inscribed 0.01 sec. after the onset of the second heart sound. Thus, his studies had indicated conclusively that U-wave enlargement is not a characteristic electrocardiographic response to the administration of customary doses of thioridazine.

Discussion

Moreover, it should be recognized that it would be imprecise to equate such a broadened bifid T-wave with a lengthening of the Q-T interval. The only currently available normal standards with respect to the Q-T interval have been derived from an analysis of normal electrocardiograms, in which the T-wave was normal not only in terms of its configuration, but also in terms of its duration. Thus, when the T-wave is broadened and notched, it is questionable whether any measurement of the Q-T interval would have any validity, if the interval is determined to be "lengthened" on the basis of a comparison with currently available normal standards. Moreover, my views, in this regard, would still pertain even though suitable corrections are made for the established influences of various heart rates of the Q-T interval ($Q\text{-}T_c$).

Similarly, my examination of the data in the report by Huston and Bell which appeared in 1966[45] indicated that the relatively minor "prolongation of the Q-T interval" in the electrocardiograms of their phenothiazine-treated patients could be ascribed entirely to the slight widening of the T-wave resulting from the administration of customary doses of such psychotropic drugs. During one phase of their studies, these investigators had correlated, in a sample of psychiatric patients receiving variable doses of thioridazine, the mean daily dose of this phrenotropic agent with both the QT_c value and the configuration of the T-wave, and found that only gross distortions of this deflection were associated with increased QT_c values. However, even then, the increase was very slight; actually it did not exceed 6 percent above the norm. Thus, according to the criteria established by a special task force of the American College of Cardiology, appointed to develop a "soundly based widely accepted uniform terminology for electrocardiographic interpretation" this degree of "prolongation of the Q-T interval" would be considered to be of no clinical significance.[63] Moreover, it is noteworthy that even Albidskov, who has investigated intensively the pathogenesis of the electrocardiographic changes identified with abnormal ventricular repolarization in the experimental animal has cautioned that "there are ambiguities in the measurement of the Q-T interval which are dependent on T-wave form."[64]

It should be recognized also that Huston and Bell[45] as well as Samet and Surawicz[47] had interpreted their data, with respect to T-wave malformations or Q-T duration in the electrocardiograms of their respective samples of phenothiazine treated patients, to be supportive of the view that such drug-induced electrocardiographic findings were neither expressive of any cardiac damage nor a counterpart of a repolarization abnormality which might be the forerunner of a sudden cardiac arrest. Thus, whenever the findings in an electrocardiogram of a phenothiazine-treated psychiatric patient signify the presence of a repolarization abnormality, one imperative must be to distinguish between the usual harmless phenothiazine-induced electrocardiographic effect from a change which is not only unrelated, etiologically, to the consumption of such a drug but also the sort which could be predictive of a sudden unexpected death.

This need was demonstrated on an occasion when this author had reviewed the electrocardiograms of two middle-aged schizophrenic women without demonstrable organic heart disease. Both had received identical medication (600 mg of thioridazine daily), but whereas one was still alive, the other had died suddenly and unexpectedly. It should be explained also that electrocardiograms had not been obtained, in either instance, before the thioridazine therapy had been instituted.

Furthermore, these two patients were different from an electrocardiographic standpoint. Thus, the only noteworthy abnormality in the electrocardiograms of the survivor was a broadened T-wave (equivalent QT_c value merely 6% to 8% above normal); clearly, this value was compatible with simply a benign thioridazine effect.[63] By contrast, in the premortem electrocardiograms of the decedent, the conspicuous change was an enlargement of the U wave easily recognizable as a deflection separate from its juxtaposed T-wave. Moreover, if the U wave had been identified, mistakenly, as part of the T-wave, the calculated QT_c value would have averaged +24%, a figure which automatically would indicate that the electrocardiographic findings, in this instance, were not related to the consumption of customary doses of thioridazine.

Therefore, it was suggested that the fatality was linked to one of the arrhythmogenic U-wave syndromes mentioned earlier in this chapter. However, since the decedent had not received quinidine salts and was not hypokalemic, it seemed likely that the enlarged U wave was the electrocardiographic counterpart of the Inherited Susceptibility to Sudden Death syndrome (see Chapter 14). Moreover, this interpretation was re-enforced when it was learned later that numerous seemingly inexplicable sudden deaths had occurred in various relatives of the decedent and that the postmortem examination had not provided any reason for her untimely death.

SERUM POTASSIUM LEVEL AND U-WAVE ENLARGEMENT

Illustrative of a different sort of U-wave enlargement in the electrocardiogram of a psychiatric patient was the prominent U-wave in the electrocardiogram of a young adult who, while receiving a daily ration of 200 mg of thioridazine, developed an intercurrent hypokalemia secondary to a severe episode of toxic gastroenteritis. On the day after his admission to the hospital, his serum potassium level was found to be 2.9 mEq; in the electrocardiogram made on that day there was an enlargement of the U-wave and, because this deflection was fused to its juxtaposed T-wave in certain leads, the net effect was an illusory "prolongation of the Q-T interval." Because of the low serum potassium level and the typical hypokalemic effect on the electrocardiogram, potassium supplements were prescribed; thus, on April 13, 1973, the second day of his hospitalization, the serum potassium level was higher (3.9 mEq) but in the electrocardiogram made on that day the U-wave still was enlarged and fused to its adjoining T-wave.

The patient continued to receive potassium supplements along with other definitive therapy and thereafter there was a gradual improvement with respect to his clinical status, serum electrolyte levels and electrocardiographic findings. On April 30, 1973, when the serum potassium level was 4.2 mEq, the electrocardiogram was normal in all respects. Moreover, during his entire period of confinement to the hospital, no cardiac arrhythmia had been observed. On July 11, 1973, approximately two months after he had resumed his customary daily dose of thioridazine, a follow-up electrocardiogram was obtained; this electrocardiogram was normal except for the presence of a truncated T-wave, a finding which correctly, was ascribed solely to the resumption of his customary dose of thioridazine.

Thus, in retrospect, the findings in this instance represented two of the three usual accompaniments of a potassium deficit. The only omission was a documented episode of ventricular arrhythmia, a feature which undoubtedly must be viewed as the most alarming complication to result from such an electrolyte disturbance. As yet, the pathogenesis of such an arrhythmia in hypokalemic patients is not entirely understood, but experiential data undoubtedly would seem to indicate that, in electrocardiographic terms, the element which can be considered to be its precursor is the enlargement of the U-wave.[19]

Moreover, there still is much to be learned with respect to the nature of the electrophysiologic complexities connected with the inscription of an enlarged U-wave. Some years ago, Lepeschkin[60] suggested that a dominant U-wave resulted from the persistence of "after potentials" during ventricular repolarization but he did not provide any experimental data which could confirm such a hypothesis. More recently, his view has been replaced by concepts advanced by Albidskov,[64] as well as by Reynolds and van der Ark.[17] These investigators postulated that it was a delay in "ventricular recovery" with a resultant incomplete "cancellation of voltages" which could account for the enlargement of this deflection. However, these respective authors also had elected to consider this electrocardiographic feature the equivalent of a "prolongation of the Q-T interval" and, correspondingly had invoked such designations as "Q-T interval syndromes" or "delayed repolarization syndromes" in order to identify the electrocardiographic hallmark of the entities discussed in their respective articles.

There also are other intriguing features which pertain to the U-wave enlargement phenomenon in man and these are discussed in articles by

Surawicz and Lepeschkin,[61] by Kerhunen et al,[27] by Moss and Mc Donald,[28] by James[87] and by Schwartz et al.[65] Moreover, with the exception of the publication by Surawicz and Lepeschkin (which was concerned primarily with the electrocardiographic correlates of hypokalemia and hypocalcemia),[61] these reports pertained to the behavior of the U wave identified with the presence of an inherited repolarization disorder likely to favor the occurrence of a life-threatening ventricular tachyarrhythmia (see Chapter 15).

In their investigations, Kerhunen et al[27] had noted that the slow intravenous infusion of potassium chloride sufficient to raise the serum potassium value from 4.2 mEq (a normal level) to 5.7 mEq resulted in "increased amplitude of the T-wave but the amplitude of the U wave remained unchanged and there were no changes in the Q-T and Q-U intervals." By contrast, Surawicz and Lepeschkin had remarked that the primary effect of potassium supplementation in patients with hypokalemia was to reduce the size of the U wave without, at the same time, increasing the altitude of the adjoining T-wave.

On the other hand, the investigations of Moss and Mc Donald[28] and of Schwartz et al[65] were confined to observations concerning the effects of surgically achieved inhibition of adrenergic activity. In this connection, Moss and Mc Donald reported, for the first time, that when a susceptibility to recurrent attacks of ventricular arrhythmia represented an inherited trait, the excision of the left stellate ganglion not only was followed by cessation of these arrhythmic episodes but also by a disappearance of the enlarged U wave which, prior to the stellectomy, was a characteristic feature in the interarrhythmic electrocardiograms.

Similar results were described by Schwartz et al[65] who also commented that whereas the noteworthy electrocardiographic change preceding the stellectomy was a "prolonged Q-T interval", such a procedure was followed not only by a *"shortening of the Q-T interval"* but also by a *"great increase in the ventricular fibrillation threshold."* Moreover, inasmuch as Schwartz et al had equated "prolongation of the Q-T interval" with enlargement of the U wave, it can be inferred that a conspicuous U wave is an electrocardiographic finding which is expressive of electrophysiologic alterations in ventricular muscle which are especially prone to favor a decrease in the ventricular fibrillation threshold. A similar correlation between U wave enlargement and a lowering of the ventricular fibrillation threshold was demonstrated by Kliks et al[85] in connection with their canine studies. Thus, there are sufficient data to indicate that it is an enlargement of the U wave which must be considered a major electrocardiographic forerunner of a life-threatening ventricular tachyarrhythmia.

By contrast, it is equally well established that ventricular arrhythmias are not identified with the sort of Q-T prolongation which is a characteristic electrocardiographic counterpart of hypocalcemia.[17] Thus, inasmuch as U-wave enlargement is not a feature of the hypocalcemic electrocardiogram, it seems evident that whereas magnified "U-wave potentials" can be an electrocardiographic "risk factor" with respect to the occurrence of a life-threatening ventricular arrhythmia, simply a lengthening of the Q-T interval, in the strict sense of the term, should not be so considered.

In this same connection, it should not be overlooked that although hypocalcemia alone does not favor the occurrence of life-threatening ventricular arrhythmias[17] it has been observed that arrhythmias have developed when both hypocalcemia and hypopotassemia were present together.[66,67] Thus, since potassium depletion characteristically is responsible for enlargement of the U-wave, such an observation would seem to provide further confirmation of the thesis that, of the various electrocardiographic components, it is a conspicuous augmentation of the U-wave which is most likely to be associated with the development of a life-threatening ventricular tachyarrhythmia.

In addition, it has been found by Surawicz that when the blood calcium level was lowered by administering EDTA to patients with supraventricular and ventricular ectopic beats, there actually was a suppression of such arrhythmias; moreover, ectopic beats suppressed in this manner reappeared after calcium administration.[66,67] In view of this correlation, it was suggested that such a hypocalcemic antiarrhythmic effect could be ascribed to a concurrent increase in the duration of the effective refractory period secondary to a delayed completion of ventricular repolarization exemplified by the hypocalcemic lengthening of the Q-T interval.[66,67] In any case it would seem correct to conclude that unequivocal prolongation of the Q-T interval, which is the electrocardiographic counterpart of calcium depletion, in man, should be linked coordinately with a physiologic change which actually inhibits rather than enhances ventricular ectopic activity.

Moreover, whereas it has been established that an inherited variety of U-wave enlargement (see Chapter 14) is not affected by the administration of a potassium compound[27] and that a quinidine-induced U-wave enlargement will persist despite the administration of a nitrate compound,[68] it has been found that either of these interventions regularly will abolish completely a primary phenothiazine-induced T-wave malformation[38-41,46,48,52,69-71] as well as other nonspecific "functional" T-wave abnormalities.[69-71,73,97]

In order to achieve this sort of result in normokalemic thioridazine-treated patients, it should be certain first, that both such interventions should not be employed on the same day; second, that both the control electrocardiogram and subsequent electrocardiograms be obtained during a single testing session; third, that when the response to the nitrate is being evaluated, all electrocardiograms should be made with the subject both supine and erect; fourth, that the nitrate compound should be one which is incorporated in a rapidly soluble tablet suitable for placement into the sublingual pouch; and fifth, that the potassium mixture, which is swallowed as a single draught, should consist of 5 grams of potassium acetate and 5 grams of potassium citrate dissolved in 100 cc of water. Timewise, the post-nitrate electrocardiograms should be obtained 10 to 20 minutes after the nitrate triturate tablet (either 0.6 mg of glyceryl trinitrate or 10 mg of isosorbide dinitrate) has dissolved in the mouth and the post-potassium electrocardiograms should be obtained both 60 and 90 minutes after the potassium mixture has been swallowed.

Ideally, the subject should omit breakfast on the morning when the response to potassium is being studied. Ordinarily, the maximal effect produced by the potassium solution is discernable 60 minutes after it is swallowed but since the absorption factor may be a slightly variable element, it has been found advantageous to record electrocardiograms both 60 and 90 minutes after the use of this intervention.[69] Moreover, it is simple to correlate the nature of the electrocardiographic response with the serum potassium level by an assay of such values in blood samples drawn before and 60-90 minutes after the potassium solution has been administered. My own data pertaining to such a procedure have shown that, on average, the serum potassium level rose from 4.0 mEq. to 5.5 mEq. concurrently with the normalization of the T-wave;[69] occasionally, slightly higher levels were reached but, even then, no arrhythmias or other adverse effects developed.

Contraindications to Potassium Therapy

The only unquestionable contraindication to this type of pharmacologic intervention is the presence of renal impairment, or a recent myocardial infarction. Therefore, it is recommended that it not be employed if, during a preliminary medical screen, laboratory studies have confirmed an elevation of the urea nitrogen or serum creatinine level. Moreover, certain authors have reported serious adverse cardiac effects following the administration of a bolus of potassium salts to patients who have experienced a recent myocardial infarction.[72] Thus, it would be prudent to avoid administering a peroral preparation of potassium salts if the purpose is solely to ascertain the effect of such an intervention on a primary T-wave abnormality resulting from an acute myocardial lesion. So far, my own experiences[69] and those of Wasserburger and Corliss[73] have indicated that such a peroral preparation of potassium salts will not produce any harmful effects in subjects with varied types of chronic myocardial disease.

In this connection, it is noteworthy that following the administration of

10 gm of potassium perorally to a series of psychiatric patients whose electrocardiograms were characterized by the presence of T-wave abnormalities due to some form of structural heart disease, it was my experience that no adverse effects resulted from this intervention.[69] Coincidentally, it was noted that primary T-wave abnormalities due to structural heart disease were not abolished by the administration of such a potassium mixture.[69,71,73] Thus, it now is evident that whereas, in normokalemic individuals, the administration of potassium salts will abolish neither a U-wave enlargement unassociated with organic heart disease[27] nor a T-wave distortion due to cardiac pathology,[69,71,73] such an intervention will regularly completely normalize those electrocardiograms which would be considered to be abnormal only by virtue of the presence of a phenothiazine-related T-wave abnormality.[69,71]

ERGOTAMINE TARTRATE ADMINISTRATION

Another preparation which has succeeded in normalizing the T-wave in phenothiazine-treated psychiatric patients without demonstrable organic heart disease has been the commercially available ergotamine tartrate, administered intravenously as a single bolus.[38,41,71,74] For this purpose, the effective dose of this ergot alkaloid was found to be 0.5 mg, dissolved in 1 cc of diluent. However, in three important respects, the T-wave transformation produced by this substance was different from the normalization of the T-wave which followed the sublingual administration of a rapidly acting nitrate.

Thus, whereas the favorable nitrate effect on the T-wave was evident usually when the electrocardiogram was made with the subject erect,[38,39,70] the normalization of the T-wave after ergotamine administration generally occurred while the subject remained supine.[39] This ergotamine-induced normalization of the T-wave was maximal between 15 and 30 minutes after its injection and the duration of this effect generally persisted for 30 minutes longer.

Equally impressive was the observation tha although the T-wave was normalized by either the ergot preparation or the nitrate compound, this effect could not be correlated with the heart rate or blood pressure response following the administration of these two respective substances. Thus, coincident with normalization of the T-wave achieved by the injection of ergotamine tartrate, the heart rate was slowed and the blood pressure rose slightly whereas orthostatic rectification of the T-wave after nitrate administration was associated with a moderate rise in the heart rate and a modest drop in the blood pressure.

Moreover, it it is noteworthy that my studies have shown that the administration of this same ergot preparation actually induced an anginal episode along with an "ischemic" sagging of the ST segment only in subjects with a known anginal syndrome secondary to occlusive coronary artery disease.[75] Also, in this connection, it should be explained that data now are available to indicate that an existing T-wave abnormality due to any type of structural cardiac abnormality will not be normalized by a similar dose of this ergot derivative.[54-56] Presumably, when this ergot alkaloid causes the ST segment depression in the electrocardiogram of known coronary patients, this effect can be ascribed to its coronary-constricting property.

This view seems to be supported by the results of arteriographic studies which have demonstrated that a kindred ergot alkaloid will produce such a vasoconstrictive action in patients of this genre; during these investigations it was noted also that after this drug was injected, the coronary constriction and associated anginal symptoms abated quickly following sublingual administration of glyceryl trinitrate.[76]

Correspondingly, on the basis of data of this sort, it would seem improper to suppose that because a nitrate compound can abolish the T-wave abnormality produced by customary doses of a phenothiazine compound, the abnormality is related to an impairment in coronary blood flow. Conversely, it is likely that the repolarization abnormality and its electrocardiographic counterpart which is produced by phenothiazine administration, is corrected by ergotamine and by nitrate compounds because these two particular interventions can produce extravascular effects still incompletely understood. Conceivably, disturbed autonomic activity may play an important role in the pathogenesis of a phenothiazine induced T-wave abnormality and correspondingly the action of the ergot compound and the nitrate preparation may be related to their respective effects on the neural pathways to the heart.

In this connection, it is noteworthy that certain investigations have shown that an injection of ergotamine tartrate will augment vagal influences on cardiac conduction,[77-78] and thus it can be perceived as a drug which indirectly can inhibit adrenergic influences. Moreover, to postulate that autonomic influences may contribute to a meaningful degree to the production of a phenothiazine-induced T-wave abnormality would be to provide some understanding of the reason that a beta blocker such as propranolol will abort or abolish the T-wave distortion which results from the consumption of customary doses of a phenothiazine derivative.[53] Furthermore, this view would seem to be supported by the results of earlier studies which have shown that the intravenous administration of a single dose of ergotamine tartrate will abolish the "functional and harmless primary type of T-wave abnormality commonly present in the routine electrocardiograms of nonphenothiazine-treated emotionally unstable persons.[54-56]

CARDIAC EFFECTS OF QUINIDINE AND THIORIDAZINE

Another set of meaningful studies, with respect to phenothiazine-induced T-wave abnormalities were those conducted by Samet and Surawicz.[47] Essentially, the purpose of their investigation was to compare the electrocardiographic effects and changes in ventricular function produced by therapeutically equivalent doses of quinidine and thioridazine in subjects without any demonstrable organic heart disease. Accordingly, their data included observations pertaining to the duration of the QRS and Q-T intervals, measurements of the systolic time intervals, and the response to beta adrenergic stimulation achieved by the intravenous infusion of a suitable amount of isoproterenol.

Altogether, 60 adults, all seemingly free of organic heart disease, were admitted to their study. Twenty were chronic schizophrenics who had received uninterrupted long-term phenothiazine therapy (Group I subjects); 14 were schizophrenics who were receiving short-term phenothiazine therapy and who were studied by similar techniques both while they were receiving customary doses of the drug and after its use had been studied by similar techniques both before and after the administration of customary peroral doses of quinidine (Group IV subjects.)

Results

The results of their studies then showed that quinidine changed the a morphology of the T-wave, depressed ventricular function, and "prolonged the Q-T interval." (note: actually the resulting enlargment of the U-wave was interpreted by them as a "prolonged Q-T interval.") On the other hand, they observed that customary doses of thioridazine and comparable phenothiazine preparations produced merely a configurational change of the T-wave; these drugs did not produce any depression of the ventricular function and did not produce a "prolongation of the Q-T interval." (Note: there was no enlargement of the U-wave following phenothiazine administratration).

Moreover, Samet and Surawicz had observed that, in the phenothiazine-treated subjects, the infusion of isoproterenol was not followed by the appearance of a cardiac arrhythmia. Consequently, inasmuch as experimental studies have shown that adrenergic stimulation ordinarily enhances inhomogeneous dispersion of refractoriness throughout the ventricular muscle mass and thereby lowers the ventricular fibrillation threshold,[88-92] the findings reported by Samet and Surawicz suggest that it would be inappropriate to suppose that a phenothiazine-induced T-wave change is the electrocardiographic correlate of that type of repolarization disturbance which would be expected to favor the occurrence of a life-threatening ventricular tachyarrhythmia.

EFFECTS OF LITHIUM TREATMENT

There is another drug-related T-wave abnormality of a controversial nature which has been observed in the electrocardiograms of normokalemic psychiatric patients; this abnormality is the readily reversible T-wave change which often follows the consumption of therapeutic amounts of lithium.[79-82] This drug-induced electrocardiographic effect was observed originally by Schou[79] and it is his view that it merely signifies the presence of a benign asymptomatic repolarization disorder, and that "if lithium would be discontinued merely becuse this cation had produced a change in the electrocardiogram, many patients would, without justification, be deprived of a valuable treatment."[79] Moreover, this interpretation also agrees with the views of Demers and Heninger.[81-82]

In addition, the results of a study undertaken by Tilkian et al[83] would seem to confirm the benign nature of lithium-induced T-wave changes. Primarily, the purpose of these investigators was to determine whether any adverse cardiac effect, including a proneness to arrhythmias would be a sequel to the continued use of therapeutic amounts of lithium, even when this substance was administerred to persons with some form of organic heart disease.

Therefore, in connection with the cardiac evaluation of their subjects, they included observations concerning the response to treadmill testing and during continuous Holter monitoring both before and after the administration of customary amounts of a lithium salt. The results of their study showed that the lithium did not produce any type of adverse cardiac effects in this sample of patients and so they were able to conclude that the effects of customary doses of this cation on the heart were entirely innocuous.

On the other hand, Kochar et al[84] who showed that the T-wave in the routine electrocardiograms of two lithium-treated patients was distorted, drew a different conclusion. These authors considered the change to be a hypokalemic effect even though all the serum electrolyte levels including lithium and potassium were well within normal limits. Moreover, my examination of the figures included with that article clearly indicated that the nature of the abnormality was simply a broadening and notching of the T-waves of the sort which characterizes a phenothiazine induced T-wave abnormality; in neither instance was the U wave enlarged nor was the QT_c value disproportionately increased. Thus, even though Kochar et al had advanced the view that lithium produces a hypokalemia-like electrocardiographic effect, there is not, as yet, any substantiating evidence to support such a thesis. Moreover, inasmuch as there is still some disagreement regarding the meaning of a lithium-induced T-wave change, it would be of interest to determine whether a lithium induced T-wave abnormality could be abolished by either a nitrate compound or potassium mixture in the same manner that such interventions were able to normalize a phenothiazine induced T-wave malformation.

U-WAVE PROMINENCE AND ARRHYTHROGENIC CARDIAC ARREST

Basically, so far, the data pertaining to the electrocardiograms of psychiatric patients would seem to indicate that, in general, it would be proper to regard a minor readily reversible nonspecific T-wave abnormality as an expression of simply a benign non-alarming repolarization disorder. On the other hand, there is a substantial body of experimental and experiental data to show that an enlargement of the U wave can be, indeed, an ominous finding. To a large extent, this connotation with respect to a dominant U-wave stems from an awareness that it is an electrocardiographic deviant which could be the portent of a life-threatening ventricular tacharrhythmia. Thus, it would be advantageous, at this juncture, to examine the observations which have investigated this particular association between U-wave prominence and the occurrence of an arrhythmogenic cardiac arrest.

Within such a context, it would seem proper to begin with an examination of the observations reported in 1975 by Kliks et al[85] however, inasmuch as their experiments constituted an extension of earlier studies conducted by Yanowitz et al,[86] it would be preferable to discuss, first, the findings described by the latter group of investigators.

Surgically-Induced Sympathetic Outflow

The canine experiments undertaken by Yanowitz et al were designed to demonstrate the changes in ventricular repolarization which result from surgically induced modification of sympathetic outflow to the heart. To achieve this objective, they obtained electrocardiographic recordings after the right and left stellate ganglia were removed, separately, and in this way they were able to show that a significant change occurred only when the right ganglion was removed and the left remained intact and unopposed.

ECG Results

The nature of the electrocardiographic effects resulting from right stellate ganglion exclusion, a circumstance akin to left stellate ganglion stimulation, was described by them as a prolongation of the Q-T interval but it was evident from an inspection of their data that such a label was a misnomer; semantically, it would have been more correct if they had indicated that the most impressive electrocardiographic effect of this intervention was an enlargement of the U wave.

Later, Kliks et al[85] utilized a slight modification of this same experimental model to determine whether augmented adrenergic influences reaching the heart from the left stellate ganglion, would simultaneously enlarge the U wave and lower the ventricular fibrillation threshold. In order to measure this threshold, these investigators determined the milleamperage required to produce an episode of ventricular fibrillation by the delivery to the ventricle of a constant current stimulus with a frequency of 100 Hertz and a duration of 2 milliseconds after every 9th basic driven cycle. Then, having established control values with the use of such a procedure, they demonstrated clearly that stimulation of the left stellate ganglion lowered the ventricular fibrillation threshold by an average of 42% below control values whereas after the left stellate ganglion had been removed, the ventricular fibrillation threshold was raised to an average of 31% above control values.

On the other hand, Schwartz et al,[65] who also studied the effects of sympathetic stimulation on the ventricular fibrillation threshold, employed an experimental model which permitted the delivery of a train of gated stimuli scanning the entire vulnerable period of the ventricle. These shocks were applied to the right anterior or left posterior ventricular surface of anesthetized and vagotomized dogs and in this manner it was possible to establish the intervention which, reciprocally, lowered and elevated the ventricular fibrillation threshold.

Heart rate was held constant by atrial pacing. Measurements were obtained in control conditions and after surgical removal of one stellate ganglion. To avoid the shortcomings associated with an irreversible procedure like stellectomy, control fibrillation threshold measurements were also alternated with determinations during reversible blockade by cooling of one stellate ganglion. The results were similar with both techniques. In nine animals, ablation or cooling of the left stellate ganglion increased ventricular threshold by $72 \pm 35\%$ compared with control values ($p < 0.001$).

By contrast, in 11 animals, ablation or cooling of the right stellate ganglion lowered the threshold by $48 \pm 14\%$ compared with control values ($p < 0.001$). Electrode location did not influence the results. The observed changes depended solely upon unilateral removal of cardiac sympathetic activity and were not demonstrable if such activity was low. It was also suggested by them that these observed differences with respect to the specific effects of the right and left cardiac sympathetic nerves on cardiac excitability could contribute to an understanding of the pathogenesis of the entity frequently termed "the long Q-T syndrome"[22,65,87] in this monograph, is has been subsumed under the rubric of "The Inherited Susceptibility to Sudden Death" (see Chapter 14).

Thus, an apposition of the data derived from these three separate experimental models would indicate that interventions which augmented adrenergic stimuli reaching the myocardium could be responsible simultaneously for an enlargement of the U wave and a lowering of the ventricular fibrillation threshold. Correspondingly, inasmuch as earlier observations have indicated that heightened sympathetic activity can stimulate ectopic impulse formation and favor the reentry of ventricular ectopic beats,[88-92] it would seem proper to consider most enlargements of the U wave to be the electrocardiographic representation of sympatheticogenic electrophysiologic events likely to increase the prospect of a life-threatening ventricular tachyarrhythmia.

This conclusion, with respect to the connotation of an exaggerated U wave, would seem to be supported by the results of other experiments as well. In this connection, the findings reported by Fastier adnd Smirk in 1948[93]; by Moore and Swain in 1960[94]; by Hutcheon and Laffan in 1963[95]; and by James and Bear in 1968[96] would seem to be particularly meaningful.

EFFECTS OF EPINEPHRINE AND AMARIN

The studies conducted by Fastier and Smirk[93] were designed to determine the cardiac responses in open-chest dogs to infusions of epinephrine following prior sensitization to amarin. Invariably, when they were used in this manner, these two pharmacologic agents promptly produced a ventricular tachyarrhythmia. Moreover, when this effect was monitored in a conventional electrocardiogram, it was observed that shortly before the arrhythmia developed, a "hypertrophy of the T-wave became visible"; soon afterward, the "R wave of the preceding normally conducted beats climbed up the greatly hypertrophied T-wave in successive cardiac cycles until at one point the R wave was about 2/3 of the way up whereupon ventricular flutter supervened." However, if the figures accompanying the text are examined closely, it will be evident that "the hypertrophied T-wave" actually is a T-wave fused to an enlarged juxtaposed U wave.

EFFECTS OF EPINEPHINE AND PROPIOPHENONE

The experiments conducted by Moore and Swain[94] also employed anesthetized open-chest dogs and the life-threatening ventricular tacharrhythmia was produced by the intravenous injection of a modified propiophenone and a small dose of epinephrine. During a preliminary phase of the study, these animals were monitored after intravenous administration of a small dose of the propiophenone compound and it was observed that such an intervention produced only "a conspicuous lengthening of the Q-T interval and a variable change in the T-wave configuration." Moreover, this T-wave effect was maximal from 2 to 5 minutes following the injection; within 20 to 30 minutes after the injection, the electrocardiogram resembled the control electrocardiogram. However, it should be explained that, actually, the "variable change in the T-wave configuration" was a fusion of an enlarged U wave with its juxtaposed T-wave. Thus, the reported "conspicuous lengthening of the Q-T interval" was an incorrect description of the electrocardiographic changes which had been observed.

Moreover, when small amounts of epinephrine were injected 2 to 5 minutes after the injection of a small dose of the propiophenone compound into these anesthetized animals, an electrocardiogram confirmed the development of ventricular fibrillation. Generally, this arrhythmia appeared about 5 seconds after the epinephrine was injected. A figure showing the electrocardiographic effects accompanied the text and thus it could be seen that several seconds before the onset of the ventricular fibrillation, when a normal sinus mechanism still controlled the cardiac rhythm, there was a marked increase in the size of the repolarization deflection; apparently, this electrocardiographic effect was due to a fusion of the T-wave with an enlarged juxtaposed U wave.

In this experimental situation, Moore and Swain[94] seemingly had again demonstrated that the three essential features of the pharmacologically-induced syndromes they had described included adrenergic stimulation, a consequent enlargement of the U wave, and a subsequent life-threatening ventricular tacharrhythmia. In this same connection, it is also of considerable interest that when, in the anesthetized animal, either levarterenol, isoproterenol, stellate ganglion stimulation, or electrically-driven tachycardia was substituted for the epinephrine, the result was similar to that produced by the epinephrine.

These investigators[94] also noted that, in unanesthetized animals, a different situation prevailed with respect to the induction of this arrhythmia. Thus, in such animals, the supplemental injection of epinephrine was not required to induce an episode of ventricular fibrillation; instead, the injection of the propiophenone compound alone was sufficient to produce this arrhythmia. However, pretreatment with reserpine (a catecholamine depleting agent) prevented this propiophenone efffect in the unanesthetized animal and pretreatment with propranolol prevented the propiophenone-epinephrine induced ventricular fibrillation in the anesthetized animal.

The nature of the repolarization deflections in the electrocardiograms of the propranolol-treated animals were neither described nor shown; accordingly, it is unknown whether this adrenergic blocking agent prevented the ventricular fibrillation primarily, because this pharmacologic intervention was not followed by the appearance of a large U wave in the electrocardiogram of the animals which had received both the epinephrine and the propiophenone compound. However, it would seem reasonable to suppose that there was, indeed, such a connection.

EFFECTS OF INHALED PETROLEUM ETHER AND INJECTED EPINEPHRINE

Another relevant experimental study was the one conducted by Hutcheon and Laffan in 1963.[95] Essentially, the object of their investigation was to provide electrocardiographic data during and just beore episodes of ventricular tachycardia and ventricular fibrillation were induced by exposing anesthetized felines to inhalation of petroleum ether and then injecting epinephrine or norepinephrine. Following these interventions, the cardiac responses were monitored with an electrocardiograph and thus it could be seen that there was a transitional change which preceded the onset of the ventricular tachyarrhythmia. The nature of this transitional change was described by the authors as a "prolongation of the Q-T interval" but it is evident from an inspection of the electrocardiograms included with the text of this report, that the so-called lengthening of the post-depolarization period actually was the result of a fusion of a relatively obscure T-wave with an enlarged U wave. Equally significant was the observation that, in the control electrocardiogram obtained before these interventions were employed, the T-waves and Q-T intervals were normal and no U waves were visible.

EFFECTS OF ALDEHYDE INFUSIONS

Comparable in importance to the experiments already cited is the one reported by James and Bear.[96] The purpose of their study was to determine the effects on the electrocardiogram and the cardiac rhythm of infusions of aldehyde compounds into the myocardium of canine hearts via the sinoatrial nodal branch of the intramural coronary arterial circulation. Of particular interest to them were the responses to the perfusion of the myocardium with solutions of either formaldehyde or glutaraldehyde, both of which were introduced also into the anterior descending coronary artery and into the right atrium.

With the use of this animal model, the primary effect produced by such an intervention actually was an enlargement of the U wave, but James and Bear chose to describe the finding as a "prolonged Q-T interval." The secondary effect, which followed soon afterward was a sudden cardiac arrest. Moreover, it was observed by them that in the 30 formaldehyde "treated" dogs, the terminal event was a ventricular fibrillation in 26 instances and "complete cessation of all electrical cardiac action in the remaining four." In addition, when the perfusate was a solution of glutaraldehyde, the primary effect was similar and, regularly, the secondary effect was a terminal ventricular fibrillation.

CONCLUSIONS

Thus, it seems evident that despite the use of separate experimental models by James and Bear,[96] by Fastier and Smirk,[93], by Moore and Swain,[94] and by Hutcheon and Laffan,[95] respectively, these various investigators had noted a connection between U-wave enlargement and a life-threatening ventricular tachyarrhythmia. Clearly, then, it would seem likely that when a T-wave in a human electrocardiogram is distorted because of a juxtaposed enlargement of the U wave, such a circumstance could reflect concurrent changes in myocardial physiology which, conceivably, could facilitate the re-entry of propaged beats and thereby the occurrence of an epiosde of cardiac arresting ventricular fibrillation. On the other hand, it would seem reasonable to conclude, on the basis of such experimental observations that simply a primary T-wave malformation, expecially if it is abolished readily by the testing methods already described, should not be viewed as a "risk factor" with respect to the occurrence of a sudden life threatening ventricular tachyarrhythmia.

REFERENCES

1. Julian, D.G. Toward preventing coronary deaths. Circulation 54:360 (1976).
2. Frank, C. et al. Angina pectoris in man. Prognostic significance of selected medical factors. Circulation 47:509 (1973).
3. Kronenberg, M.W. et al. S-T segment variations after myocardial infarction. Relationship to clinical status. Circulation 54:756 (1976).
4. Kotler, M.N. et al. Prognostic significance of ventricular ectopic beats with respect to sudden death in the late post-infarction period. Circulation 47:959 (1973).
5. Chiang, B.N. et al. Premature systoles and sudden death. Ann. Int. Med. 70:1159 (1969).
6. Vismara, L.A. et al. Relation of ventricular arrhythmias in the late hospital phase of acute myocardial infarction to sudden death after hospital discharge. Am. J. Med. 59:6 (1975).
7. Coronary Drug Project Research Group: Prognostic importance of premature beats following myocardial infarction. Experience in the Coronary Drug Project. J.A.M.A. 223:1116 (1973).
8. Lawrie, M. et al. A coronary care unit in the routine management of the acute myocardial infarction. Lancet 2:109 (1967).
9. Schwartz, P.J. and Wolf, S. Q-T interval prolongation as predictor of sudden death in patients with myocardial infaction. Circulation 57:1074 (1978).

10. Guttierez, M.B. et al. Significance of T-wave interruption by premature beats as a cause of sudden death. Can. M.A.J. 98:144 (1968).
11. Lown, B. and Wolf, M. Approaches to sudden death from coronary heart disease. Circulation 44:130 (1971).
12. Abildskov, J.A. et al. The electrocardiogram and the central nervous system. Progr. Cardiovasc. Dis. 13:210 (1970).
13. Hugenholtz, P.G. et al. Electrocardiographic abnormalities in cerebral disorders. Report of 6 cases and review of the literature. Am. Heart J. 63:451 (1962).
14. Shuster, S. The electrocardiogram in subarachnoid hemorrhage. Brit. Heart J. 22:316 (1960).
15. Surawicz, B. and Lasseter, K.C. Effects of drugs on the electrocardiogram. Progr. Cardiovasc. Dis. 13:26 (1970).
16. Surawicz, B. Relationship between electrocardiogram and electrolytes. Am. Heart J. 73:814 (1967).
17. Reynolds, E.W. and Van der Ark, C.R. Quinidine syncope and the delayed repolarization syndromes. Mod. Concepts Cardiovasc. Dis. 45:117 (1976).
18. Mullican, W.S. and Fisch, C. Post-extrasystolic alternans of the U wave due to hypokalemia. Am. Heart J. 68:383 (1964).
19. Scherf, D. et al. Ectopic ventricular tachycardia, hypokalemia, and convulsions in alcoholics. Cardiologia 50:129 (1967).
20. Bashour, T. et al. U-wave alternans and increased ventricular irritability. Chest 64:377 (1973).
21. Weaver, W.F. and Burchell, H.B. Serum potassium and the electrocardiogram in hypokalemia. Circulation 21:505 (1960).
22. Vincent, C.M. et al. Q-T interval syndromes. Progr. Cardiovasc. Dis. 16:523 (1974).
23. Jervell, A. and Lange-Nielsen, F. Congenital deaf-mutism, functional heart disease with prolongation of Q-T interval and sudden death. Am. Heart J. 54:59 (1957).
24. Levine, S. and Woodworth, C. Congenital deaf mutism, prolonged Q-T interval, syncopal attacks, and sudden death. New Eng. J. Med. 259:412 (1958).
25. Garza, L.A. et al. Heritable Q-T prolongation without deafness. Circulation 41:39 (1970).
26. Lipp, H. et al. Recurrent ventricular tachyarrhythmias in a patient with a prolonged Q-T interval. Med. J. Aust. 1:1296 (1970).
27. Karhunen, P. et al. Syncope and Q-T prolongation without deafness. The Romano-Ward syndrome. Am. Heart J. 80:820 (1970).
28. Moss, A.J. and Mc Donald, J. Unilateral cervicothoracic sympathetic ganglionectomy for the treatment of long Q-T interval syndrome. New Eng. J. Med. 285:903 (1971).
29. Ratshin, R.A. et al. Q-T interval prolongation, paroxysmal ventricular arrhythmias, and convulsive syncope. Ann. Int. Med. 75:919 (1971).
30. Mathews, E.C. et al. Q-T prolongation and ventricular arrhythmias, with and without deafness, in the same family. Am. J. Cardiol. 29:702 (1972).
31. Johansson, B.W. and Jorming, B. Hereditary prolongation of Q-T interval. Brit. Heart J. 34:744 (1972).
32. Csanady, M. and Kiss, Z. Heritable Q-T prolongation without congenital deafness (Romano-Ward syndrome). Chest 64:359 (1973).
33. Moothart, R.W. et al. The heritable syndrome of prolonged Q-T interval, syncope and sudden death. Chest 70:263 (1976).
34. Ban, T.A. and St. Jean, A. The effect of phenothiazines on the electrocardiogram. Can. M.A.J. 91:537 (1964).
35. Fowler, N.O. et al. Electrocardiographic changes and cardiac arrhythmias in patients receiving psychotropic drugs. Am. J. Cardiol. 37:223 (1976).
36. Gottschalk, L.A. et al. Plasma concentrations of thioridazine metabolites and electrocardiographic abnormalities. J. Pharm. Sci. 67:155 (1978).

37. Wendkos, M.H. Thioridazine and electrocardiographic abnormalities. *Can. M.A.J.* 89:1297 (1963).
38. Wendkos, M.H. The significance of electrocardiographic changes produced by thioridazine. *J. New Drugs* 4:322 (1964).
39. Wendkos, M.H. Cardiac changes related to phenothiazine therapy with special reference to thioridazine. *J. Am. Geriat. Soc.* 15:20 (1967).
40. Wendkos, M.H. A functional myocardial aberration in phenothiazine treated psychiatric patients. *Excerpta Med.* International Congress Series 150 (1967).
41. Wendkos, M.H. *Experiments With Thioridazine, in Toxicity and Adverse Reaction Studies in Neuroleptics and Antidepressants,* H.E. Lehmann and T.A. Ban, eds. Quebec Psychological Research Association, Verdun (1968).
42. Wendkos, H.H. and Thornton, C.C. An electrocardiographic survey of thioridazine treated patients. *Behav. Neuropsych.* 1:18 (1969).
43. Thornton, C.C. and Wendkos, M.H. Electrocardiographic T-wave distortions among thioridazine treated in-patients. *Dis. Nerv. Sys.* 32:320 (1971).
44. Graupner, K.I. and Murphree, O.D. Electrocardiographic changes associated with the use of thioridazine. *J. Neuropsych.* 5:344 (1964).
45. Huston, JR. and Bell, G.E. The effect of thioridazine hydrochloride and chlorpromazine on the electrocardiogram. *J.A.M.A.* 198:16 (1966).
46. Alvarez-Mena, S.C. and Frank, MJ. Phenothiazine-induced T-wave abnormalities. Effects of overnight fasting. *J.A.M.A.* 224:1730 (1973).
47. Samet, J.M. and Surawicz, B. Cardiac function in patients treated with phenothiazines. Comparison with quinidine. *J. Clin. Pharmacol.* 14:588 (1974).
48. Alexander, S. et al. Electrocardiographic effects of thioridazine hydrochloride. *Lahey Clin. Found. Bull.* 16:207 (1967).
49. Lapierre, Y.D. et al. Phenothiazine treatment and electrocardiographic abnormalities. *Can. Psychiatr. A.J.* 14:517 (1969).
50. Kelly, H.G. et al. Thioridazine hydrochloride (Mellaril): Its effect on the electrocardiogram and a report of 2 fatalities with electrocardiographic abnormalities. *Can. M.A.J.* 89:546 (1963).
51. Burda, C.D. Electrocardiographic abnormalities induced by thioridazine. (Mellaril). *Am. Heart J.* 76:153 (1968).
52. Tetreault, L. et al. Comparative study of TPS-23, chlorpromazine and placebo in chronic schizophrenic patients. *Dis. Nerv. Sys.* 30;74 (1969).
53. Arita, M. et al. Effects of propranolol on electrocardiographic abnormalities induced by phenothiazine derivatives. *Jap. Circul. J.* 34:391 (1970).
54. Wendkos, M.H. The influence of autonomic imbalance on the human electrocardiogram: Unstable T-waves in emotionally unstable persons. *Am. Heart J.* 28:549 (1944).
55. Wendkos, M.H. and Logue, R.B. Unstable T-waves in leads II and III in neurocirculatory asthenia. *Am. Heart J.* 31:711 (1946.)
56. Wendkos, M.H. and Nadler, H. Observations concerning the instability of the T-wave in the Wolff-Parkinson-White syndrome. (Abstracted) *Proc. Am. Fed. Clin. Res.* 3:621 (1947).
57. Dolara, A. Early premature ventricular beats, repetitive ventricular response, and ventricular fibrillation. *Am. Heart J.* 74:332 (1967).
58. Smirk, F.H. and Palmer, D.G. A myocardial syndrome: With particular reference to the occurrence of sudden death and premature systoles interrupting antecedent T-waves. *Am. J. Cardiol* 6:620 (1960).
59. Palmer, D.G. Interruption of T-wave by premature QRS complexes and the relationship of this phenomenon to ventricular fibrillation. *Am. Heart J.* 63:367 (1962).
60. Lepeschkin, E. The U wave of the electrocardiogram. *Arch. Int. Med.* 96:600 (1955).

61. Lepeschkin, E. and Surawicz, B. The duration of the Q-U interval and its components in electrocardiograms of normal persons. *Am. Heart J.* 46:9 (1953).
62. Kalbian, V.V. Q-T prolongations associated with the use of thioridazine hydrochloride (Mellaril). *West Virg. Med. J.* 67:296 (1971).
63. Surawicz, B. et al. Task Force I: Standardization of terminology and interpretation. *Am. J. Cardiol.* 41:130 (1978).
64. Abildskov, J.A. Adrenergic effects on the Q-T interval of the electrocardiogram. *Am. Heart J.* 92:210 (1976).
65. Schwartz, P.J. et al. The long Q-T syndrome. *Am. Heart J.* 89:378 (1975.)
66. Surawicz, B. and Lepeschkin, E. The electrocardiographic pattern of hypopotassemia with and without hypocalcemia. *Circulation* 8:801 (1953).
67 Surawicz, B. Arrhythmias and electrolyte disturbances. *Bull. N. Y. Aced. Med.* 43:1160 (1967).
68. Wendkos, M.H. (Unpublished observations).
69. Wendkos, M.H. The effects of a potassium mixture on abnormal cardiac repolarization in hospitalized psychiatric patients. *Am. J. Med. Sci.* 249:412 (1965).
70. Wendkos, M.H. Electrocardiographic evidences of nitrate activity in man. *Postgrad. Med.* 39:132 (1966).
71. Wendkos, M.H. The use of pharmacologic agents to differentiate between "functional" and "organic" T-wave abnormalities. *Triangle* 7:177 (1966).
72. Dodge, H.T. et al. The effects of induced hyperkalemia on the normal and abnormal electrocardiogram, *Am. Heart J.* 45:725 (1953.)
73. Wasserburger, R.H. and Corliss, R.J. Value of oral potassium salts in differentiation of functional and organic T-wave changes. *Am. J. Cardiol* 10:673 (1962).
74. Wendkos, M.H. The electrocardiographic effects of ergot alkaloids in anginal patients and in subjects without demonstrable organic heart disease. *Circulation* Suppl. 3, 34:237 (1966).
75. Wendkos, M.H. The anti-anginal effect of rapidly acting nitrates in subjects with ergot-induced angina. *Am. J. Med. Sci.* 253:39 (1967).
76. Schroeder, J.S. et al. Provocation of coronary spasm with ergonovine maleate. New test with result in 57 patients undergoing coronary arteriography. *Am. J. Cardiol.* 40:487 (1977).
77. Wendkos, M.H. Supplemental use of ergotamine tartrate in eliciting transient disturbances of rhythm in acute rheumatic fever. *Proc. Soc. Exper. Biol. Med.* 58:303 (1945).
78. Wendkos, M.H. The influence of food intake and ergot alkaloids upon vagogenic atrio-ventricular heart block of the Wenckebach type. *Vascular Dis.* 5:21 (1968).
79. Schou, M. Electrocardiographic changes during treatment with lithium and drugs of the imipramine type. *Acta Psychiatr. Scand.* 38:331 (1962).
80. Schou, M. Normothymotics, "mood normalizers," *Brit. J. Psychiatr.* 109:803 (1963).

81. Demers, R.G. and Heninger, G.R. Electrocardiographic changes during lithium treatment. *Dis. Nerv. Sys.* 31:674 (1970).
82. Demers, R.G. and Heninger, G.R. Electrocardiographic T-wave changes during lithium carbonate treatment. *J.A.M.A.* 218:381 (1971).
83. Tilkian, A.G. et al. Effect of lithium on cardiovascular performance: Report on extended ambulatory monitoring and exercise testing before and during lithium therapy. *Am. J. Cardiol* 38:701 (1976).
84. Kochar, M.S. et al. Electrocardiographic changes simulating hypokalemia during treatment with lithium carbonate. *J. Electrocardiol.* 4:371 (1971).
85. Kliks, B.R. et al. Influence of sympathetic tone on ventricular fibrillation threshold during experimental coronary occlusion. *Am. J. Cardiol.* 36:45 (1975).

86. Yanowitz, F. et al. Functional distribution of right and left stellate innervation to the ventricles. Production of neurogenic electrocardiographic changes by unilateral alteration of sympathetic tone. *Circ. Res.* 18:416 (1966).
87. James, T.N. Q-T prolongation and sudden death. *Mod. Concepts Cardiovasc. Dis.* 38:35 (1969).
88. Han, J. et al. Adrenergic effects on ventricular vulnerability. *Circ. Res.* 14:516 (1964).
89. Hageman, G.R. et al. Cardiac dysrhythmias induced by autonomic nerve stimulation. *Am. J. Cardiol.* 32:823 (1973).
90. Vassalle, M. et al. On the sympathetic control of ventricular automaticity, the effects of stellate ganglion stimulation. *Circ. Res.* 23:249 (1968).
91. Maling, H.M. and Moran, N.C. Ventricular arrhythmias induced by sympathomimetic amines in unanesthetized dogs following coronary artery occlusion. *Circ. Res.* 5:409 (1957).
92. Harris, A.S. et al. The induction of arrhythmias by sympathetic activity before and after occlusion of a coronary artery in the canine heart. *J. Electrocardiol.* 4:34 (1971).
93. Fastier, F.N. and Smirk, F.H. Some properties of Amarin with special reference to its use in conjunction with adrenaline for the production of idioventricular rhythms. *J. Physiol.* 107:318 (1948).
94. Moore, J.I. and Swain, H.H. Sensitization to ventricular fibrillation. I. Sensitization by a substituted propiophenone, U-0882. *J. Pharmac. Exp. Ther.* 128:243 (1960).
95. Hutcheon, D.E. and Laffan, R. Electrocardiographic changes preceding catecholamine-induced arrhythmias. *Proc. Soc. Exp. Biol. Med.* 113:557 (1963).
96. James, T.N. and Bear, E.S. Effects of ethanol and acetaldehyde on the heart. *Am. Heart J.* 74:243 (1967).
97. Wendkos, M.H. Pharmacologic studies in a hitherto unreported benign repolarization disturbance among schizophrenics. *J. New Drugs* 4:98 (1964).

CHAPTER 14

The Inherited Susceptibility To Sudden Death

Sudden deaths due solely to the presence of an inherited cardiac disorder affecting ventricular repolarization were described for the first time in a report by Jervell and Lange-Nielson which appeared in 1957.[1] These authors indicated that the findings in a routine electrocardiogram were primarily responsible for their discovery that such an inherited trait was responsible for such fatalities. In these instances, the electrocardiographic abnormality was an enlargment of the U wave which was termed by them an "elongation of the Q-T interval."

Since the time these original observations were reported, much additional data with respect to this fatal syndrome have been provided by others.[2-45,47-48] Consequently, it can now be agreed that there are chiefly two diagnostic features of this unique inherited fatal malady. These include a past or family history of syncopal "spells" combined with the presence of the electrocardiographic hallmark just described. For this reason, in this chapter, those fatalities linked primarily to an inherited aberration of ventricular repolarization have been discussed under the rubric of an "Inherited Susceptibility to Sudden Death" syndrome.

CLINICAL FEATURES AND CLUES

Although a single attack of fatal cardioplegic ventricular arrhythmia often may be the first clinical manifestation of this inherited cardiac disorder, it is known also that in some of its victims, recurrent prodromes of arrhythmogenic thanatoid syncope (see Chapter 2) may precede a terminal episode of fatal syncope.[1,2,8,10,16,22,44] Usually, this type of clinical pattern has been observed in children but it has been shown also that some persons whose electrocardiograms are characterized by the presence of a genetically determined enlargment of the U wave can survive until early or late adulthood before they develop such a thanatoid or fatal episode of syncope.[20,44]

It has been observed also that syncopal episodes due to this inherited syndrome often can be initiated by an emotional disturbance or by excessive physical exertion.[1,2,10,16,35,44,47] Nevertheless, without an awareness of the electrocardiographic findings prior to the time of death or without a thorough knowledge of the past medical and family history, it clearly would be difficult to identify with certainty those fatalities for which an inherited repolarization anomaly can be basically held responsible.

The presence of an inherited hearing deficit may also provide a clue to the existence of an inherited susceptibility to sudden-death syndrome. It should be recognized, however, that several large-scale surveys among children in schools for the deaf have uncovered only a very small number of students whose routine electrocardiograms were characterized by the presence of conspicuous U waves, larger than their juxtaposed T-Waves.[18,28,33]

Family History

A detailed family history which concentrates on familial physical handicaps in maternal and paternal relatives, may help to establish whether a sudden, seemingly inexplicable, death should be considered to be the result of an inherited susceptibility to sudden death. In this connection, it would be important to determine whether relatives in the same or preceding generations may have suffered from a hearing impairment or "spells" and whether any had died suddenly at a relatively young age for reasons which were not altogether clear.

Chromosome Studies

In addition, it is of interest that even though the inherited susceptibility to sudden death is a genetically determined entity, chromosome studies have not demonstrated any chromosomal aberrations. However, such a finding is of questionable importance inasmuch as it was based on a chromosomal study in only a single genotype.[9]

Postmortem Examination

Generally, too, it has been observed that a routine autopsy of decedents with an Inherited Susceptibility to Sudden Death will not provide an explanation for the sudden death.[12,14,20,22] On the other hand, more elaborate examinations of the pacemaker sites and conducting tissues of the heart may disclose meaningful changes.[8,22,26] Obviously, then, because of this circumstance, it would be proper to conjecture that some previously reported autopsy-negative fatalities of psychiatric patients, which have been categorized as enigmatic sudden deaths, actually may have been due to such a previously unsuspected inherited susceptibility to sudden death.

Mode of Inheritance

Also unsettled, as yet, is the mode of inheritance of this genetically determined entity. Some articles which have discussed this aspect have favored the view that it is an autosomal recessive trait[28] but, on the other hand, there are many authors who have perceived it to be an autosomal dominant characteristic.[11,23,45,48]

The evidence in favor of either view has been questioned by James[20] who emphasized that, at the present time, any final conclusions concerning the mode of inheritance must be held in abeyance. As far as can be determined, James' position, in this regard, is based on a conviction that normal findings in the routine electrocardiograms of parents of "affected" children do not necessarily exclude the presence of an inherited repolarization anomaly inasmuch as the evidences of this anomaly sometimes may be visible only if the electrocardiogram is made after exercise.[20,24,25] However, genealogic studies which have been undertaken in auditionally normal and auditionally abnormal children afflicted with a congenital anomalous repolarization syndrome seemed to show--at least in those with normal hearing--that it is inherited as an autosomal nonsex-linked dominant trait.[3,11,48]

NEUROGENIC RISK FACTORS

As yet, the functional aberration of repolarization and the clinical manifestations of this inherited fatal malady are not completely understood; it is conceivable, however, that a disturbance of the autonomic nervous system may be an important underlying "risk factor."

Results of Neurologic Manipulation

Studies in canines have already demonstrated that manipulation of sympathetic nerve supply to the heart will result in an enlargement of the U wave in the electrocardiogram[50] and also, coordinately, in a lowering of the ventricular fibrillation threshold.[51] Moreover, as will be discussed more fully in a subsequent section of this chapter, excision of the left stellate ganglion[29] or the administration of propranolol[35,44,45,43] can prevent recurrent ventricular arrhythmias and their companionate syncopal episodes in persons afflicted with the inherited susceptibility to sudden death. As a result of such interventions, these patients have remained asymptomatic despite the performance of excessive physical exertion or the development of emotional arousal, either of which ordinarily augment adrenergic traffic to the heart[55-57] and frequently precede an attack of thanatoid or fatal syncope in patients of this genre.[1,10,37,44,45,47]

Results of Hemodynamic Studies

Also compatible with the view that neurogenic factors underlie the various features of the "Inherited Susceptibility to Sudden Death" syndrome have been the results of hemodynamic studies which have indicated that ventricular function is normal despite the characteristic arrhythmogenicity of the heart associated with this inherited cardiac disorder.[27,29] However, it should be explained also that organic changes in the coronary microcirculation may represent an additional risk factor with respect to the occurrence of life-threatening ventricular tachyarrhythmias in persons afflicted with this fatal malady.

Results of Histologic Studies

The first to discuss this possibility were Fraser et al[8] whose observations were based on a method of histologic examinations of the heart advocated by T.N. James (see Appendix). The findings Fraser et al had described were a narrowing of the nutrient artery of the sinoatrial node and the presence of infarcted areas in the node and adjacent atrial wall. Subsequently, Phillips and Ichinose[22] (who also utilized the technique developed by James) observed the heart of a single auditionally normal child who had the same type of inherited susceptibility to sudden death. They found fibrotic changes that involved the conducting branches, as well as degenerative changes in the small arterioles located in this area.[22]

Thus, although both Fraser et al and Phillips and Ichinose conceded that a basic element in the pathogenesis of the sudden deaths of their respective patients may have been a life-threatening ventricular tachyarrhythmia, both postulated that the "trigger" which actually provoked the final syncopal episode in these respective decedents may have been ischemic effects on strategically important tissues in the heart secondary to an angiopathy of the coronary microcirculation. The findings reported by Lipp[26] also are in accord with this view.

The cause of such vascular lesions still is uncertain and their relationship to the inherited susceptibility to sudden death has not yet been clarified. Nevertheless, the detection of these nonspecific abnormalities affecting the coronary microcirculation in instances of sudden death associated with the Inherited Susceptibility to Sudden Death syndrome has validated the view of James[12] that "there is now abundant evidence that a detailed study of the cardiac conduction system may provide a convincing explanation of seemingly mystifying sudden deaths" and that "the failure to include such a study in any case of otherwise unclarified sudden death must be considered an inexcusable oversight."

Family Case Study

The data in an article by Green et al[17] also emphasize the importance of such an anatomical study in postmortem examinations of individuals who have died suddenly and unexpectedly.

Family Data

These authors described the sudden deaths of two young siblings who were part of a family in which, for three successive generations, unexplained sudden deaths at an average age of 26 years represented a familial trait. Moveover, many of these relatives had been considered to be epileptic because they had suffered from episodic syncopal attacks prior to the time of death.

A genealogic survey undertaken by Green et al with respect to these three generations also indicated an absence of hearing impairment. Because electrocardiographic data pertaining to members of this family were available, it was possible to exclude the presence of an inherited repolarization anomaly or conduction defect at any time prior to their respective sudden and unexpected deaths.

Equally impressive were the postmortem findings Greeen et al had described insofar as these pertained to the hearts of the two young siblings whose biographical data they had documented in considerable detail.

Sibling No. 1

He was a 15-year-old boy who always had been in excellent health. Two weeks before his unexpected and untimely death a thorough physical examination revealed no abnormalities. Nevertheless, although he had been adequately conditioned for competitive track he died suddenly at the end of a 100-yard sprint.

Sibling No. 2

The other case was this boy's sister who had been examined at the Shands Teaching Hospital one year prior to the time of her sudden death at age 15, and, at that institution, no abnormalities with her cardiovascular system were detected. The physical examination of the heart disclosed no abnormalities; the findings in the chest roentgenogram were within normal limits; the electrocardiographic findings were considered to be normal. However, it was noted that there was a history of occasional seemingly inexplicable brief syncopal episodes from which she made rapid uncomplicated recoveries. Nevertheless, when she was informed of her brother's death, she fainted and when it was evident to the family that she had suffered a cardiac arrest, attempts to resuscitate her were made but were unsuccessful. Shortly after the cardiac arrest, an electrocardiogram was made in the office of her family physician; it confirmed the presence of ventricular fibrillation but further efforts to resuscitate her, including electrical defibrillation, proved to be futile.

Sibling No. 3

The anamnestic data with respect to this family also indicated that another sister died suddenly and unexpectedly at the age of 10 years while she had been playing on the beach; prior to this unfortunate event, she had been considered to be in perfect health.

The Mother

The family history also indicated that the mother of these three children had had frequent fainting episodes and, on one occasion, when she was exercising on a bicycle ergometer, she developed frequent ventricular premature contractions but no other noteworthy cardiac abnormalities.

Postmortem Findings

Until the conduction system in the heart of the 14-year-old decedent and his 14-year-old sister had been studied with the use of the semiserial conduction method of Lev (see Appendix) as modified by Shanklin and Laite,[60] the autopsy findings were insufficient to provide an explanation for the sudden deaths of these two siblings. Thus, it was found that in the heart of the 15-year-old boy there was a conduction bundle "with a number of spurious blind-end branches as it passed through the pars membranacea which had no attachment or insertion to the ventricular myocardium. The hypoplastic bundle continued into the ventricular myocardium and the atrioventricular node was indistinct and the approach tissue seemed to give rise to the bundle of His itself. The nodal artery could not be identified." A faulty development of the bundle of His, the atrioventricular node, and the bundle branches was also noted in the heart of the 15-year-old girl.

Conclusions. Accordingly, it was the conclusion of Green et al that a congenital defect with respect to the conducting tissues could be the explanation for the sudden deaths of these two youngsters and presumably might have accounted for the sudden unexpected death of their younger sister as well.

FATAL FAMILIAL CARDIAC ARRHYTHMIAS

In certain respects, the data pertaining to these two fatalities would seem to indicate that the underlying cause was an entity subsumed by Gault et al in 1972 under the rubric of "Fatal Familial Cardiac Arrhythmias."[49] As Gault et al had explained, this cognomen had been chosen to identify a subset of individuals who belonged to a single family characterized by a predisposition to develop life-threatening ventricular tachyarrhythmias and to die suddenly, despite an absence of Q-T prolongation in their electrocardiograms.

Postmortem Findings

The postmortem examination of the heart of one member of this family (a 16-year-old child) demonstrated cardiac hypertrophy (heart weight = 370 gm) and focal endocardial fibroelastosis of the left ventricle; also, detailed histologic studies of the interventricular septum and adjacent conducting tissues confirmed the presence of fatty changes and mononuclear cell infiltration in the A-V conduction system and main left bundle branch. Thus, in this instance, as in the cases described by Green et al, the sudden deaths were ascribed to a fatal ventricular tachyarrhythmia linked to the presence of genetically determined defects involving the conduction system in the heart.

INHERITED ECG ANOMALY, SUDDEN DEATH, AND CONGENITAL HEARING DEFECT

A somewhat different group of fatalities were those which have been described in the original report by Jervell and Lange-Nielson[1] and in a number of other articles which have appeared since 1957.[2-48] The three decedents discussed by Jervell and Lange-Nielson were siblings whose ages at the time of death were 4, 5, and 9 years, respectively. The surviving members of the family were three other siblings and both parents.

Familial Features

Since their births, the three decedents and one of the surviving siblings had been affected with a severe hearing impairment; the hearing of the other two surviving children and both parents (who were still alive) was unaffected. Thus congenital deafness was present in four of the six children and only these four deaf children had experienced repeated episodes of thanatoid or simple syncope on various occasions since infancy. For this reason, even though these repeated nonfatal attacks of syncope generally were induced by physical effort only, these "seizure prone" children had been considered to be epileptics as well until the results of a subsequent electrocardiographic survey in this family unit had suggested that the syncopal attacks were due to episodic ventricular arrhythmias in hearts with an inherited repolarization anomaly likely to favor the occurrence of such an arrhythmia.

ECG Findings

Particularly noteworthy was the nature of the findings Jervell and Lange-Nielson had observed during their electrocardiographic survey of this family. Thus, abnormalities expressive of abnormal repolarization were present regularly in intersyncopal electrocardiograms of the four deaf children; similar abnormalities were not present in the remaining members of the family who were neither deaf nor afflicted with syncopal attacks. Moreover, serum electrolyte levels were normal in those with either an abnormal or normal electrocardiogram.

Uniformly, the nature of the electrocardiographic deviation was listed by Jervell and Lange-Nielson as a "prolongation of the Q-T interval," but in one section of their article they conceded that, actually, "the delay in repolarization was manifested by a prominent U wave with a possible merging of the T and U waves." The figures which accompanied the text of their paper would seem to corroborate the latter interpretation.

In one instance, when an exercise test was employed, it accentuated the U wave in an intersyncopal electrocardiogram. No synsyncopal electrocardiographic studies were obtained and so Jervell and Lange-Nielson were not able to establish with certainty that such seizures were characteristic of a physiogenic variety of epilepsy.

Genesis of Inherited ECG Anomaly

Another aspect of this syndrome which Jervell and Lange-Nielson found to be puzzling was the genesis of the inherited electrocardiographic anomaly they had observed. Regarding this feature, they speculated that it was due to a "congenital anomaly of the myocardial metabolism with delay of the repolarization phase caused by some enzymatic deficiency." However, they did not provide any additional details and did not discuss the possible genetic mechanisms which might account for the inherited physiologic abnormality and the congenital hearing defect.

Postmortem Findings

The postmortem data supplied by Jervell and Lange-Nielson pertained to only one of their decedents. In this instance, a routine autopsy disclosed normal findings with regard to the heart. This organ "weighed 195 gm and was well contracted. The coronary orifices were normal, as were the 5 major branches of the coronary artery. There was no hypertrophy or visible lesion of the myocardium. Some small atheromatous streaks were seen in the intima of the aorta just distal to the aortic valve. There was no patentcy of ductus arteriosus or foramen ovale. The endocardium had a normal appearance, with normal orifices and normal heart valves. Microscopically, the heart and other organs were normal."[1] However, it should be noted that the pathologist had not examined the conducting tissues or pacemaker sites of the heart, in the manner advocated by Lev or James (see Appendix).

In the following year, Levine and Woodworth[2] reported another case of sudden unexpected death in a deaf "epileptic" child whose repeated premortem "resting" intersyncopal electrocardiograms indicated the presence of prolonged repolarization despite the absence of any demonstrable organic heart disease.

Case Study

The siblings of this decedent were auditionally normal, seizure-free, and not prone to sudden death; similarly, his parents were neither deaf nor seizure-prone. This child developed an attack of fatal syncope when he was 13 years of age but ever since the age of 3, he had manifested repeated attacks of thanatoid syncope which, mistakenly, were considered to be manifestions of epilepsy. Accordingly, anticonvulsants were prescribed but, as in the case of the children in the family reported by Jervell and Lange-Nielson, these agents proved to be ineffective in preventing the recurrent "fits." Moreover, it was observed that "psychic problems seemed to have an important role in precipitating spells of syncope." The photographs of this child's "resting" electrocardiograms which were included with the text showed clearly that the important change was a conspicuous enlargement of the U wave (a so-called "prolongation of the Q-T interval").

Conclusions

The presence of this electrocardiographic anomaly prompted Levine and Woodworth to speculate that the attack of fatal syncope was the result of an irreversible ventricular tachyarrhythmia. They made it clear, however, that they did not believe the recurrent episodes of thanatoid syncope, which occurred when he was younger, were due to a similar paroxsysmal ventricular arrhythmia. Moreover, these authors did not offer any explanation for the "lengthened Q-T interval" and, instead they mentioned a communication from Dr. Frank N. Wilson who had suggested that the electrocardiographic anomaly might be ascribed to a malfunction of the vegetative nervous system. After the patient died, a routine autopsy was performed and this "failed to throw any light on the condition. Grossly and microscopically, nothing significant was found in the heart or brain." However, the technique advocated by Lev or James (see Appendix) was not employed.

Other Cases

Following the appearance of the article by Levine and Woodworth in 1958, there have been relatively few additional reports of sudden unexpected death in young pseudo-epileptics with impaired hearing and a "prolongation of the Q-T interval." As far as can be determined, only five additional cases of this sort have been described. Of these, there were three which were mentioned in the article by Fraser et al;[8] another was reported by Lisker and Finkelstein[10] and the fifth by Van Bruggen et al.[19]

Emotionality and Syncopal Attacks

The publications by these three respective sets of authors are noteworthy also because they emphasized a connection between emotionality and the development of syncopal attacks in their respective patients, thus confirming an association previously observed by Levine and Woodworth[2] with regard to the "fits" which are such a characteristic feature of this syndrome. The report by Van Bruggen et al was important in one other respect; this was the documentation it provided that a ventricular tachyarrhythmia was responsible for an episode of thanatoid syncope and, later, for an attack of fatal syncope. In the words of these authors: "The patient was a deaf 8-year-old child who was admitted to an epileptic center for further examination. While an electroencephalogram was being recorded, the patient had an attack and the pulse became irregular. A simultaneously recorded electrocardiogram showed the characteristics of ventricular tachycardia turning into ventricular fibrillation. Subsequently, on the 8th day, the child suffered a fatal attack. The electrocardiographic features were those of ventricular fibrillation. Immediate attempts at resuscitation with electrical defibrillation failed."[19]
Features of ECG. The text of the article by Van Bruggen et al was accompanied by a photograph of an intersyncopal conventional "resting electrocardiogram." Thus, it could be seen that the most important change was a broadening and inversion of the T-waves resulting from a fusion of the T and U waves; superficially, therefore, this finding resembled a lengthened Q-T interval (see Chapter 14).

Nonfatal Hereditary Abnormal Ventricular Repolarization

Despite the various reports which have emphasized the lethality of an inherited repolarization anomaly in congenitally deaf seizure-prone children without demonstrable organic heart disease, several other publications have shown also that deaf children with these same additional attributes still can remain alive. Articles of this nature are those by Jervell, Thingstad, and Endsjo[9] by Olley and Fowler[27] and by Van der Straaten and Bruins.[39]

Case Study No. 1

The paper by Jervell et al[9] summarized observations of three such children ranging in ages from 7 to 13 years. Each had experienced recurrent episodes of thanatoid syncope which were "triggered" by either physical exertion or an emotional reaction such as fear or anger.
ECG Findings. Uniformly, conspicuous U waves (mistakenly termed a lengthened Q-T interval by the authors) were present in their respective "resting" intersyncopal electrocardiograms. It is also of interest that these U waves disappeared following complete digitalization and became more pronounced following an exercise test.
Chromosomal Findings. Of these three children, the chromosomes of only the 7-year-old boy was studied and this investigation "did not show any abnormalities."

Case Study No. 2

The paper by Olley and Fowler[27] described the findings in two congenitally deaf pseudo-epileptic boys whose recurrent attacks of syncope were provoked by "fright, anger, or excitement." One boy was 5 years of age and the other was 9 years old.
ECG Findings. Their respective "resting" intersyncopal electrocardiograms were characterized by the presence of conspicuous U waves (mistakenly interpreted by the authors to be an indication of a lengthened Q-T interval). On one occasion, a synsyncopal electrocardiogram of the younger child was obtained and this indicated that the cardiac mechanism at the time was a ventricular tachyarrhythmia.
Physiologic Findings. With respect to both children, the physical examination as well as hemodynamic and angiographic studies during the intersyncopal periods did not demonstrate the presence of any structural cardiac lesion or any type of myocardiopathy known to predispose to episodes of syncope, ventricular tachyarrhythmia, or sudden death.

Case Study No. 3

The case reported by Van der Straaten and Bruins[39] was a 10-year-old boy who, following audiometric testing, was found to have a mild perceptive type of deafness but his major affliction was his proneness to develop frequent syncopal attacks. The results of the physical examination, teleroentgenogram of the chest and a phonocardiogram did not confirm the presence of any organic cardiac abnormality.

ECG Findings. In a routine "resting" intersyncopal electrocardiogram there was an alleged "prolongation of the Q-T interval, the duration of which measured 0.60 second compared to a predicted normal value of 0.38 second." A photograph of this electrocardiogram was not included with the text but, in all likelihood, it was an unrecognized conspicuous U wave which was responsible for the increased duration of repolarization.

Conclusions. This publication is important because it provided data pertaining to numerous relatives of the deaf 10-year-old seizure-prone child which could be meaningful in relation to considerations concerning the pattern of genetic transmission of this particular malady.

Their investigation showed that the routine "resting" electrocardiograms of the patient's father, paternal aunt, and paternal uncle along with three surviving first cousins of the patient were normal except for an alleged "prolongation of the Q-T interval;" none of these relatives, except one of the cousins, had experienced syncopal attacks. Moreover, sudden and unexpected deaths for which "the cause could not be ascertained" had terminated the lives of the patient's paternal grandfather and his grandfather's brother at the ages of 39 and 29 years, respectively.

ROMANO-WARD SYNDROME—STUDIES OF AUDITIONALLY NORMAL CASES

Another subgroup of those with an inherited susceptibility to sudden death includes those persons who, except for the hearing impairment, resemble in all particulars congenitally deaf individuals prone to die suddenly and unexpectedly.

Case Study No. 1—Romano

The first to report such a case were Romano et al whose observations were first published fully in 1963 in an Italian journal[3] and in 1965, in condensed form.[11] The "affected" individual was 3 months of age when she came to the attention of these authors and, already then, she had been experiencing recurrent syncopal attacks for one month.

ECG Results and Conclusions

While in the hospital, both intersyncopal and synsyncopal electrocardiograms of this auditionally normal infant were obtained. In this way, it was possible to establish, first, that syncope and a ventricular tachyarrhythmia were companionate phenomena and, second, that when the infant was conscious there were "abnormal alternate complexes and lengthening of the Q-T interval with broad diphasic T-waves." However, in the photograph which accompanied the text, the prolonged repolarization phase actually appeared to be the result of a conspicuous U wave giving the impression of a "broad diphasic T-wave."

Case Study No. 2—Ward

In 1964, a report by Ward[6] affirmed an affiliation between syncopal attacks and a ventricular tachyarrhythmia in a 6-year-old auditionally normal girl whose younger brother, like herself, had been considered to be an epileptic. The synsyncopal ventricular tachyarrhythmia was demonstrated when, during an exercise test, this child developed an attack of unconsciousness. Her history indicated that ever since the age of 16 months, she had experienced episodes of unconsciousness, generally after exertion, and for this reason, she had been treated for epilepsy until her seizures were demonstrated to be physiogenic in nature.

ECG Findings

A noteworthy finding in an intersyncopal "resting" electrocardiogram was "an abnormally long Q-T interval." A photograph of this electrocardiogram was not included with the text but it is suspected that the "abnormally long Q-T interval" was the result of a conspicuous U wave. A similar "prolongation of the Q-T interval" was observed in an intersyncopal electrocardiogram of an infant brother who exhibited recurrent syncopal attacks, during one of which he died. Another brother age 6 years was healthy and his electrocardiogram was normal. The father's electrocardiogram was normal also but "there was some lengthening of the Q-T interval in the mother's electrocardiogram" (electrocardiogram not shown). A deceased maternal aunt of the patient was also known to lose consciousness repeatedly during her lifetime; "she died during one of those episodes at the age of 30."

Use of Adrenergic Blocking Agents

Ward's report is of interest for another reason: as far as can be determined, he was the first to employ an adrenergic blocking agent (pronethalol) to reduce the frequency of syncopal attacks in a person afflicted with the combination of an inherited repolarization anomaly and a pseudo-epileptic syndrome. Moreover, in his patient, there was a dramatic reduction in seizure frequency as a result of this therapy.

Thus, Ward had also provided indirect evidence of a link between heightened adrenergic activity and the patient's recurrent arrhythmogenic seizures—a percept which would be in accord with anamnestic data which indicated that her "fits" were regularly provoked by physical exertion, a type of activity known to augment the effects of the sympathetic neuroendocrine apparatus in the body.[55]

Additional Observations

Several subsequent reports also have attested to the partial or complete control of syncopal attacks in patients afflicted with a Romano-Ward syndrome when they were treated with a beta-blocking drug.[6,7,16,27,35,37,43,45,48] However, despite the beneficial antiarrhythmic effect resulting from propranolol in these instances, it was also noted that such a preparation did not simultaneously abolish the U wave or "shorten the Q-T interval" in the electrocardiograms of this group of pseudo-epileptics.[7,35]

Demographic Observations

Demographic observations with respect to this unique arrhythmic syndrome are also of interest. In this connection, it is noteworthy that, since 1970, there have been rapidly increasing number of reports concerning this entity in many civilized countries.[21-27,30-45] Supposedly, then, the past indifference to the prevalence of this syndrome can be attributed less to its rarity and more to a belated awareness that there can be, indeed, a genetic basis for certain deaths which formerly were somewhat mystifying.

Variant of Syndrome - "Familial Syncope"

A slight variant of the Romano-Ward syndrome was the one described by Barlow et al;[4] the data in their article pertained to a familial type of pseudo-epilepsy which clearly could be traced to a maternal ancestry alone. Involved were five auditionally normal siblings ranging in age from 11 to 19 years. Of these, four were still alive; the fifth, when 12 years of age, had died suddenly during one of his "seizures." The 37-year-old mother of these five siblings had "attacks of unconsciousness" since the age of 3 years and as a child had witnessed fatal episodes in her 37-year-old mother and in an 18-year-old sister.

ECG Findings

The findings in the intersyncopal electrocardiograms of the four surviving siblings and their mother provided the proof that such attacks of "familial syncope" were due to an inherited repolarization anomaly. Thus, "as in Ward's patients, electrocardiograms revealed prolonged Q-T intervals and T-waves which were often broad with a slow ascending limb and a rapid descending limb."

Physiogenic Seizures

Moreover, Barlow et al had observed that the syncopal attacks "usually took place after a fright, an emotional shock, or strenuous exercise." Therefore, even though no synsyncopal electrocardiograms had been obtained to determine the nature of the cardiac mechanism at such times, it is likely that the circumstances had "triggered" the development of a ventricular tachyrrhythmia which, in turn, had caused a physiogenic seizure.

Other Studies: Gamstorp

Under the title of "Congenital Cardiac Arrhythmia," Gamstorp et al[5] described the clinical findings and the results of cardiac studies in a 35 year-old woman and a young son, which clearly indicated that although both were auditionally normal, each, otherwise, had exhibited all the characteristics of pseudo-epilelpsy associated with an inherited repolarization anomaly.

The boy's mother, at the age of 6 years, had experienced a few syncopal attacks while bathing at the beach; "these were so severe that it was necessary to employ resuscitative measures." Thereafter, she remained in good health until the age of 35, when at variable intervals, she began to develop brief attacks of unconciousness from which she would recover spontaneously. Synsyncopal electrocardiograms were never obtained and so it could only be presumed that a ventricular tachyarrhythmia was present during such attacks.

Intersyncopal ECG findings. An intersyncopal electrocardiogram showed "low T-waves and large U waves but mistakenly, because of low normal values with respect to the serum potassium level (3.2-3.8 mEq), this electrocardiographic finding was attributed to hypopotassemia.

Moreover, despite the administration of potassium supplements, repeated follow-up "resting" intersyncopal electrocardiograms sometimes were normal and at other times "showed flattened or slightly negative T-waves and a pronounced positive after potential following the second heart sound" (evidently, an enlargement of the U wave). Also, during a two-year follow-up period, whenever the "resting" conventional electrocardiogram was normal or "mildly abnormal" the effect of exercise was to markedly accentuate the U wave and thus produce an illusory lengthening of the Q-T interval.

The Son

Unfortunately, her son's clinical course was less benign. Nonfatal attacks of syncope developed for the first time when he was 3 years of age and they continued intermittently until the age of 9 years when, suddenly, he developed an episode of fatal syncope. A physical examination and electroencephalographic study several years before he died had not disclosed any abnormalities. When he was 5 years of age, a routine "resting" intersyncopal electrocardiogram was obtained and, at that time, the presence of "low and broad T-waves" was noted. No other details with respect to this decedent were supplied.

Conclusions

In retrospect it would appear that both the auditionally normal mother and her son were seizure-prone because each was afflicted with an inherited type of repolarization anomaly which favored the development of recurrent arrhythmogenic seizures.

Discussion

Generally, these seizures reported by Gamstorp et al[5] were spontaneously self-limiting except for the one which occurred when the youngster was 9 years of age. Conceivably, the more benign course of this inherited malady in the mother can be ascribed to the fact that the repolarization abnormality in her case was present in only a latent form; this supposition was supported by the observation that it became manifest only after the performance of an exercise test. Clearly such a response to exercise also implies that reliance cannot be placed exclusively on the findings in a single or even in more than one routine "resting" electrocardiogram in order to identify all persons who are "at risk" in terms of an inherited susceptibility to sudden death.

A somewhat similar view is implicit in some of the statements made by T.N. James.[20] In this connection the reference is to his discussion of the electrocardiographic data pertaining to a 33-year-old auditionally normal woman who did not develop syncopal episodes until she was 30 years of age. Her family history indicated that three of her four children and her father and five of her siblings had "fainted" occasionally and even at times had developed a typical epileptiform seizure. Thus, even though her "spells" had not appeared until a relatively late period of her life, this circumstance could not vitiate the diagnosis of an inherited susceptibility to sudden death.

Synsyncopal electrocardiograms were obtained during several of her "fits" and thus it was possible to demonstrate that her "seizures" and a ventricular tachyarrhythmia were companionate events. On the other hand, when routine "resting" intersyncopal electrocardiograms were obtained at various times, it could be seen that there was "more Q-T prolongation on some days than on others"; also, inasmuch as James believed that "there seems little doubt that a major component of the Q-T prolongation was due largely to a generous U wave" this variability of the so-called Q-T interval could be attributed to corresponding differences in the magnitude of the U wave.

James also suggested that the spontaneous variability in the duration of the Q-T interval in the "resting" electrocardiograms of seizure-prone individuals with an inherited repolarization anomaly may account for a lesser likelihood of such persons to develop physiogenic seizures and thus there may be a reduced prospect that death will result from a sudden episode of fatal syncope.

Surely, this concept is an intriguing one but, on the other hand, without an adequate number of long-term studies of seizure-prone subjects whose electrocardiograms have signified the presence of an inherited repolarization anomaly, no firm conclusions in this respect can be made as yet.

Approach to Therapeutic Management

Noteworthy observations in auditionally normal persons with an inherited susceptibility to sudden death were made also by Garza et al[16,23] and, later, by Mathews et al.[35]

In their publication, Garza et al not only described the clinical and electrocardiographic findings in several members of a single family with this malady but they also reported the results of a unique series of experiments which were undertaken with the hope that thereby a rational form of therapy could be devised to improve the prognosis for those afflicted with this type of inherited seizure disorder.

Electrocardiographic Data: Garza

The opportunity to conduct such an investigation presented itself to Garza et al when they were consulted regarding the care of a 3-year-old child with residual brain damage following his recovery from an episode of cardiac arrest. In this instance, his 38-year-old auditionally normal mother, (who, herself, had "fainted" after vigorous exercise when she was 12, 16, and 36 years of age) was able, by means of emergency procedures, to restore normal cardiac action. However, because of the resulting cerebral anoxia during the episode of cardiac arrest, the child never regained consciousness and he remained comatose during the entire time he was confined to the hospital.

It is of some interest that the Q-T interval was prolonged in routine "resting" electrocardiograms of a surviving auditionally normal seizure-prone brother and of his mother; also, it had been noted that the Q-T interval became further prolonged in the surviving brother's electrocardiogram following a simple exercise test. (It was known that the brothers seizures were associated with such activities as swimming, running, or bicycling.)

During the first two weeks of the childs hospitalization, 85 episodes of ventricular fibrillation" were observed while he was attached to a cardiac monitor. Twice the arrhythmia disappeared spontaneously within a few seconds; on other occasions, normal sinus rhythm was restored by defibrillation techniques. During six separate 10-hour sessions when the cardiac rhythm was normal, "the Q-T interval remained prolonged without change in the QRS complex; the T-wave changed from tall and peaked to low voltage and notched." However, it is evident from an inspection of a representative intersyncopal electrocardiogram included with the text of this article that the so-called lengthening of the Q-T interval was the result of an accentuated U wave.

During the first phase of their studies, Garza et al sought to determine whether the response to catecholamine administration in their test subject would be comparable to the effects observed earlier in experimental animals by Fastier and Smirk[54] whose investigations were confined to the relationaship between a pharmacologically-induced "prolongation of the Q-T interval" and a catecholamine-induced ventricular tachyarrhythmia. Accordingly, they monitored electrocardiographically in this child (a) the responses to three different compounds capable of producing adrenergic stimulation and (b) the effects of epinephine following prior administration of a beta blocking agent (propranolol).

Photographs showing the electrocardiographic repsonses to epinephrine, phenylephrine and isopoterenol were included with the text and thus, it could be seen that when the intervention was an infusion of epinephrine, the initial response was a progressive accentuation of the U wave at the expense of the T-wave. This effect, which first appeared 6 seconds after the infusion was begun, was not associated with any cardiac acceleration. Then, approximately 10 seconds after the infusion was started, the first effect was the development of three coupled ventricular premature contractions; immediately after, the rhythm changed abruptly to ventricular flutter. At that point, the ectopic rhythm was abolished promptly by the use of defibrillation equipment.

It could be seen also that a somewhat similar response followed the administration of phenylephrine whereas isoproterenol produced only a sinus tachycardia and a "rate related shortening of the Q-T wave interval." Moreover, propranolol given intravenously prior to the administration of epinephrine proved effective in preventing the ventricular tachyarrhythmia this catecholamine had produced previously.

Value of Pharmacologic Studies

Thus, the pharmacologic studies undertaken by Garza et al in their test subject were meaningful in several important respects. First, by showing that a ventricular tachyarrhythmia can follow an augmentation of adrenergic stimulation in an individual with an inherited physiologic anomaly involving ventricular repolarization, they reproduced in man a phenomenon which was essentially the same as that encountered previously in the experimental model employed by Fastier and Smirk.[54] Second, they demonstrated that a prodrome of the ventricular tachyarrhythmia was the appearance of a conspicuous U wave. Third, inasmuch as increased catecholamine release is known to follow either physical overexertion[55] or emotional overload[56,57] their results have helped to explain why either of these circumstances has been noted to be an important exogenous "risk factor" in terms of "triggering" a syncopal attack in individuals with an inherited repolarization anomaly. Fourth, their findings with respect to the effects of propranolol confirmed earlier observations by Ward[6,7] who had determined empirically that syncopal attacks in children with this inherited repolarization defect could be prevented by the use of such a preparation.

Evaluation of Persistent Ventricular Tacharrhythmia - A Case Study

The report by Mathews et al[35] showed that these authors had made observations somewhat comparable to those of Garza et al but their test subject was an 18-year-old seizure-prone auditionally normal woman without demonstrable organic heart disease, many of whose close relatives had manifested various combinations of perceptive deafness, syncopal attacks, and Q-T interval prolongation in the electrocardiogram.

Originally, she had been referred to the Medical College of Virginia on October 15, 1968 for evaluation of persistent ventricular tachycardia. She had been in good health until December 1967 when, in another hospital 12 hours following her first delivery after an uneventful pregnancy, she had a cardiac arrest requiring resuscitation. No electrocardiogram was obtained at that time. General physical examination, cardiac examination, and neurologic examination in October of 1968 revealed no significant abnormalities.

The subsequent electrocardiogram, showed a prolonged Q-T interval and a prominent U wave. A vectorcardiogram was normal and a phonocardiogram showed a normal mechanical systolic ejction period in spite of the "prolonged electrical systole." A chest roetgenogram showed no abnormality.
ECG responses to pharmacologic agents. During this hospitalization, observations were made with repsect to the electrocardiographic repsonses to various pharmacologic agents. Thus, following an intravenous injection of atropine (1.5 mg) there was an increase in the heart rate to 115 per minute and a reduction of the Q-T interval to 0.30 second which was well within the normal limits. On another occasion, phenylephrine (10 mg in 500 cc of distilled water given by slow infusion) increased systolic blood presssure from 120 to 150 mm of mercury, decreased the heart rate from 75 to 60 per min. and produced ventricular flutter. Intravenous administration of lidocaine promptly restored normal sinus rhythm. At a different time, digoxin 2.5 mg orally in 60 hours, produced no change in the Q-T interval.
Ninety six hours after discontinuation of all medication, the patient experienced a sudden attack of ventricular fibrillation confirmed by a synsyncopal electrocardiogram. The prompt use of cardioversion equipment successfully restored normal rhythm.

Subsequently, oral treatment with propranolol, 20 mg four times daily and diphenylhydantoin, 100 mg three times daily, was instituted and with this therapy the electrocardiogram continued to show a marked prolongation of the Q-T interval and a sinus arrhythmia, but for one year there was no recurrence of ventricular arrhythmia or syncope.

Conclusions

The results of the investigations and drug trials conducted by Garza et al[16,23] and by Mathews et al,[35] respectively, seem to have shown 1) that repolarization "after potentials" (the electrocardiographic hallmark of after potentials is a conspicuous enlargement of the U wave) and adrenergic augmentation are the elements which, together, favor the development of ventricular tachyarrhythmia in persons with an inherited repolarization anomaly associated with seizure-proneness; and 2) that a preparation which inhibits sympathetic stimulation of the heart in such individuals can be effective in reducing the frequency of life-threatening arrhythmias and, thus, the companionate syncopal attacks, as well.

LINKS BETWEEN ADRENERGIC ACTIVITY and SUDDEN DEATH

There are also other data with respect to the Inherited Susceptibility to Sudden Death syndrome which confirm the close links between adrenergic activity and both electrocardiographic and clinical features of this genetically determined entity. These are the findings described by Moss and McDonald[29] who, aware of the observations of Yanowitz et al[50] (that excision of the right stellate ganglion in canines resulted in enlargement of the U waves in the electrocardiogram), excised the left stellate ganglion in a non-epileptic female who at the age of 39 began to develop recurrent syncopal attacks presumably related to a "Q-T interval syndrome." Afterwards, it was noted by them that both the U-wave enlargement and the syncopal attacks in this patient disappeared.

Clearly, then, inasmuch as subsequent experimental investigations in canines, reported by Kliks et al[51] and by Schwartz et al,[44] have demonstrated that right stellate ganglion excision lowered and left stellate ganglion excision raised the ventricular fibrillation threshold, respectively, it is evident that there are now an adequate body of animal data to show that the measure employed by Moss and McDonald in a patient with an inherited susceptibility to sudden death was scientifically sound. Moreover, their data would seem to provide further corroboration of the view that augmented adrenergic traffic along the autonomic fibers supplying the heart contributes materially to the pathogenesis of all the features characteristic of this inherited fatal syndrome.

Correspondingly, such a perspective would suggest that a possible variant of the Inherited Susceptibility to Sudden Death syndrome might account for the ventricular arrhythmias which were encountered in the case described by Wellens et al in 1972.[58] Their patient was a young girl who,

> "when she was 14 years of age suddenly lost consciousness during one night when there was a severe rain storm accompanied by considerable thunder. When she regained consciousness a few minutes later, it was noted that she had been incontinent of urine. Thereafter, similar episodes occurred always on waking up, usually following the noise of the

alarm clock. She was admitted elsewhere four years later because of a tentative diagnosis of epilepsy. The attending cardiologist at that institution found that during her fainting spells, ventricular fibrillation was present and that the attacks could be provoked by setting off an alarm clock. Subsequently she was referred for evaluation and the physical examination did not disclose any abnormalities with repsect to the cardiovascular system. Similarly, the results of blood and urine laboratory tests, and encephalogram, and electromyogram, and audiometric testing were within normal limits. The routine electrocardiogram showed sinus rhythm, with normal P-Q interval and QRS width. However, in a routine EKG there were slight S-T segment changes associated with marked enlargement of the U waves. The family history was unremarkable. The electrocardiograms of the parents and five siblings of the patient showed normal Q-T segments at rest and following exercise. During the observation period of this patient it was repeatedly possible to evoke ventricular fibrillation by awakening her with an auditory stimulus. T-wave inversion appeared 8 seconds after the alarm signal and this was followed by premature beats and further bizarre changes in the Q-T segment. The combination of these Q-T segment abnormalities and ectopic activity resulted in ventricular premature beats following shortly after the summit of the T-wave leading to ventricular fibrillation. Seven of these episodes were recorded but all ended spontaneously. The longest one lasted 2 minutes and 11 seconds. These attacks could not be provoked by exercise, hyperventilation, the Valsalva maneuver, carotid sinus massage, or frightening her when she was awake. No arrhythmia occurred when she awakened spontaneously. Right and left sided heart catheterization revealed normal hemodynamics during both rest and exercise. No abnormalities were noted in cineangiograms of the left ventricle and coronary arteries. The functional properties of the A-V conduction system as measured by the extrastimulus method were normal.

"Following the completion of these investigations it was decided to prescribe 80 mg of propranolol daily. While she was receiving this drug, arousal with the alarm clock resulted only in Q-T changes but not in ectopic ventricular activity. Accordingly, she was discharged with the recommendation that she continue with the regular use of propranolol. Three months following her discharge, she suffered another attack of ventricular fibrillation and transient unconsciousness. Therefore, she was advised to supplement the propranolol with 50 mg of diphenylhydantoin four times daily. Since then she has remained free from attacks for the past 11 months."[58]

VENTRICULAR ECTOPIA and REM SLEEP

It is possible also that the recurrent episodes of ventricular fibrillation described by Lown et al in 1976[59] may be related to another variant of the Inherited Susceptibility to Sudden Death Syndrome. His patient was a 39-year-old educator who suddenly developed an episode of thanatoid syncope while he was at home. His wife, who was a registered nurse, was nearby and immediately initiated cardiopulmonary resuscitation and normal cardiac activity was resumed. Soon after, the patient was transported to a community hospital where the presence of intermittent ventricular fibrillation was confirmed. Accordingly, countershock therapy was instituted promptly but "defibrillation was achieved with some difficulty": consciousness returned 12 hours afterward.

There was no history of any previous cardiac illness and the results of a series of sophisticated cardiac studies including cardiac catheterization excluded any type of underlying organic heart disease. During his rather lengthy hospitalization, various monitoring devices were utilized to detect the frequency of recurrent ventricular arrhythmias in a variety of stressful situations, including psychiatric interviews. A similar modality was used to determine the incidence and nature of these arrhythmias during various phases of sleep and during programmed meditation sessions. Moreover, it was demonstrated that digitalis in combination with beta blocking drugs was especially effective in preventing further episodes of a life-threatening ventricular tachyarrhythmia.

Findings from Psychologic Testing and Sleep Studies

The results of psychologic testing and several psychiatric interviews indicated that the patient was a person with a great deal of underlying hostility who tended to use denial and other defenses to overcome violent impulses and anxiety.

The findings derived from sleep studies showed that during REM sleep, ventricular premature contractions increased in number and on one occasion an episode of actual cardioplegic ventricular fibrillation occurred,: the latter was "abolished promptly by appropriate treatment."

Results from Programmed Meditation

The results obtained from programmed meditation were especially intriguing inasmuch as monitored cardiac activity during such sessions demonstrated clearly that relaxation achieved in this manner succeeded in reducing the frequency of ventricular premature beats. Moreover, on several occasions when "he was harboring great emotional tension and was beginning to exhibit advanced grades of arrhythmias he was able to abolish them by meditation." Thus, it was the view of the authors of this article that their observations indicated that, despite the absence of any demonstrable organic heart disease or any supposed genetic predisposition to develop life-threatening ventricular arrhythmias, the occurrence of ventricular ectopic activity and, sometimes, even episodes of a life-threatening ventricular tachyarrhythmia could be not only "neurally mediated" but, more specifically, could be considered to be the result of augmented traffic moving along the sympathetic outflow pathways to the heart.

Observations Summarized

In support of this concept Lown et al cited, first, the beneficial effects of meditation—an act which in their view produces a generalized decrease in sympathetic nervous activity and perhaps also an increase in parasympathetic discharge; second, the increase in ventricular ectopic activity during the early morning hours of sleep which is the time when the REM phase with its usual disruption of autonomic activity is at its height: and third, the reduction in ventricular ectopic activity by drugs known either to augment vagal activity or to inhibit adrenergic influences reaching the heart.

CONCLUSIONS

It must be acknowledged, on the basis of the material discussed in this chapter, that whenever a premortem cardiac evaluation or a postmortem examination has not demonstrated the presence of organic heart disease in an individual who has died suddenly, it always must be considered that such a fatality could be due to a cardioplegic ventricular arrhythmia resulting from an augmentation of traffic along the sympathetic nervous pathways to the heart. Moreover, in this connection, the data in the article by Lown et al have emphasized the importance of a detailed family history in order to differentiate among such sudden deaths, those which could be linked to an inherited susceptibility to sudden death from those which could be neurogenic and yet not genetically determined. Particularly noteworthy, too, were the findings reported by Lown et al[59] with respect to the close temporal relationship between the occurrence of ventricular ectopia and REM sleep: conceivably, such an observation could help to explain some of the seemingly mystifying synsomnial sudden deaths which have occurred among the mentally ill (see Chapter 6).

REFERENCES

1. Jervell, A. and Lange-Nielson, F. Congenital deaf-mutism, functional heart disease with prolongation of Q-T interval and sudden death. *Am. Heart J.* 54:59 (1957).
2. Levine, S.A. and Woodworth, C.R. Congenital deaf-mutism, prolonged Q-T interval, syncopal attacks, and sudden death. *New Eng. J. Med.* 259:412 (1958).
3. Romano, C. et al. Aritmie cardiache rare del'eta pediatrica. *Clin. Pediatr.* 45:656 (1963).
4. Barlow, J.B. et al. Congenital cardiac arrhythmia. *Lancet* 2:531 (1964).
5. Gamstorp, I. et al. Congenital cardiac arrhythmia. *Lancet* 2:965 (1964).
6. Ward, O.C. A new familial cardiac syndrome in children. *J. Irish Med. Assoc.* 54:103 (1964).
7. Ward, O.C. The electrocardiographic abnormality in familial cardiac arrhythmia. *Irish J. Med. Sci.* 491:553 (1966).
8. Fraser, G.R. et al. Congenital deafness associated with electrocardiographic abnormalities, fainting attacks and sudden death. *Quarterly J. Med.* 33:361 (1964).
9. Jervell, A. et al. The surdocardiac syndrome. Three new cases of congenital deafness with syncopal attacks and Q-T prolongation in the electrocardiogram. *Am. Heart J.* 72:582 (1966).
10. Lisker, S.A. and Finkelstein, D. The cardio-auditory syndrome of Jervell and Lange-Nielson: Report of an additional case with radioelectrocardiographic monitoring during exercise. *Am. J. Med. Sci.* 252:458 (1966).
11. Romano, C. Congenital cardiac arrhythmia. *Lancet* 2:531 (1964).
12. James, T.N.-Apoplexy of the heart. *Circulation* 57:385 (1978).
13. Jervell, A. and Sivertssen, E. Surdo-cardialt Syndrom. *Nord. Med.* 78:1443 (1967).
14. James, T.N. Congenital deafness and cardiac arrhythmias. *Am. J. Cardiol.* 19:627 (1967).
15. Kallfelz, H.C. Ueber ein neues EKG syndrom bei kindern mit syncopalen anfallen und plotzlichem tod. *Dtsch. Med. Wochenschr.* 93:1046 (1968).
16. Garza, L.A. et al. Familial repolarization myocardiopathy. *Am. J. Cardiol.* 23:112 (1969).
17. Green, R. et al. Sudden unexpected death in three generations. *Arch. Int. Med.* 124:359 (1969).
18. Sanchez Cascos, A. et al. Cardio-auditory syndromes. Cardiac and genetic study of 511 deaf mute children. *Brit. Heart J.* 31:26 (1969).
19. van Bruggen, H.W. et al. Convulsive syncope resulting from arrhythmia in a case of congenital deafness with electrocardiographic abnormalities. *Am. Heart J.* 78:81 (1969).
20. James, T.N. Q-T prolongation and sudden death. *Mod. Concepts Cardiovas. Dis.* 38:35 (1969).
21. Gale, G.E. et al. Heriditary Prolongation of the Q-T Interval (Study of Two Families). *Brit. Heart J.* 32:505 (1970).
22. Phillips, J. and Ichinose, H. Clinical and Pathologic Studies in the Hereditary Syndrome of a Long Q-T Interval, Syncopal Spells and Sudden Death. *Chest* 58:236 (1970).
23. Garza, L.A. et al. Heritable Q-T prolongation without deafness. *Circulation* 41:39 (1970).
24. Karhunen, P. et al. Syncope and Q-T prolongation without deafness. The Romano-Ward syndrome. *Am. Heart J.* 80:820 (1970).
25. Motte, G. et al. The long Q-T interval and syncope. *Arch. Mal. Coeur* 63:831 (1970).
26. Lipp, H. et al. Recurrent ventricular tachyarrhythmias in a patient with a prolonged Q-T interval. *Med. J. Aust.* 1:1296 (1970).
27. Olley, P.M. and Fowler, R.S. The surdo-cardiac syndrome and therapeutic observations. *Brit. Heart J.* 32:467 (1970).
28. Fraser, G.R. et al. Genetical aspects of the cardio-auditory syndrome of Jervell and Lange-Nielsen (Congenital Deafness and Electrocardiographic Abnormalities) *Ann. Hum. Genet.* 28:133 (1964).

29. Moss, A.J. and Mc Donald, J. Unilateral cervicothoracic sympathetic ganglionectomy for the treatment of long Q-T interval syndrome. *N. Eng. J. Med.* 285:903 (1971).
30. Wennevold, A. and Kringelback, J. Prolonged Q-T interval and cardiac syncopes. *Acta. Paediatr. Scand.* 60:239 (1971).
31. Ratshin, R.A. et al. Q-T interval prolongation, paroxysmal ventricular arrhythmias, and convulsive syncope. *Ann. Int. Med.* 75:919 (1971).
32. Choussat, A. et al. Familial cardio-auditory syndrome *J. Arch. Mal. Coeur* 63:1715 (1970).
33. Fay, J.E. et al. Surdo-Cardiac Syndrome: Incidence Among Children in School for Deaf. *Can. Med. Assoc. J.* 105:718 (1971).
34. Csanady, M. and Kiss, Z. Hereditary protraction of the Q-T distance in the electrocardiogram without congenital deafness (Romano-Ward syndrome). *Orv. Hetil.* 113:2840 (1972).
35. Mathews, E.C. et al. Q-T prolongation and ventricular arrhythmias with and without deafness in the same family. *Am. J. Cardiol.* 29:702 (1972).
36. Diewitz, M. et al. Uber ein Familiaries Syndrom, mit Q-T Zeit-Verlangerung und Synkopalen Anfallen (Romano-Ward syndrom). *Med. Welt* 23:1377 (1972).
37. Johansson, B.W. and Jorming, B. Hereditary prolongation of Q-T interval. *Brit. Heart J.* 34:744 (1972).
38. Gallez, A. Allongement de Q-T et syncopes, sans surdite: le syndrome de Romano-Ward. *Giorn. It.* 2:218 (1972).
39. Van der Stratten, P.J.C. and Bruins, C.L.D. A family with heritable electrocardiographic Q-T prolongation. *J. Med. Genet.* 10:158 (1973).
40. Hanozono, N. et al. Heritable Q-T prolongation without deafness: The Romano-Ward syndrome. *Jap. Heart J.* 14:479 (1973).
41. Csanady, M. and Kiss, Z. Heritable Q-T prolongation without congenital deafness (Romano-Ward syndrome) *Chest* 64:359 (1973).
42. Langslet, A. and Sorland, S.J. Changes in ECG and cardiac rhythm with epilepsy-like attacks and sudden death in childhood. *T. Norske Laegeforen* 94:632 (1974).
43. Crawford, M.H. Prolonged Q-T interval syndrome: Sucessful treatment with combined ventricular pacing and propranolol. *Chest* 68:369 (1975).
44. Schwartz, P.J. et al. The long Q-T syndrome. *Am. Heart J.* 89:378 (1975).
45. Roy, P.R. et al Hereditary prolongation of the Q-T interval: Genetic observations and management in three families with twelve affected members. *Am. J. Cardiol.* 37:237 (1976).
46. Reynolds, E.W. and Vander Ark, C.R. Quinidine syncope and the delayed repolarization syndromes. *Mod. Concepts Cardiovas. Dis.* 45:117 (1976).
47. Vincent, C.M. et al. Q-T interval syndromes. *Progr. Cardiovasc. Dis.* 16:523 (1974).
48. Moothart, R.W. et al. The heritable syndrome of prolonged Q-T interval, syncope, and sudden death. *Chest* 60:263 (1976).
49. Gault, J.H. et al. Fatal familial cardiac arrhythmias: Histologic observations on the cardiac conduction system. *Am. J. Cardiol.* 29:548 (1972).
50. Yanowitz, F. et al. Functional distribution of right and left stellate inervation to the ventricles. Production of neurogenic electrocardiographic changes by unilateral alteration of sympathetic tone. *Circ. Res.* 18:416 (1966).
51. Kliks, B. et al. The Influence of sympathetic tone on ventricular fibrillation threshold during experimental coronary occlusion. *Circulation* 46:II - 115 (1972).
52. Kralios, F. et al. Effects of sympathetic nerve branch stimulation on ventricular recovery properties and cardiac rhythm. *Am. J. Cardiol.* 31:142 (1973).
53. Albidskov, J.A. Adrenergic effects on the Q-T interval of the electrocardiogram. *Am. Heart J.* 92:210 (1976).

54. Fastier, F.N. and Smirk, F.H. Some properties of amarin with special reference to its use in conjunction with adrenalin for the production of idioventricular rhythms. *J. Physiol.* 107:318 (1948).
55. Raine, A.E.G. and Pickering, T.G. Cardiovascular and sympathetic response to exercise after long-term beta adrenergic blockade. *Brit. Med. J.* 2:90 (1977).
56. Nestel, P.J. Catecholamine secretion and sympathetic nervous system responses to emotion in man with and without angina pectoris. *Am. Heart J.* 73:227 (1967).
57. Wolf, S. Emotions and the autonomic nervous system. *Arch. Int. Med.* 126:1024 (1970).
58. Wellens, H.J.J. et al. Ventricular fibrillation occurring on arousal from sleep by auditory stimuli. *Circulation* 46:661 (1972).
59. Lown, B. et al. Basis for recurring ventricular fibrillation in the absence of coronary heart disease and its management. *New Eng. J. Med.* 294:623 (1976).
60. Shanklin D.R. and Laite M.B. - Pickett-Sommer film strip technique. *Arch. Path.* 75:91 (1963).

CHAPTER 15

Psychotropic Agents

Elsewhere in this monograph it has been shown that in chronic alcoholics sudden deaths sometimes can follow the use of recommended doses of a substance primarily designed to benefit patients of this genre (see Chapter 4), and that when it is improperly used, a psychotropic agent like methadone can be responsible for a sudden death in narcotic addicts (see Chapter 11). Thus, it would seem proper, at this juncture, to examine some of the available data pertaining to the prospect that a different group of remedial phrenotropic substances may be inculpated in instances of sudden death among psychiatric patients whose illnesses are not considered to be primarily related to the misuse of either alcoholic beverages or narcotic drugs. Consequently, this chapter will deal mainly with the problem of sudden deaths which can be linked either to overdoses of the phenothiazines or to overdoses of tricyclic antidepressant compounds.

THE ROLE OF PHENOTHIAZINES IN SUDDEN DEATH

Historically, the article by Hollister which appeared in 1957[1] was one of the first to advance the view that phenothiazines might be linked to the occurrence of sudden deaths in psychiatric patients. The fatalities described in that paper were attributed to postconvulsive asphyxia, in the belief that phenothiazines lower the seizure threshold in seizure-prone psychiatric patients, particularly when the doses of the phenothiazines are excessive and when the phenothiazine administered was chlorpromazine. (See Chapter 5). However, it is currently recognized that a lowering of the seizure threshold cannot adequately explain the occurrence of a sudden death in psychiatric patients who have consumed customary amounts of a phenothiazine and who were not already seizure prone. Thus, alternatively, it has been suggested by certain observers[2] that, perhaps, a sudden death in psychiatric patients treated with phenothiazines, without a seizure diathesis, might be ascribed to a cardiotoxic property of the drug. However, as yet, no one has been able to provide any meaningful data to show that customary doses of any phenothiazine will indeed lower the ventricular fibrillation threshold or, in any other way, exert a cardiotoxic effect. Actually, there is now a body of data which seems to indicate that even though thioridazine, in customary doses, often will alter the morphology of the T-wave, this drug in ordinary doses does not produce any adverse cardiac effects.[3-21]

Effects of Thioridazine: Case Reports

Moreover, although it has been established already[3-21] that it is simply a pharmacogenic benign readily reversible repolarization alteration which is the physiologic counterpart of a thioridazine-induced T-wave change in the electrocardiograms of otherwise healthy psychiatric patients who have received customary amounts of this drug (see Chapter 13), certain reports in the medical literature have suggested that the administration of this particular phenothiazine preparation may be followed by a sudden death due to a drug-induced cardioplegic ventricular arrhythemia. However, after the data in these respective publications had been scrutinized by me it became evident that those who had postulated the existence of such a cardiotoxic effect of thioridazine had not given sufficient consideration to other variables including overdoses of the drug, concurrent administration of other psychotropics, the behaviorial traits of the decedent, the nature of the underlying psychiatric illness, and the postmortem findings.

This circumstance was emphasized in my previous discussion of the fatality reported by Kelly et al (see Chapter 12), and such a criticism would seem to be valid with respect to the six fatalities mentioned in the article by Hollister and Kosek.[22] Thus, an epicritical examination of their data seemed to indicate that the death, in one instance, could be ascribed to alimentary strangulation (see Chapter 5); in a second, to occlusive coronary artery disease (see Chapter 3); in a third, to fatty liver disease (see Chapter 4). Furthermore, even the data pertaining to the three remaining sudden deaths described by Hollister and Kosek, and the three fatalities reported by others[29,32-33] which are discussed in the succeeding section of this review, seem to show that a thioridazine treated patient is not at increased risk of dying suddenly, unless other extenuating factors are operative.

With respect to these six fatalities, it is noteworthy that in five instances, the dose of thioridazine consumed prior to the time of death was excessive; the exception was a patient who had received 400 mg of thioridazine but, concurrently, he had been consuming 1600 mg of chlorpromazine daily. In three instances the occurrence of at least one episode of life-threatening ventricular tachyarrhythmia, shortly before the time of death, was demonstrable. Five of the six decedents were adult schizophrenics ranging in age from 19 years to 44 years; the sixth decedent was a 35-year-old woman with a depressive reaction and a history of suicidal attempts. Anecdotal data pertaining to the first three of this group of six thioridazine treated decedents can be found in the article by Hollister and Kosek[22]

Case Report No. 1

One decedent was a 44-year-old schizophrenic man without a seizure history who died on the 52nd day of his hospitalization. He was extremely disturbed and assaultive and in order to control his aggressive behavior, increasing amounts of chlorpromazine were required. Accordingly, by the 40th day of his hospitalization he was receiving 1600 mg of this drug each day. On the 48th day of hospitalization thioridazine (400 mg daily) was added to the treatment program. On the 52nd day of hospitalization, the patient "had to be held by three nursing assistants while cuff restraints were applied. As this was being done, he suddenly stopped struggling, respirations stopped, and he was observed to become cyanotic and pulseless. Efforts at resuscitation were fruitless." The authors mentioned also that a postmortem examination was performed and added that the autopsy "could not ascertain the cause of death."

Discussion.

Thus, it is evident that the circumstances associated with this fatality are congruent with fatalities which have been observed formerly in patients with the syndrome of acute exhaustive mania (see Chapter 10). Consequently, it is conceivable, in this instance, that the forcible restraint during an episode of agitated behavior, and not *only* the drugs the patient had received prior to the time of death, could have been responsible for triggering the abrupt onset of a seeming cardioplegic ventricular arrhythmia.

Case Report No. 2

Another of the three allegedly autopsy-negative decedents was a 33-year-old man who had been confined to the hospital from January 16, 1961 to the day of his death on August 31, 1964. Throughout most of his hospitalization he received large doses of chlorpromazine (1600 to 1050 mg daily) but during the few weeks before his death, the daily dose of chlorpromazine had been reduced to 400 mg daily. During the time he received 1050 mg of chlorpromazine daily he was also given 1200 mg of thioridazine daily to control his hyperactivity and agitation. However, when the dose of chlorpromazine had been reduced to 400 mg daily, all thiordazine simultaneously had been discontinued. During his prolonged hospitalization, he had not shown any indication of a seizure state and anticonvulsant drugs had not been prescribed. Nevertheless, the anecdotal data pertaining to this decedent had indicated that two electroencephalograms had been made while he was receiving the combined thioridazine-chlorpromazine therapy; these studies disclosed diffuse paroxysmal slowing considered to be due to the influence of the phenothiazines on cerebral activity. The changes were not considered to be indicative of a seizure diathesis. By mid-August 1964 his disturbed behavior was less evident and along with this improvement he required smaller doses of the chlorpromazine. Nevertheless, on August 31, 1964, while he was with his group in the occupational therapy shop, he developed a typical attack of fatal syncope. "A physician who saw him soon afterward could detect no sign of life. A postmortem examination was made and this did not reveal any obvious cause for death."

Discussion.

Aside from this brief statement with respect to the postmortem findings, no information was supplied regarding the results of the necropsy. Presumably, the heart was judged to be normal on the basis of both gross and microscopic examination but undoubtedly it would have been helpful if the heart weight had been stated and the condition of the coronary arteries had been described in detail. Also, in view of the relatively young age of this patient, it would have been most desirable to obtain sections of the heart made in accord with the technique recommended by Lev (see Appendix) and by James[23,30] in order to exclude the possibility that the sudden cardiac arrest may have been the result of occlusive lesions of the coronary microcirculation or of some structural change located in the bundle of His or adjacent conduction tissues. The advantages of such a procedure in cases of sudden death are indisputable, inasmuch as meaningful data which have been assembled during the past two decades have shown clearly that a variety of such lesions can be a cause of a seemingly unexplained or mystifying sudden death.[23-24]

Also, it should be recognized that even though Moritz and Zamchek[25] had already shown, in 1946, that simple atherosclerotic luminal reduction of extramural coronary arteries could account for seemingly mystifying sudden deaths in military personnel (see Chapter 3), a pathologist who does not subscribe to this view could, understandably, disregard the significance of such coronary changes during an autopsy of a young adult who has died suddenly. Thus, it would be important to know whether, in this instance, the statement "postmortem examination revealed no obvious cause of death" meant that even simple constrictions along the course of the extramural coronary arteries had not been in evidence.

Moreover, since it generally is acknowledged that the majority of sudden deaths, even in psychiatric patients, are coronary-related fatalities (see Chapter 3), it would be equally advantageous to be certain that the prosector, in this instance, had made a meticulous examination of the coronary arteries throughout their course, and thus be able to affirm, with reasonable certainty, the absence of any arteriosclerotic narrowing of the extramural or intramural coronary vessels.

In this connection, Rodriguez et al[26] have made some particularly noteworthy observations. In their paper, which appeared in 1964, these investigators summarized their views:

"Schlesinger's work has shown that unaided dissection of non-injected coronary arteries may fail to disclose many of the occlusions present in a given series of specimens and this we have confirmed. If one assumed the number of occlusions found in our injected hearts to be similar to that in the non-injected control hearts, the proportion of occlusions missed in the latter comprises as much as two thirds of the total and the number of control hearts in which occlusions were found underestimates the correct figure by more than half. As might be expected, the occlusions not shown by routine methods of study, appear to be mostly those far from the coronary ostia and in the coronary branches rather than in the mainstems. Nevertheless, we share Schlesinger's view that the disparity in the results obtained with the two methods is less a matter of the care with which specimens are processed than it is of the adequacy of the technique of examination. With non-injected hearts, our own experience has been that it is practically impossible even with the most painstaking care to dissect and fully expose for study more than a fraction of the coronary arterial tree. Unless the examination of hearts in routine autopsies is done much more adequately than appears to have been true in our laboratory, it would seem safe to assume that the autopsy data now on record which bear on the incidence and topography of coronary occlusions include gross inaccuracies."

Thus, even if the pathologist, in this instance, may not have observed a meaningful degree of narrowing of the extramural coronary arteries, it would be uncertain whether the postmortem examination, indeed, had excluded the possibility that the fatality was ascribable to arteriosclerotic coronary artery disease. On the other hand, inasmuch as the postmortem data had not established a vascular basis for the death, it could be postulated that the dramatic instantaneous sudden death of this decedent may have resulted from the presence of a syndrome described elsewhere in this monograph under the rubric of the Inherited Susceptibility to Sudden Death (see Chapter 14). Usually, the postmortem examination, in persons who have died because of this inherited entity, does not indicate the presence of any structural cardiac abnormality. It has been observed, however, that when the coronary microcirculation is examined in detail with the aid of a specialized sectioning technique, occlusive lesions of the vessels supplying the specialized pacemaker sites of the heart have been discerned.[23,27]

Of some importance, also, is the fact that the anecdotal data with respect to this decedent had indicated that two electroencephalograms had been made during his prolonged hospitalization and that neither had confirmed the presence of epilepsy. Ordinarily, an electroencephalogram is not requested unless a patient has exhibited syncopal or other manifestions suggestive of a convulsive disorder and therefore it can be postulated that those responsible for the care of this decedent during his lengthy hospitalization had observed recurrent episodes of syncope prior to his untimely death.

Thus, inasmuch as spontaneously reversible pseudo-epileptic prodromes preceding a subsequent abrupt irreversible life-threatening ventricular tachyarrhythmia in a person without an evident structural cardiac abnormality represent a feature commonly observed in persons afflicted with the inherited susceptibility to sudden-death syndrome, the available anecdotal data in this instance would not conflict with the proposition that the sudden death of this decedent may have been due to such an inherited life-threatening entity. Frequently, this diagnosis can be confirmed by means of electrocardiographic data (see Chapter 14); but, it is clear that in this instance electrocardiograms had not been made when the electroencephalograms had been obtained. Nevertheless, in view of the syncopal prodromes exhibited by this patient prior to the time of death, it would seem improper to exclude the possibility that such an inherited entity was responsible for his sudden death.

Case Report No. 3

A third sudden death reported by Hollister and Kosek was a 40-year-old schizophrenic woman who had always been in good physical health. There was no history of seizures and she had never received any anticonvulsant drugs. Her last hospitalization lasted only 47 days, but throughout that relatively short period she received unusually large doses of phenothiazine drugs in order to control her psychotic behavior. The nature of the behavioral disturbance was not described but, in wiew of the large doses of the phenothiazines which were prescribed, it can safely be assumed that she was very hyperactive and assaultive.

The first phenothiazine she received was chlorpromazine; the maximum daily dose was 2400 mg. This maximum amount was reached six days before her death; but after this dose level was reached, the drug was then withdrawn abruptly and 1600 mg of thioridazine was substituted. Also, coincident with the onset of thioridazine therapy, a daily dose of 20 mg of trifluoperazine was prescribed. This daily dosage of thioridazine and trifluoperazine was continued for six days until she developed an attack of cardiac syncope.

Six days after the thioridazine-trifluoperazine therapy had been started, she was found unconscious in her room; resuscitation was attempted but she remained unconscious although her vital signs were normal when measured 30 minutes after the unsuccessful resuscitation attempt. So far as could be determined from the anecdotal data, no one had any knowledge of what, specifically, had transpired immediately before the onset of this syncopal episode and there was no history of prior episodes of syncope. Because of her persistent coma, she was transferred to the medical ward and, thereafter, no further phenothiazines were administered. It was unknown whether she had swallowed a large overdose of any of the drugs available to her in the hospital.

Soon after she had been transferred to the medical ward, she vomited and aspirated some of the vomitus. At this time, neither pulse, heart sounds, respirations, nor blood pressure were perceptible. Her vital signs were restored promptly but only by the use of mouth-to-mouth breathing and supplemental external cardiac massage.

The second attack of syncope occurred 3 hours after the first one and during the next 14 hours, 45 episodes of ventricular fibrillation were recorded on the monitor (clips of these electrocardiograms did not accompany the text). Treatment of these life-threatening ventricular tachyarrhythmias consisted of the administration of digitalis, procaineamide, dilantin, molar lactate, levarternol, and various antibiotics along with the supplemental use of defibrillatory electric countershocks. However, such treatment was successful in abolishing all but the 45th and final episode of ventricular fibrillation.

Following the patient's death, which occurred 17 hours after the first syncopal episode, a postmortem examination was performed; this examination revealed "a severe aspiration bronchopneumonia, left ventricular dilatation, and some histological myocardial changes secondary to electrodefibrillation."

Discussion. Thus, on the basis of all these data, it must be presumed that the initial episode of unconsciousness was, in fact, due to an episode of sudden cardiac arrest incidental to the development of either ventricular tachycardia or ventricular fibrillation. Accordingly, the persistent unconsciousness thereafter, until the patient finally died, can be attributed to the severe anoxic effects on her brain, resulting from the initial cardiac arrest. In turn, the recurrent episodes of documented ventricular fibrillation can be ascribed, either in part or entirely, to the effects of myocardial anoxia secondary to the initial cardiac arrest or to the presence, disclosed by the autopsy, of multiple areas of microscopic myocardial necrosis which may have antedated the first episode of life-threatening ventricular tachyarrhythmia.

However, it must be acknowledged that with respect to the pathogenesis of the life-threatening ventricular arrhythmia in this instance, the role of the phenothiazines cannot be minimized, inasmuch as it is known that the patient had received excessive doses of these drugs before the catastrophic event had occurred. In this connection, it should be noted that six days before the onset of the first syncopal episode, the decedent had received 2400 mg of chlorpromazine daily and then, without time having elapsed for the excretion of this drug (or its metabolites) from the various tissue sites (including the myocardium), a daily intake of 1600 mg of thioridazine and 20 mg of trifluoperazine simultaneously were immediately substituted for the previous dose of chlorpromazine; thereafter these drugs in these amounts, continued to be consumed until the patient was found unconscious in her room, 6 days after the shift to thioridazine and trifluoperazine. It is also conceivable that she may have swallowed, not long before the onset of her first syncopal episode, an overdose of one of these drugs prior to her first episode of syncope. The results of toxicologic studies of the body fluids had seemingly excluded such a possibility; but it is still uncertain whether serum levels of thioridazine can provide a reliable means of excluding the consumption of an overdose of these drugs.

Aside from such considerations, however, which are based exclusively upon current percepts regarding the pharmacology of the phenothiazines, it is necessary to consider another important possibility. The disruption of the autonomic equilibrium engendered by the underlying emotional disturbance for which the large doses of phenothiazines were administered in the first place, may have been responsible, at least in part, for the development of the cardiac arrhythmias which were in turn responsible for the initial episode of cardiac syncope and the recurrent attacks of life-threatening ventricular tachyarrhythmias. The events described by Hollister and Kosek with respect to this decedent may have thus supervened not so much because of the phenothiazines she had received, but in spite of them. Correspondingly, it is conceivable that the areas of myocardial necrosis disclosed at the time of the necropsy, which were ascribed by the on-site pathologist to "histological myocardial changes secondary to electrode-fibrillation" may have instead been actually stress-induced zones of myocardial necrosis (see Chapter 12).

In this connection, the observations of B.R. Pugh et al[28] are especially noteworthy. These authors reported their findings with respect to the myocardial effects of repeated application of D.C. countershock to the chest wall of several dogs. Each of two animals were given, every 5 minutes, as many as 10 shocks consisting of 400 watt-seconds each, and each of three other animals received five shocks at 5-minute intervals each consisting of 200 watt-seconds. After myocardial scintigrams with technetium-99 stannous pyrophosphate were obtained, the animals were sacrificed and skeletal muscle tissue near the sites of electrode placement as well as myocardial tissue from the right ventricle and anterior and posterior regions of the left ventricle were removed for histologic examination.

These histologic studies demonstrated that small isolated areas of myocardial necrosis were present in the hearts of only one of the three animals which had received, at 5-minute intervals, five shocks of 200 watt-seconds each and in the heart of one of the two animals which had received, at 5-minute intervals, ten shocks of 400 watt-seconds each. Moreover, in these two hearts the microscopic zones of myocardial necrosis were limited to the subepicardial area and it was noted also that deposits of calcium were present in these necrotic areas.

Pugh et al did not explain, however, the absence of myocardial necrosis in the other three animals, even though they had received equally large doses of D.C. current applied at frequent intervals to their chest walls, which clearly are much thinner than the chest wall of humans. Nevertheless, on the basis of their experimental findings, Pugh et al, postulated that when considerable electrical energy is applied over a short time period, myocardial necrosis of the sort they had described might also occur in man. However, they qualified this assumption by adding that this is a subject that will need additional prospective evaluation.

Thus, although the anecdotal data which Hollister and Kosek had provided with respect to this decedent had indicated that 44 episodes of ventricular fibrillation over a 14-hour period were terminated by external defibrillation *or* massage, it would be helpful to know specifically the magnitude of each shock in terms of watt-seconds, the number of shocks actually applied, and the time interval between each shock. Otherwise, it would be difficult to determine whether the experimental findings reported by Pugh et al concerning the pathogenesis of the myocardial necrosis in their animals would be relevant to the observations of Hollister and Kosek, who had considered that the repeated countershocks they had employed to abolish the ventricular tachyarrhythmia were responsible for the zones of myocardial necrosis the autopsy had disclosed. Moreover, in this same connection, it would be important to learn whether the histologic changes Hollister and Kosek had observed were limited to the subepicardium and whether they contained deposits of calcium like those reported by Pugh et al. Clearly, then, without such additional information it is difficult to determine whether, in this instance, the myocardial necrotic lesions, indeed, antedated or followed the onset of the life-threatening ventricular tachyarrhythmias.

Moreover, it should be evident that the clinical and postmortem findings in this instance resemble, to a large degree, the attributes described by Kelly, Fay, and Laverty[2] with respect to one of their decedents. Thus, in both instances, the following features were observed: (a) marked and persistent agitation despite the administration of excessive doses of phenothiazine compounds; (b) pre-terminal episodes of life-threatening ventricular tachyarrhythmias; (c) the presence of myocardial necrosis without associated occlusive coronary artery disease; (d) ultimately, a sudden cardiac arrest presumably due to an irreversible cardioplegic ventricular arrhythmia. Clearly, the only feature which differentiated these two decedents pertain to the use of a defibrillator; this was employed to manage the cardiac arrhythmia exhibited by Hollister and Kosek's patient, whereas it was not employed in connection with the treatment of the patient whose case history was included in the report by Kelly, Fay, and Laverty.

Thus, it is conceivable that the myocardial necrosis in the two respective decedents discussed by Kelly, Fay, and Laverty and by Hollister and Kosek was, mainly, a response to the severe emotional turmoil and its companionate excessive release of adrenergic hormones (see Chapter 12). Correspondingly, in accord with such a perspective, it would be reasonable to suppose that the myocardial necrosis in both instances antedated the first episode of ventricular fibrillation. Hence, the myocardial necrosis in the decedent reported by Hollister and Kosek could be viewed also as a major risk factor with respect to the development of the first and subsequent episodes of life threatening ventricular tachyarrhythmias which ultimately were responsible for an irreversible cardiac arrest.

Case Report No. 4

Subsequently, in 1968, Giles and Modlin[29] reported an allegedly autopsy-negative sudden death in a 19-year-old psychiatric patient who was treated with thioridazine. In this instance, the decedent was a soldier who had been admitted to the hospital on June 24, 1967 with a diagnosis of schizophrenic reaction of an undifferentiated type. At the time of his admission, he was highly agitated and assaultive and therefore was given increasing amounts of chlorpromazine over the next two months. By mid-August of 1967, he was receiving 3600 mg of this drug daily; in addition, he received large doses of perphenazine (32 mg daily) and large doses of trihexyphenidyl hydrochloride.

On September 1, 1967, for reasons which are not stated, the chlorpromazine was discontinued and was replaced with a daily dose of 3600 mg of thioridazine hydrochloride. Moreover, the other 2 drugs were continued in the same dose as before. On September 2, 1967, the patient experienced a brief episode of syncope while in the bathroom. He recovered spontaneously and suffered only a minimal amount of injury.

On September 5, 1967, he developed another episode of syncope and at that time it was noted that he was "cyanotic apneic, and pulseless." Therefore, those in the vicinity, immediately applied "blows on the chest which resulted in a resumption of the heart beat and respiration" and a return of consciousness. Also, at the time of this second syncopal attack, he vomited some gastric contents which supposedly were aspirated when his respirations returned. At the same time, it was noted that the abdomen was distended and an x-ray study confirmed the presence of an "adynamic ileus."

ECG Findings. After he had recovered from the second syncopal episode, an electrocardiogram was obtained; in this electrocardiogram, the significant finding was an enlargement of the U wave (this was evident in the electrocardiogram which accompanied the text of this article.) Apparently, no prior electrocardiograms had been obtained during this patient's hospitalization so that it was uncertain, first whether the prominent U-wave would have been present on a previous occasion as well and, second, whether the prominent U-wave was linked to the two episodes of syncope. Also, it should be noted that there was no evidence of a cardiac arrhythmia in this electrocardiogram.

Clinical findings after second attack. Also noteworthy was the finding that "values with respect to serum potassium, chlorides, carbon dioxide, calcium and phosphorous were normal" soon after the patient's recovery from the second syncopal attack. Nevertheless, the patient was considered ill enough at that time to be treated in an intensive care unit where he was attached to a cardiac monitor. Soon after his transfer to this unit, he had an "explosive bowel movement and soon afterward became cyanotic." Coincidentally, "the cardiac monitor revealed the presence of a ventricular tachycardia." (This arrhythmia was evident in the photograph of the electrocardiogram which accompanied the text.) Accordingly, a bolus of lidocaine was injected intravenously and thereafter the patient received a continuous intravenous drip of the same substance. With this treatment, a normal sinus rhythm was maintained except for the occasional bursts of ventricular tachycardia which were abolished by the use of D.C. countershocks.

Features of third attack. Sometime afterward (the time was not specified) the patient developed a third episode of apnea and syncope. However, attempts to resuscitate him were only partially successful because although normal sinus rhythm was restored, consciousness did not return; thereafter, he remained comatose until his sudden death 13 days after the third syncopal attack.

Following his third syncopal episode, an electrocardiogram was obtained and in that recording "the Q-T interval was normal even though there were evidences of ventricular irritability, particularly noticeable during the act of defecation." Moreover, soon after he had recovered from the third syncopal episode, the "values for serial chemical determinations including blood electrolytes and serum enzymes remained within normal limits." Repeated chest x-ray films confirmed an aspiration pneumonia and the patient was given antibiotics and fluids intravenously. Nevertheless, suddenly, on September 18,1967, he "became apneic, there was no cardiac electrical activity, and he was pronounced dead."

Postmortem findings. A postmortem examination was made and the following statements represent a summary of the pathologist's findings:

"The brain was severely edematous (presumably due to anoxia). The pericardium contained 20 cc of clear fluid and the myocardial surface was clear and glistening. The heart weighed 300 gm and was normal in size, shape, and position. The endocardium and valves were normal. The coronary arteries were normal in origin and distribution and free from atherosclerosis. Multiple microscopic sections of the heart were taken from the left atrium and ventricle, the mitral, tricuspid, and aortic valves, and from the interventricular and interatrial septa in the region of the conducting system. These showed the myocardial fibers to be normal in size with normal sized nuclei. However, there were scattered areas in which cytoplasmic fragmentation was prominent and in all areas, there was variable loosening of the intercellular connective tissue. This was prominent around the small arterioles and capillaries and was accompanied by an infiltrate of mononuclear cells with occasional drop out of myocardial fibers and pigment laden macrophages. No lesions were found without the conducting system itself."

Discussion. The anecdotal data pertaining to this auditionally normal decedent have described the occurrence of a sudden death in a normokalemic, thioridazine-treated, floridly psychotic, young adult schizophrenic who, prior to the time of death, developed anoxic brain damage and persistent coma seemingly after an attack of cardiac syncope initiated by an episode of ventricular fibrillation. Also, it is noteworthy that the postmortem examination had not disclosed any organic cardiac pathology except for a zone of myocardial necrosis which the pathologist seemingly had not considered to be responsible for the recurrent life-threatening ventricular arrhythmias and their companionate episodes of thanatoid syncope. Other meaningful features pertaining to this decedent's terminal illness included recurrent arrhythmic prodromes before he had expired and along with these arrhythmic prodromes, the intermittent appearance of an enlarged U wave in his electrocardiogram. Clearly, then, the sequence of events in this instance could be explained by either a U wave syndrome of an inherited variety which is described in this monograph under the rubric of an Inherited Susceptibility to Sudden Death (see Chapter 14), or by a U-wave syndrome due either to the consumption of excessive doses of thioridazine or to the presence of a myonecrotic lesion in the heart resulting from a companionate catecholamine excess incidental to the marked emotional disturbance for which the decedent had been hospitalized (see Chapter 12).

Actually, Giles and Modlin[29] also had considered the possibility that an inherited entity associated with a lowered ventricular fibrillation threshold might explain the occurrence of this fatality but after some deliberation, they deemed it unreasonable to suppose that it was, indeed, the basis for this patient's sudden death. The reasons Giles and Modlin had advanced for rejecting such a possible relationship were, first, the lack of any associated hearing disturbance; second, the lack of any family history of sudden unexpected deaths; third, the disappearance of a "Q-T prolongation" in electrocardiograms made subsequent to the first one; fourth, the failure on the part of their pathologist to demonstrate occlusive lesions of the intranodal coronary branches of the sort which T.N. James[30] had considered to be one of the characteristic anatomical features of this syndrome.

However, the important discoveries which have been made during the past decade concerning the variants of this life-threatening entity, make it evident that the objections of Giles and Modlin are unwarranted. It must be acknowledged that originally, the matter of an associated hearing impairment was believed to be one of the fundamental features of an inherited susceptibility to sudden death,[31] but additional observations have demonstrated that this inherited fatal entity can account for some sudden deaths in auditionally normal young persons as well (see Chapter 14). Moreover, the authors of some recent publications have emphasized the inconstancy of the characteristic electrocardiographic features of the Inherited Susceptibility to Sudden Death syndrome. (see Chapter 13)

Equally invalid is their assertion that they had dismissed any connection between this soldier's unexpected death and an inherited susceptibility to sudden death because the "family history was negative." This statement would imply that they either had questioned the patient or his relatives at the time of his admission to the hospital about such an hereditary trait or that they had made a genealogic survey of the relatives to determine first, whether any had suffered from syncopal attacks; second, whether any had died suddenly or unexpectedly; third, whether any had manifested evidences of congenital deafness; fourth, whether electrocardiograms of any relatives had demonstrated a prolongation of the Q-T interval.

However, since the patient was already "floridly psychotic and therefore unmanageable" when he was admitted to the psychiatric unit of the Army hospital where he died, it is unlikely that this decedent could have provided any relevant information in regard to such considerations. Moreover, anyone familiar with customary procedures connected with "history taking" recognizes that it is not usual to include an interrogation about such familial traits even when a close friend or relative who has accompanied a disturbed psychotic to the hospital is available for questioning with regard to details of this nature. Also, it is patently impossible to know with any degree of certainty to what extent the authors had attempted to obtain information of this sort after the patient had died.

Moreover, since this inherited fatal syndrome was first described in 1957,[31] occasional reports have been published which indicate that there may be a "negative family history" even in auditionally normal young persons with an inherited susceptibility to sudden death (see Chapter 14). In two such instances, the postmortem examination, which included special sectioning techniques of the heart, demonstrated the presence of a vasculopathy involving the small coronary branches supplying the sensitive pacemaker sites of the heart; moreover, this vasculopathy was considered to be a lesion resulting from a genetically-determined abnormality of these vessels. Thus, with regard to these two fatalities, an hereditary factor was involved in the pathogenesis not only of the vasculopathy but also of the cardiac arresting ventricular tachyarrhythmia responsible for these sudden deaths. Correspondingly, in view of such observations, it is regrettable that the conducting tissues of the heart of the decedent reported by Giles and Modlin were not studied in accordance with the method described by James[30] in order to exclude the type of inherited vasculopathy he had described.

Moreover, it cannot be denied, categorically, that the myocardial necrosis discovered by the pathologist could have resulted from the catecholamine excess induced by the psychotic turmoil (see Chapter 12) and that this lesion, in turn, was the source of the arrhythmic cardiac behavior which ultimately caused the sudden death of the patient reported by Giles and Modlin. However, in the final analysis, it would be reasonable to agree with the proposition of these authors that the electrocardiographic findings, the recurrent ventricular arrhythmias, and the sudden death of their patient were, in part, if not completely, the sequel to the combination of extreme psychotic behavior and the consumption of *excessive* doses of both thioridazine and chlorpromazine.

Case Report No. 5

Also, there was reported by Leestma and Koenig[32] (again in 1968) the sudden death of another thioridazine-treated agitated schizophrenic but in this instance the fatality was a 24-year-old woman who had received this drug for only one day before she died. Nevertheless, in certain respects, the clinical and postmortem findings linked to her sudden death resembled the corresponding features with respect to the sudden death of the highly agitated 44-year-old schizophrenic Hollister and Kosek had described in the paper they had published in 1965.[22] Thus, each of the decedents described by Leestma and Koenig and by Hollister and Kosek, respectively, had received chlorpromazine and thioridazine prior to the time of death; each remained highly disturbed despite the administration of these drugs; each developed a cardiac arrest while being restrained forcibly during an episode of violent behavior; in each instance, the postmortem examination did not disclose any anatomical changes in the heart or in any other part of the body which could explain the sudden death.

However, the sudden deaths reported by Hollister and Kosek and by Leestma and Koenig, respectively, were not identical. With regard to the sudden death described by Leestma and Koenig, there was a 10-hour interval of unconsciousness between the time of death and the onset of the syncopal prodrome which coincided with the attempt to apply the restraints whereas Hollister and Kosek's patient had died instantly when the restraints were applied. On the other hand, this may not be an important difference inasmuch as it was only the patient reported by Leestma and Koenig who received prompt external cardiac massage coincident with the onset of her syncopal episode.

Anecdotal data. The anecdotal data provided by Leestma and Koenig concerning the drugs their patient had consumed prior to the time of death indicated that on day #1 of her hospitalization she received 400 mg of chlorpromazine but over the ensuing five days, the dose gradually was increased, presumably because of a progressive deterioration of her psychotic state along with increasing difficulties in controlling her agitation. Accordingly, between day #6 and day #9, inclusive, she was receiving more than 2000 mg per day of chlorpromazine. However, on day #10, she received 2100 mg of thioridazine instead of her usual dose of chlorpromazine.

Nevertheless, during the evening of day #10, she became markedly agitated and assaultive and for this reason the attendants on duty at that time attempted to restrain her forcibly. However, during this procedure, she became unconscious and cyanotic and those nearby could not hear her heart sounds. Immediately thereafter, they instituted external cardiac massage but although audibility of the heart beat was restored, she remained comatose and an electrocardiogram obtained 30 minutes after the onset of the syncopal episode confirmed the presence of a ventricular tachycardia along with nonspecific T-wave and ST segment changes. Other unspecified laboratory studies "were interpreted as normal." Despite supportive measures to maintain her blood pressure during the ensuing period of persistent coma, "she died 10 hours after her collapse without regaining consciousness." No studies were done to determine the phenothiazine blood levels.

Discussion. Thus, it would seem reasonable to suppose that, in this instance, several factors in unison were operating to produce the syncopal episode which was not immediately fatal only because of the prompt institution of external cardiac massage. Certainly, it cannot be denied that one of these factors could have been the excessive amounts of the thioridazine the decedent had received on day #10 summated with the large amounts of chlorpromazine she had received during the preceding four days. However, in view of the experience reported earlier by Hollister and Kosek[22] and the indication that the onset of both the arrhythmic and syncopal episodes of Leestma and Koenig's patient occurred simultaneously with attempts to restrain her forcibly while she similarly was in the throes of a highly agitated state, it would seem proper to emphasize that "restraint stress" with its secondary augmentation of catecholamine activity (see Chapter 10) may, in a patient already highly agitated, lower the ventricular fibrillation threshold and thus favor an arrhythmogenic cardiac arrest.

Case Report No. 6

In 1976, eight years after the paper by Lesstma and Koenig had appeared, Fowler et al reported another sudden death in a thioridazine treated psychiatric patient without demostrable organic heart disease.[33] The decedent, who was a 35-year-old woman, had been admitted to the hospital on August 17, 1968 because of a psychotic depressive reaction and after "an attempted suicide."

At the time of her admisssion, there was no history of a seizure diathesis, or any form of heart disease. Initially, the phrenotropic drugs which were prescribed for her included the following phenothiazine prepartions; 1000 mg of thioridazine daily; 40 mg of trifluoperazine daily; a 300 mg spansule of chlorpromazine daily. There was no information to indicate whether any medication changes had been made prior to the day she died. Moreover, from the anecdotal data which these authors had provided, it could not be ascertained whether or not the administration of these drugs had been followed by an improvement or worsening of her depressive state. Also lacking was any indication of the nature of her behavioral traits while she was receiving these drugs.

Clearly, during her confinement to the hospital, the most alarming and dramatic change in her condition occurred on the 36th day following her admission. On that day, she developed, suddenly, a series of convulsive episodes. In addition, at the time of the first seizure, a "physician observed her pulse to be irregular" but an electrocardiogram presumably obtained soon afterward and possibly after she had received such antiarrhythmic drugs as lidocaine and procaine amide, had confirmed the presence of (a) a normal sinus mechanism with the heart rate of about 80 per minute; (b) "a prolonged Q-T interval"; (c) "prominent U waves in limb and precordial leads." An electrocardiogram obtained shortly afterward demonstrated the presence of a ventricular tachycardia followed by restoration of a normal rhythm by means of a "blow to the chest."

Subsequently, the attending physicians observed recurrent episodes of recurrent tachyarrhythmia which, generally, were abolished by the use of such measures as lidocaine and procaine amide infusions, countershock therapy, and the insertion of a transvenous pacemaker; however, before the day had ended, the decedent developed an irreversible cardiac arrest. A postmortem examination was made and according to the coroner who performed the autopsy, "there was no gross or microscopic cardiac abnormality."

Discussion. Lacking in the case history extract was any information with respect to the nature of the decedent's depressive reaction. Thus, it is unknown whether her depression was accompanied by considerable agitation for which the conglomeration of phenothiazines had been prescribed and if, before the onset of the initial seizure and its companionate arrhythmia, she had become overly agitated and consequently was restrained forcibly. This consideration has been introduced inasmuch as the experience reported earlier by Leestma and Koenig[32] as has been explained already, had indicated that such restraints were the proximate cause of a presumed arrhythmogenic cardiac arrest.

Another noteworthy omission from the anecdotal data pertaining to the fatality reported by Fowler et al[33] was any reference to toxicologic studies which could have helped to determine whether, shortly before the onset of the initial seizure, the decedent had swallowed impulsively a megadose of thioridazine or any of the other drugs she had been receiving during her relatively brief period of hospitalization. This consideration is mentioned primarily for three reasons. First, it is recognized that depressed patients who are known suicidal risks, frequently and surreptitiously will swallow overdoses of any drugs which are within reach and will devise various strategies in order to make it possible for them to perform such an act.[34] Second, during electrocardiographic monitoring of a patient who survived after swallowing an overdose of thioridazine in connection with a suicidal attempt[35] the noteworthy findings included periods of normal sinus rhythm associated with an enlargement of the U wave alternating with episodes of ventricular tachycardia and ventricular fibrillation; moreover, in these instances, the conspicuous U wave was no longer present after the patient had recovered. Third, it has been observed that the consumption of a megadose of thioridazine with suicidal intent can be followed by the sudden onset of seizures and, soon afterward, by an irreversible cardiac arrest, even though the autopsy indicated that the heart was sound structurally.

Conclusions. Thus, in retrospect, inasmuch as the cluster of findings preceding the sudden death described by Fowler et al included an abrupt onset of seizures, an enlargement of the U wave in the electrocardiogram and the occurrence of a life-threatening ventricular tachyarrhythmia prior to the time of death, it would seem proper to consider a phenothiazine overdose to be one of the possible causes for that fatality.

However, it would be necessary to exclude also the presence of an acute intracranial lesion as the basis for her unexpected death and for the various prodromes which preceded the cardiac arrest. For this reason, it would be helpful to know whether, at the time of the necropsy, the prosector (the local medical examiner) had opened the skull and had examined carefully the intracranial contents. Actually, the anecdotal data pertaining to this decedent indicated merely that "there was no gross or microscopic cardiac abnormality"; no other details were provided with respect to the autopsy findings.

POSSIBLE PHYSIOLOGIC MECHANISMS FOR VENTRICULAR ARRHYTHMIA

The connection between an acute intracranial lesion and the development of seizures, and an enlargement of the U wave, and a companionate life-threatening ventricular arrhythmia has been discussed thoroughly in a paper by Cruickshank et al.[36] These British investigators had measured total body exchangeable potassium, catecholamine excretion, serum cortisol, and potassium levels and had correlated these findings with electrocardiographic data in a large sample of patients with subarachnoid hemorrhage and they had noted that even when there was little lowering of the serum potassium levels, the characteristic features of a potassium deficit were present in the electrocardiogram. These changes consisted primarily of T-wave inversion and tall U waves (a so-called long Q-T interval); moreover, despite the normal serum potassium level, the measurements of body exchangeable potassium indicated an intracellular potassium deficit. The concurrent increase in catecholamine excretion was ascribed by them to hypothalamic stimulation secondary to an acute intracerebral insult; therefore, they proposed that the electrocardiographic abnormalities in such instances could be a release of catecholamines secondary to hypothalamic stimulation in conjunction with the rise in corticosteroid activity and an associated potassium deficiency. Inferentially, then, such a combination of circumstances might have been the explanation for the occurrence of the ventricular arrhythmias and even of the presumed arrhythmogenic cardiac arrest in the decedent reported by Fowler et at.[33]

THE ROLE OF TRICYCLIC ANTIDEPRESSANTS IN SUDDEN DEATH

Like the phenothiazines, the tricyclic antidepressants also represent a group of remedial phrenotropic substances which, in customary doses, can be of great benefit to the psychiatric patient but, in overdoses, can be not only poisonous but lethal as well. The first to describe such a drug-related fatality were Michon et al, whose paper was published in 1959.[37] Since then, many other reports have appeared which either have cited or described fatal as well as non-fatal episodes of tricyclic antidepressant poisoning in adult psychiatric patients who, willfully, have swallowed an overdose of such a drug in connection with a suicidal attempt.[37-64,78-83]

Moreover, the data in these numerous reports have delineated the typical features of tricyclic antidepressant intoxication in psychiatric patients without preexisting heart disease. Thus, it is now generally agreed that the usual clinical syndrome resulting from tricyclic antidepressant overdosage includes, on the one hand, certain neurologic manifestations (rapid onset of coma, delirium, convulsions) and, on the other hand, a variety of electrocardiographic abnormalities.[42] Of the latter, the most important are the evidences of delayed intraventricular conduction, sometimes followed by major cardiac arrhythmias (atrial or ventricular); in addition, in the fatal cases, such cardiac effects usually are followed by a bradycardia and an asystolic cardiac arrest rather than a cardioplegic ventricular fibrillation.[40,42,64] Also it is noteworthy that when there was no preexistent cardiac disease, the postmortem findings pertaining to such fatalities generally have excluded the presence of any cardiac pathology.[43,64,48]

However, it should be recognized that although abnormal cardiac behavior is the usual basis for a fatal outcome in cases of tricyclic antidepressant poisoning, not all fatalities associated with overdoses of tricyclic antidepressants are due solely to this cause. On rare occasions, such drug related deaths allegedly have been the result of an "adult respiratory distress syndrome"[57,58] or one due to a disseminated intravascular coagulopathy associated with a fatal hyperpyrexia syndrome.[57] Most often, there is no detectable visceral or other pathology.[56]

As yet, it has not been possible to establish the exact incidence of sudden deaths due to poisoning from tricyclic antidepressants in psychiatric patients, but there is no doubt that these psychotropic drugs have been responsible for ever increasing numbers of fatal as well as non-fatal poisonings in patients of this genre.

This conclusion seems to be supported by the findings reported by Larcan et al from France,[50] by Newton from Scotland,[61] and by Vohra et al from Australia.[51] Larcan et al noted that between 1958 and 1962 tricyclic antidepressant poisoning accounted for only 3% of the 102 cases of drug-induced intoxications admitted to a hospital in the environs of Paris, whereas throughout the single year of 1968, when drug intoxications accounted for 222 admissions to that same hospital, the proportion who had been poisoned by an overdose of tricyclic antidepressants had risen to 8.5%. The data provided by Newton indicated that in 1965 the tricyclic antidepressants were implicated in only 1% of the poisoning cases admitted to the Regional Poisoning Center in Edinburgh, (the special unit set aside to serve a population of three quarters of a million persons) whereas, between 1965 and 1973, when 2104 poisonings were treated there, 10% of these cases were found to be the result of tricyclic antidepressant overdosage. Although the findings of Vorha were based on a more limited survey, their data, in this regard were even more impressive. Thus, they noted that "during an 18-month period (June 1971 to December 1972) 340 cases of self poisoning were admitted to the Royal Melbourne Hospital and of these, 76 (22%) were due to the ingestion of tricyclic antidepressants."

Effects of Megadoses

Larcan et al[50] attempted also to ascertain the dose of a tricyclic antidepressant (imipramine or amitriptyline) required to produce a characteristic episode of fatal tricyclic antidepressant poisoning. For this purpose, they examined all the available evidence pertaining to a sample of 24 patients who, impulsively, had swallowed a megadose of the drug. Thereafter, they made the following observations: "of the 14 patients who had consumed less than 1.5 gm of the drug, all survived; of the 5 who had consumed between 1.5 gm and 2.5 gm, one died; in the remaining 3, the size of the overdose was not known." However, these investigators did not supply any information regarding the survivability of these 3 additional patients.

Also, it was mentioned by Larcan et al that when megadoses of a tricyclic antidepressant are involved, measurements of the blood levels of these compounds or their metabolities cannot provide meaningful information with respect to the dose which had been consumed or the severity of the intoxication. In this regard, their findings seemed to be in accord with the observations of Lewis and Oswald[62] and of Spiker et al.[47] Accordingly, Larcan et al suggested that the amounts removed during gastric lavage when the patient is admitted to the hospital for treatment of an episode of tricyclic antidepressant intoxication, probably would provide a better estimate of the amount of the tricyclic antidepressant which had been ingested prior to the onset of the clinical evidences of intoxication than could be determined from toxicologic studies of the body fluids.

Furthermore, Larcan et al postulated that the severity of the abnormalities in an electrocardiogram obtained during an episode of tricyclic antidepressant intoxication might be an index of the size of the dose responsible for the intoxication. In order to test the validity of this hypothesis, they compared the findings in the electrocardiograms obtained in 14 patients whose intoxication had followed the consumption of no more than 1 gm of the drug with the findings in the electrocardiograms of 12 patients who had ingested 1.5 gm or more prior to the time of admission to the hospital. The results of this phase of their survey showed that changes indicative of abnormalities of conduction were present in the electrocardiograms of 3 of the 12 patients who had swallowed 1.5 gm or more whereas the usual electrocardiographic responses following the consumption of less than 1.5 gm of a tricyclic antidepressant was a sinus tachycardia, sometimes associated with evidences of an abnormality of repolarization (a nonspecific T-wave change and an occasional companionate enlargement of the U wave).

Thus, it is evident that these observations reported by Larcan et al are essentially in accord with the results of an earlier survey conducted by Gaultier et al.[64] In connection with their undertaking, these investigators had analyzed the data in the case records of 100 patients who had been admitted, prior to 1965, to the Widal Hospital in Paris, France because of "acute intentional poisoning" following the ingestion of an overdose of a tricyclic antidepressant. Although imipramine was the drug which was involved chiefly (73 instances) there were 17 instances of poisoning due to amiptryline and 10 due to trimeproprimine. Moreover, Gaultier et al found that 56 of these 100 patients had consumed between 500 and 1100 mg during the suicidal attempt, whereas 44 had swallowed more than 1100 mg. These differences proved to be meaningful especially in relation to the mortality data. In this connection, it is noteworthy that 9 fatalities had occurred exclusively as a result of tricyclic antidepressant intoxication but these had swallowed more than 1100 mg of the drug.

Finally, on the basis of a sizeable body of animal data[64,65,66] and because of the electrocardiographic findings in the patient sample they had investigated, Gaultier et al concluded that "serious acute poisoning with imipramine and related compounds owes its grave prognosis to a specific cardiotoxicity. The latter appears only with doses of more than 1 gm which relieves therapeutic doses of this risk, apart from "individual contraindications." However, in their article, these observers did not identify precisely what they had considered to be an "individual contraindication." Supposedly, in view of the results of the prospective human studies undertaken by Muller et al prior to 1961[67] and because of the anecdotal data reported in 1959 by Freyhan[68] and by Malitz et al[69] they were concerned about the possibility that the administration of even customary doses of a tricyclic antidepressant to elderly depressives with established cardiovascular disease might be followed by an adverse cardiac effect and even a sudden coronary related cardiac arrest.

Effects of Customary Doses in Coronary Patients

Similar considerations concerning the possible adverse cardiac effects of *customary doses* of a tricyclic antidepressant were responsible for the prospective and longitudinal study undertaken by Moir et al in Scotland.[70] Their entire patient sample consisted of 312 persons and these were divided into 2 groups. Presumably, the patients in both subsets were depressed and were being treated concurrently for their underlying "cardiac disease", but one subset, which comprised 162 such persons, were not receiving amitriptyline; these were labelled the "controls" because, allegedly, they were the "match" of the remaining 150 patients (the index group), in terms of age, sex, and the proportion with a past history of myocardial infarction. Thus, Moir et al considered the index group to be different from the "controls", only because the former were the patients with "cardiac disease" who had been receiving a daily ration of amitriptyline; the dose and duration of the therapy with this tricyclic antipressant were not mentioned but it can be assumed that the dose was the usual one.

Although Moir et al did not state clearly that both the index group and the "matched controls" were individuals with atherosclerotic coronary artery disease, it can be presumed that the cardiac impairment of their subjects was due to this type of degenerative heart disease. Moreover, the data in their publication did not provide any information to indicate that the two groups did, indeed, resemble each other with respect to the following characteristics: (a) the extent of coronary stenosis; (b) equal proportions with a history of more than a signle myocardial infaction; (c) equal proportions with "malignant" ventricular premature contractions; (d) equal proportions with ventricular asynergy; (e) equal proportions who continued to smoke; (f) equal proportions who continued to drink alcoholic beverages to excess; (g) equal proportions who remained obese; (h) equal proportions who were diabetic; (i) equal proportions who were hypertensive; (j) equal proportions with cardiac enlargement.

Clearly, inasmuch as the primary goal of their study was to compare the incidence of sudden deaths in an amitriptyline treated subset of coronary patients with the incidence of such fatalities in "matched controls" who were not receiving amitriptyline it would seem proper to be certain that the two subsets were indeed alike with respect to such particular traits. These particular attributes have been selected because there is now a substantial body of data to indicate that any combination of such variables could favor the occurrence of sudden deaths in persons with an authenticated diagnosis of atherosclerotic coronary artery disease[71-76,91-95,98-101]

Another criticism with respect to the report of Moir et al pertains to the ambiguity of their statement that, unlike the "matched controls", the "majority of the amitriptyline treated patients in the present study had been acute emergencies admitted to the hospital." Surely, if the amitriptyline-treated patient sample had been hospitalized more often then the "controls" because of the development of an acute coronary complication, it must be acknowledged that they represented a group of persons who, aside from any regard to tricyclic antidepressant therapy, already were at increased risk of dying suddenly (see Chapter 3). Correspondingly, then, the observation by Moir et al that "there were 13 sudden unexpected deaths in the group of 119 amitriptyline treated patients compared with only three in a carefully matched control group" would not mean, necessarily, that the prospect of a sudden death is enhanced fourfold when amitriptyline, in customary doses, is prescribed for a coronary patient who is also in need of treatment for a depressive reaction. Moreover, in this same connection, it is noteworthy that the findings of the Boston Collaborative Drug Study pertaining to the effects of tricyclic antidepressants in hospitalized patients with cardiovascular disease[77] contradicted completely the views of Moir et al regarding the cardiotoxicity of "amitriptyline when given in therapeutic doses patients with preexisting heart disease."

Effect of Single Megadose on the Heart

Additional meaningful insights, but of a somewhat different sort, have been provided by Spiker et al,[47] by C Thorstrand[41,44] and by Biggs et al,[47] with respect to the cardiac toxicity produced by single megadoses of tricyclic antidepressants. The patient samples studied by these respective observers varied in size but all comprised psychiatric patients without demonstrable organic heart disease, who, prior to their admission to the hospital, had developed some degree of coma following a suicidal attempt by swallowing an overdose of a tricyclic antidepressant compound.

The report by Spiker et al[47] was based on observations in 15 adults who had been intoxicated due to consumption of an overdose of tricyclic compounds, but who had survived after they had received appropriate treatment for their drug intoxication at the Barnes Hospital in St. Louis. The particular drugs were amitriptyline alone (10 cases); amipryline plus protriptyline (1 case); desipramine alone (1 case); desipramine plus imipramine (1 case); imipramine alone (1 case); and doxepin alone (1 case). In seven instances the amount ingested was known; in the remainder, the amount was uncertain.

Moreover, it should be explained that these investigators established the gravity of the intoxication on the basis of serometric values and not on the depth of the coma. Thus, the primary purpose of their study was to correlate the electrocardiographic findings during the first 24 hours of hospitalization with the plasma levels of the tricyclic antidepressant, as measured by "gas chromatography-mass fragmentography." However, in each instance, such toxicologic studies were not confined to the first 24 hours following the patient's admission to the hospital; they were performed for a period of six days or until the time of discharge if this occurred sooner than six days following admission to the hospital. A similar program was adopted with respect to the electrocardiographic studies.

Electrocardiographic Findings

The findings in the electrocardiograms which these investigators considered to be of particular importance were the following: (a) evidences of an intraventricular conduction defect; (b) nonspecific ST-T-wave abnormalities; (c) evidences of a sinus tachycardia. However, it should be noted that these observers had not described precisely the nature of the changes they had categorized as "nonspecific ST-T-wave abnormalities."

An examination of their data indicated also that a diagnosis of sinus tachycardia was made in eight instances; in five of these eight instances, the respective heart rates were 140, 110, 130, 120, and 125 beats per minute, and in the remaining three it was 100 per minute. It is noteworthy that no other arrhythmia ever was observed in either the initial or serial electrocardiograms of any of these 15 surviving tricyclic-intoxicated subjects. Evidence of an intraventricular conduction defect, which was the electrocardiographic abnormality of greatest concern to Spiker et al, was found in the initial electrocardiograms of only 4 of the 15 patients. However, it also was observed that the abnormality disappeared when the patients had receovered from the intoxicating effects of the drug overdose. Also, in these four instances, the abnormal intraventricular conduction was associated with nonspecific ST-T abnormalities only once. In four other patients, the initial electrocardiogram was reported to be "within normal limits."

Moreover, inasmuch as it was the view of Spiker et al[47] that the severity of the drug intoxication should not be gauged by the neurologic findings (depth of coma, pupillary reactivity, seizures, etc.) but rather by the level of tricyclic antidepressant drugs in the plasma, their electrocardiographic data were examined by them to determine whether the presence of electrocardiographic abnormalities could be correlated with the levels of the drugs in the blood. In this connection, it should be noted that, on this basis, severe intoxication was associated with a blood level of the tricyclic antidepressants which was in excess of 1000 nannograms per cc during the first 24 hours of hospitalization. Thus, in six of the patients who could be classified as severely intoxicated individuals, the respective blood levels were 1560, 1190, 1860, 1130, 2190, and 2080 nannograms per cc. Correspondingly, the electrocardiographic data with respect to these six individuals indicated that an intraventricular conduction defect was present in five; in the sixth patient, the plasma level was 1860 nannograms per cc and the electrocardiogram disclosed merely a heart rate of 100 per minute associated with non-specific ST-T-wave abnormalities which were not described.

In five other instances, the initial blood levels of the antidepressant compound ranged between 90 and 690 nannograms per cc and, in this particular subset, the only observed deviation in the initial electrocardiogram was a "nonspecific ST-T abnormality" associated, with one exception, with a sinus tachycardia (heart rates ranging from 100 to 130 per minute). In four other instances, when the initial blood levels of the antidepressant compound ranged between 220 and 640 nannograms per cc, the findings in the initial electrocardiogram were "within normal limits."

Grades of unconsciousness at the time of admission to the hospital ranged from I to IV but no correlation could be established between the depth of the coma and the level of the drug in the plasma. Clearly, then, electrocardiographic evidence of delayed intraventricular conduction correlated best with the gravity of the tricyclic antidepressant poisoning only when blood levels of the drug were employed to estimate the seriousness of the intoxication. Nevertheless, the experiential data reported by Spiker et al seemed to indicate that the prognosis can be favorable regardless of the extent of the electrocardiographic abnormality and the severity of the tricyclic antidepressant intoxication, judged in accordance with their criteria.

It also was observed by these authors that there was a poor correlation between the amount of drug ingested and its plasma level. Thus, when 1.5 gm or more had been swallowed (5 instances) the plasma level exceeded 1000 nannograms per cc in only three and was less than 400 nannograms per cc in the remaining two.

Conclusion. Therefore, it can be inferred that delayed absorption of even a massive dose of a tricyclic antidepressant can be responsible simultaneously for a lack of significant elevation in the plasma as well as an absence of any intracardiac conduction defect. Correspondingly, it can be concluded, on the basis of such findings that the severity or prognosis of tricyclic antidepressant toxicity cannot be determined entirely by the amount of a tricyclic antidepressant which was impulsively swallowed for suicidal purposes, even when the dose exceeds 1.5 gm.

Additional Electrocardiographic Surveys

A much larger electrocardiographic survey in psychiatric patients who were hospitalized because of tricyclic antidepressant poisoning was reported in 1976 by C. Thorstrand.[44] His total sample consisted of 153 such cases and his purposes were, first, to determine whether the extent of the electrocardiographic changes could be correlated with the severity of the intoxication and, second, to ascertain which of these drug related electrocardiographic effects might be able to identify the intoxications likely to be fatal. Accordingly, a variety of observations were made during this retrospective study, which pertained to 87 comatose patients who, because of tricyclic antidepressant poisoning, were admitted to an intensive care unity in Stockholm, Sweden, between January 21, 1968 and may 6, 1973.

Among 70 such patients, who were able to breathe spontaneously, variable pH values were found. Thus, it was less than 7.35 in 31, less than 7.30 in 14, and 7.18 in one instance; in the remainder, the pH value was either normal or indicative of a mild alkalosis. The arterial pO_2 generally was low with a mean value of 71 mm Hg; only 16 patients had values above 85 mm Hg. Nevertheless, only 35 patients required respiratory assist devices during the treatment of their intoxication.

Especially significant was Thorstrand's finding, first, that "the concentrations of tricyclic antidepressant in blood and urine showed no detectable relationship to the dose ingested or the degree of electrocardiographic changes"; second, that "in the absence of previous electrocardiographic changes, the degree of QRS prolongation is a measure of the severity of the tricylic antidepressant poisoning." Thus, their conclusions essentially are in accord with the views previously expressed by Spiker et al,[47] whose survey pertained to a much smaller sample of patients.

It also is noteworthy that Thorstrand had observed that both the Q-T interval and the P-Q time were less useful correlates of the degree of tricyclic antidepressant poisoning than was the duration of the QRS compex. He also noted that sinus tachycardia, a supposedly anticholinergic effect, was a common finding in the surviving patients regardless of the severity of the intoxication; this observation therefore is in agreement with data reported by Noble and Mathew[46] and by others.[49]

On the other hand, at the time of their admission to the hospital, the five fatal cases in Thorstrand's patient sample already exhibited cardiorespiratory complications such as arrhythmias and aspiration or acidosis. On average, the dose of the tricyclic antidepressant ingested in the fatal cases was more than three times larger than the dose ingested by the survivors. Other features which characterized the fatalities were low initial mean blood pressure; low body temperature; markedly increased average QRS and Q-T intervals (0.19

sec. and 0.55 sec., respectively); variations in the configuration of the QRS complexes; a variety of atrial and ventricular arrhythmias culminating in the development of slow idioventricular rhythms and later in an asystolic irreversible cardiac arrest.

Other impressive findings reported by Thorstrand pertained to the cardiac responses, in terms of hemodynamic effects, in 10 psychiatric patients without demonstrable organic heart disease, both during the comatose phase of a non-fatal episode of tricyclic antidepressant intoxication as well as after full consciousness had returned. The mean QRS duration in the electrocardiograms of this particular patient sample, while they were comatose, was 0.14 sec. (unequivocal evidence of delayed intraventricular conduction) whereas, after they regained consciousness, the electrocardiogram was normal in all respects and the results of hemodynamic studies likewise were normal.

Moreover, during their comatose state, the intravenous infusion of 5 mg of propranolol was not followed by any change in the duration of the QRS complex; nevertheless, the propranolol produced a pronounced but temporary drop in cardiac output which had been higher than normal before the administration of this beta blocking agent. In addition, Thorstrand observed that the central venous pressure, systemic arterial blood pressure, and pulmonary arterial pressures were normal when the patients were unconscious. Thus, his studies seemed to show that even though characteristic features of tricylic antidepressant intoxication included a delay of intraventricular conduction (prolonged QRS duration) and a companionate hyperkinetic circulation, an overdose of a tricyclic antidepressant ordinarily is not likely to produce any evidences of myocardial insufficiency.

Subsequently, in 1977, Biggs et al[45] published data concerning electrocardiographic findings and toxicologic studies in 40 psychiatric patients who had been admitted to the Barnes Hospital in St. Louis following an overdose of a tricyclic antidepressant drug. The clinical course of all except three of these patients was uneventful; these three had developed a cardiac arrest but it proved to be irreversible in only two instances. All 40 patients had been treated and studied in accordance with a similar standardized protocol; hence a daily plasma tricyclic antidepressant value and electrocardiogram were obtained and, although all were comatose at the time of admission, mechanical respiratory devices were employed only whenever they seemed to be required.

The tricyclic antidepressant plasma level was in excess of 1000 nannograms per cc in only 13 patients in this series; one of these 13 patients developed a reversible and 2 an irreversible cardiac arrest. With respect to these three patients who experienced a cardiac arrest, the intoxicating dose of the tricyclic antidepressant was in excess of 2 gm and the average plasma tricyclic antidepressant level was 1700 nannograms were cc. However, whereas a single reversible cardiac arrest occurred in conjunction with a plasma level of 1422 nannograms per cc, the two instances of irreversible cardiac arrest occurred in patients whose highest tricyclic antidepressant plasma level was 1746 nannograms per cc and 1940 nannograms per cc, respectively. However, in terms of the amounts of tricyclic antidepressant ingested prior to the time of admission to the hospital, there was little difference between the two patients who did not survive the cardiac arrest and the one who did. Thus, the two who died had swallowed 2.5 gm of amitriptyline alone or amitriptyline and doxepin together whereas the one with a reversible cardiac arrest had ingested only slightly less than this amount. Moreover, although the cardiac arrests in these three patients followed a cardiac arrhythmia, only the reversible cardiac arrest was preceded by electrocardiographic evidences of a bundle branch block.

Data pertaining to the 10 remaining patients whose tricyclic antidepressant plasma levels, on average, exceeded 1680 nannograms per cc, indicated that none in this subset developed any serious cardiac or other complication prior to the time of discharge from the hospital. However, in the three members of this group with electrocardiographic evidence of a bundle branch block, the average plasma tricyclic antidepressant level was 1870 nannograms per cc whereas in the seven without such an intraventricular conduction defect, the average plasma tricylic antidepressant level was 1600 nannograms per cc, hardly a meaningful difference. Equally impressive was the lack of correlation between the mean plasma tricyclic antidepressant level and the occurrence of an arrhythmia in these remaining 10 patients. Thus, whereas the mean level was 1385 nannograms per cc in the two patients who exhibited an arrhythmia, it was 1755 nannograms per cc in the patients whose cardiac rhythm was unaffected.

Conclusions

Nevertheless, in view of the high degree of correlation between excessive plasma levels of the tricyclic antidepressant and the occurrence of electrocardiographic evidence of delayed intraventricular conduction, the data in the report of Biggs et al would seem to support their thesis that "in the presence of a persistent increase in the duration of the QRS, normal vital signs and normal level of consciousness do not ensure that a patient (with tricyclic antidepressant intoxication) is not a potential medical risk." Correspondingly, then, their observations would seem to imply that continued careful monitoring of patients receiving treatment for tricyclic antidepressant poisoning will be required until it is certain that electrocardiographic evidences of delayed intraventricular conduction have disappeared completely. (see APPENDIX)

Salvage Rate

Still uncertain is the salvage rate, with regard to patients hospitalized because of an episode of tricyclic antidepressant intoxication. Nevertheless, there is now a substantial amount of experiential data which appeared to show that aggressive therapy often will be followed by a complete recovery from this drug-related illness. However, inasmuch as the basic principles underlying such treatment has been discussed already in considerable detail in the reviews prepared by Davis et al[43] and by others[40,42,80] it has been decided that it would be preferable to include a distillate of their recommendations in the Appendix instead of placing, in the body of this monograph, the guidelines which can serve as the basic principles to be followed with respect to the management of patients with this particular drug induced malady.

At this juncture, it also is pertinent to mention that total recovery from an episode of tricyclic antidepressant poisoning cannot be predicated always upon a disappearance of its neurologic manifestations which, in this type of intoxication, generally are ascribed to the profound anticholinergic effects exerted by overdoses of tricyclic antidepressants on the central nervous system.[81-83] Actually, it even has been observed that a delayed and unexpected sudden cardiac arrest may occur occasionally several days after such an overdosed patient has become conscious and no longer is confused.[43,59,103,104]

The reasons for such a seemingly paradoxical phenomenon can be better understood largely as a result of the electrocardiographic data reported in 1969 by Larcan et al[50] and because of the serometric findings subsequently described by Spiker and Biggs.[102] In connection with their studies, Larcan et al showed that whereas recovery from an episode of tricyclic antidepressant poisoning usually was associated with a disappearance of electrocardiographic evidences of a conduction delay within 24 hours after treatment for the intoxication was instituted, there also were exceptions to this rule. Thus, as they observed "in one case with a pattern of right bundle branch block, it took more than 4 days before this abnormality disappeared; in another case, the abnormalities indicative of conduction delay disappeared in 6 days; in a third case, the intraventricular conduction disturbance disappeared in 5 days but evidence of atrioventricular conduction delay persisted and in yet another instance, the conduction disturbance did not disappear until 6 days later." Moreover, Larcan et all noted that the long or short persistence of electrocardiographic abnormalities could not be correlated with the doses the intoxicated patient had ingested for suicidal purposes.

Equally meaningful were the data reported in 1976 by Spiker and Biggs[102] who were particularly concerned with the pharmacokinetics of the megadoses of tricyclics which had been consumed by 24 depressed adults during a suicidal attempt. In each of them, the plasma tricyclic antidepressant level was determined at the time of admission to the hospital and again each day, for a period of 144 hours. In all but six of this patient sample, the plasma level consistently was less than 1000 nannograms per ml. In these six patients, the plasma levels exceeded 1000 nannograms per ml. at the time of admission and the QRS intervals in their electrocardiograms exceeded 100 milliseconds. Moreover, during the ensuing 144 hours, the plasma level measurements in this subset varied considerably; thus, whereas within 96 hours the plasma anti-depressant level had dropped to 170 up to 640 nannograms per ml in four instances, the levels remained above 1000 nannograms per ml in two other instances. However, in one of these two patients, the level had dropped from 2190 nannograms per ml to 1280 nannograms per ml and, in the other, it had dropped merely from 1530 nannograms per ml to 1289 nannograms per ml. Conceivably, then, persistently high tricyclic antidepressant levels in the plasma in patients who have swallowed an overdose of these compounds might account for an occasional delayed sudden death. Moreover, such experiential data would suggest the importance of monitoring patients with tricyclic antidepressant poisoning not only by repeated electrocardiographic studies but also with repeated determinations of the plasma tricyclic antidepressant levels.

Electrolyte Abnormalities

Although studies already have clarified the electrophysiologic basis for the conduction delays associated with tricyclic antidepressant intoxication[51,53,84] there still is no comparable understanding of the mechanisms responsible for the ventricular arrhythmias which are a feature of the more severe episodes of this drug related syndrome. So far as is known, the only observers who have suggested that an electrolyte disorder may be involved in the pathogenesis of such arrhythmias have been Larcan et al.[50] Originally, their interest in this sort of connection was stimulated by their finding that, sometimes, the only conspicuous change in the electrocardiogram of a patient with tricyclic antidepressant intoxication was a lowering of the T-wave and S-T segment accompanied by an enlargement of the U wave. Accordingly, Larcan et al measured the serum potassium levels in all tricyclic antidepressant intoxicated patients whose electrocardiograms conformed with this particular pattern.

The results of such an endeavor showed that in 8 of 16 such instances, the serum potassium levels were normal but were 2.5 mEq and 2.7 mEq in two cases and 3.2 to 3.6 mEq in the remainder. Nevertheless, they also advanced the position that some of the cardiac arrests following the consumption of a megadose of a tricyclic antidepressant may have occurred as a result of a hypokalemic cardioplegic ventricular arrhythmia.

So far, the validity of such a thesis has not been confirmed by others and, actually, Thorstrand[41] has found that in a group of psychiatric patients who survived an episode of tricyclic antidepressant intoxication, the serum potassium levels uniformly were normal even though the electrocardiogram, in every instance, was abnormal. Moreover, it now is well established that it is the intravenous administration of sodium salts which often is responsible for the recovery of the patients with tricyclic antidepressant poisoning.[64,85] Nevertheless, it might be useful in the future, to evaluate the electrolyte behavior as well as the electrocardiographic findings in all patients of this genre.

In addition, it should be recognized that a rapidly developing degree of prostration which is followed within several hours, by a cardiac arrest sometimes can result from an incompletely understood interaction between even customary doses of a tricyclic antidepressant and customary doses of a monoamine oxidase inhibitor. Clinically, the principal features of this alarming development comprise not only a sudden circulatory collapse but also a marked rise in temperature before the time of death. Therefore, it was considered appropriate to discuss this particular drug induced life threatening syndrome in more detail elsewhere in this monograph, under the rubric of Fatal Hyperpyrexia (see Chapter 9).

Moreover, it has been observed that a monoamine oxidase inhibitor alone, in overdoses, also can be responsible for a sudden death in psychiatric patients who have consumed these large amounts of the drug in connection with a suicidal attempt. Data pertaining to this type of fatal drug intoxication can be found in several reports.[86-90] Usually, tranylcypromine was the monoamine oxidase inhibitor which was chosen for this purpose, but occasionally it was an overdose of Nialamide which was involved.

In general, intoxication caused by an overdose of a monoamine oxidase inhibitor is characterized by coma with hyperthermia, rapid respirations, tachycardia, dilated pupils, and hyperactive reflexes, but along with these manifestations, which are comparable to an episode of atropine poisoning, a variety of involuntary movements also may be present. A representative case of monoamine oxidase intoxication was the one described in the review prepared by Davis et al.[43] In this instance, the decedent was "a 49-year-old woman who had ingested 65 tranylcypromine tablets (total dose 650 mg). She was taken to a hospital where she was noted to be depressed, agitated, oriented, with normal blood pressure and temperature. Approximately 4 hours later, she began to show episodes of restlessness and thrashing about her bed and complained of flashes of hot and cold sensations. By 6 hours her temperature had risen to 105°F and her pulse had accelerated to 110 per minute. Eight hours later, her speech became incoherent and she became tremulous with generalized hyperactivity and profound perspiration. By 11 hours after ingestion, her temperature was 102°F and she showed arching of the back and clonus. Her temperature continued to rise in spite of alcohol baths until she expired less than 24 hours after the ingestion of the drug."

CONCLUSION

It has been noted also that spontaneous recovery from this sort of drug-related poisoning has occurred but, in general, as soon as the cause of the intoxication has been determined, it would be prudent to employ, as promptly as possible all the measures which customarily are employed in the management of any form of intoxication. Thus, it would be advisable to rely on good nursing care, respiratory assisting devices, anticonvulsive preparations, such as diazepam, vasopressors as needed, and even on hemodialysis as well as on a cholinergic drug such as physostigmine. The use of additional measures should be determined by the results of arterial blood gas determinations and the findings in repeated electrocardiograms. (see APPENDIX)

REFERENCES

1. Hollister, L.E. Unexpected asphyxial deaths and tranquilizing drugs. *Am. J. Psychiatry.* 114:366 (1957).
2. Kelly, H.G., et al. Thioridazine hydrochloride: Its effects on the electrocardiogram and a report of 2 fatalities with electrocardiographic abnormalities. *Can. M.A.J.* 89:546 (1963).
3. Haden, P. Thioridazine and electrocardiographic changes. *Can. M.A.J.* 69: (1963).
4. Wendkos, M.H. Thioridazine and electrocardiographic abnormalities. *Can. M.A.J.* 89:1297 (1963).
5. Graupner, K.I. and Murphree, O.D. Electrocardiographic changes associated with the use of thioridazine. *J. Neuropsych.* 5:344 (1963-1964).
6. Wendkos, M.H. Pharmacologic studies in a hitherto unreported benign repolarization disturbance among schizophrenics. *J. New Drugs.* 4:98 (1964).
7. Wendkos, M.H. The significance of electrocardiographic changes produced by thioridazine. *J. New Drugs.* 4:322 (1964).
8. Wendkos, M.H. The effects of a potassium mixture on abnormal cardiac repolarization in hospitalized psychiatric patients. *Am. J. Med. Sci.* 249:412 (1965).
9. Wendkos, M.H. Electrocardiographic evidences of nitrate activity in man. *Postgrad. Med.* 39:132 (1966).
10. Huston, J.R. and Bell, G.E. The effect of thioridazine hydrochloride and chlorpromazine on the electrocardiogram. *J.A.M.A.* 193:16 (1966).
11. Wendkos, M.H. Cardiac changes related to phènothiazine therapy with special reference to thioridazine. *J. Am. Geriat. Soc.* 15:20 (1967).
12. Alexander, S. et al. Electrocardiographic effects of thioridazine hydrochloride. *Lahey Clinic Found. Bull.* 16:207 (1967).
13. Wendkos, M.H. Observations concerning a benign myocardial disorder in phenothiazine treated psychiatric patients. *Excerpta Med.* (International Congress Series) 134:24 (1967).
14. Wendkos, M.H. A functional myocardial aberration in phenothiazine treated psychiatric patients. *Excerpta. Med.* (International Congress Series) (1967).
15. Burda, C.D. Electrocardiographic abnormalities induced by thioridazine. *Am. Heart J.* 76:153 (1968).

16. Wendkos, M.H. Experiments with thioridazine. In: *Toxicity and Adverse Reaction Studies with Neuroleptics and Antidepressants.* J.E. Lehmann, and T.A. Ban, eds. Quebec Psychopharmacological Research Association, Verdun, p. 143 (1968).
17. Lapierre, Y.D. et al. Phenothiazine treatment and electrocardiographic abnormalities. *Can. Psychiatr. A.J.* 14:517 (1969).
18. Wendkos, M.H. and Thornton, C.C. An electrocardiographic survey of thioridazine treated patients. *Behav. Neuropsychiatry* 1:18 (1969).
19. Thornton, C.C. and Wendkos, M.H. Electrocardiographic T-wave distortions among thioridazine treated psychiatric in-patients. *Dis. Nerv. Sys.* 32:320 (1971).
20. Alverez-Mena, S.C. and Frank, M.J. Phenothiazine-induced T-wave abnormalities: Effects of overnight fasting. *J.A.M.A.* 224:1730 (1973).
21. Samet, J.M. and Surawicz, B. Cardiac function in patients treated with phenothiazines; comparison with quinidine. *J. Clin. Pharmacol.* 14:588 (1974).
22. Hollister, L.E. and Kosek, J.C. Sudden death during treatment with phenothiazine derivatives. *J.A.M.A.* 192:1035 (1965).
23. James, T.N. Apoplexy of the heart. *Circulation* 57:385 (1978).
24. Schwartz, C.J. and Walsh, W.J. The pathologic basis of sudden death. *Progr. Cardiovasc. Dis.* 13:465 (1971).
25. Moritz, A.R. and Zamcheck, N. Sudden and unexpected deaths of young soldiers: Diseases responsible for sudden deaths during World War II. *Arch. Pathol. Lab. Med.* 42:459 (1946).
26. Rodriguez, F.L. et al. Postmortem angiographic studies on the coronary arterial circulation: Incidence and topography of occlusive coronary lesions. *Am. Heart J.* 68:490 (1964).
27. Fraser, G.R. et al. Congenital deafness associated with electrocardiographic abnormalities, fainting attacks, and sudden death. A recessive syndrome. *Quart. J. Med.* 33:361 (1964).
28. Pugh, B.R. et al. Cardioversion and "false positive" technetium stannous pyrophosphate myocardial scintigrams. *Circulation* 54:399 (1976).
29. Giles, T.D. and Modlin, R.K. Death associated with ventricular arrhythmia and thioridazine hydrochloride. *J.A.M.A.* 205:108 (1968).
30. James, T.N. Q-T prolongation and sudden death. *Mod. Concepts Cardiovasc. Dis.* 38:35 (1969).
31. Jervell, A. and Lange-Nielsen, F. Congenital deaf mutism, functional heart disease, with prolongation of the Q-T interval and sudden death. *Am. Heart J.* 54:59 (1957).
32. Leestma, J.E. and Koenig, K.L. Sudden death and phenothiazines: A current controversy. *Arch. Gen. Psych.* 18:137 (1968).
33. Fowler, N.O. et al. Electrocardiographic changes and cardiac arrhythmias in patients receiving psychotropic drugs. *Am. J. Cardiol.* 37:223 (1976).
34. Davis, J.M. et al. Overdosage of psychotropic drugs: A review. *Dis. Nerv. Sys.* 29:157 (1968).
35. Wendkos, M.H. (Unpublished data.)
36. Cruickshank, J.M. et al. Possible role of catecholamines, corticosteroids, and potassium in production of electrocardiographic abnormalities associated with subarachnoid hemorrhage. *Brit. Heart J.* 36:697 (1974).
37. Michon, P. et al. Voluntary fatal intoxication with imipramine. *Bull. Mem. Soc. Hosp. Paris* 75:989 (1959).
38. Pettinger, W.A. et al. *Cardiovascular Effects and Toxicity of Psychotropic Agents in Man.* Public Health Services Publication #1836, p. 589 (1968).
39. Arieff, A.I. and Friedman, E.A., Coma Following Non-narcotic Drug Overdosage: Management of 208 Adult Patients, *A.M., J. Med. Sci.* 266:405 (1973)
40. Moccetti, T. et al. Cardiotoxicity of tricyclic antidepressants. *Schweiz. Med. Wschr.* 101:1 (1971).

41. Thorstrand, C. Cardiovascular effects of poisoning with tricyclic antidepressants. *Acta Med. Scand.* 195:505 (1974).
42. Jefferson, J.W. A Review of the cardiovascular effects and toxicity of tricyclic antidepressants. *Psychosom. Med.* 37:160 (1975).
43. Davis, J.M. et al. Overdosage of psychotropic drugs: A review. Part II. Antidepressants and other psychotropic agents. *Dis. Nerv. Sys.* 29:246 (1968).
44. Thorstrand, C. Clinical features in poisonings with tricyclic antidepressants with reference to the electrocardiogram. *Acta Med. Scand.* 199:337 (1976).
45. Biggs, J.T. et al. Tricyclic antidepressant overdose. *J.A.M.A.* 238:135 (1977).
46. Noble, J. and Mathew, H. Acute poisoning by tricyclic antidepressants: Clinical features and management of 100 patients. *Clin. Toxicol.* 2:403 (1969).
47. Spiker, D.G. et al. Tricyclic antidepressant overdose: Clinical presentations and plasma levels. *Clin. Pharm. Therap.* 18:539 (1975).
48. Sedal, L. et al. Overdosage of tricyclic antidepressants. A report of 2 deaths and a prospective study of 24 patients. *Med. J. Aust.* 2:74 (1972).
49. Freeman, J.W. et al. Cardiac abnormalities in poisoning with tricyclic antidepressants. *Brit. Med. J.* 2:610 (1969).
50. Larcan, A. et al. Ionic disturbances and electrocardiographic changes in the course of intoxications due to thymoleptics. In: *Heart and Toxicity* (Ed. by Masson and Cie) Paris. 1969.
51. Vohra, J. et al. Intracardiac conduction deflects following overdose of tricyclic antidepressant drugs. *Europ. J. Cardiol. Excerpta Med.* 2/4:453 (1975).
52. Barnes, R.J. et al. Electrocardiographic changes in amitriptyline poisoning. *Brit. Med. J.* 3:222 (1968).
53. Burrows, G.D. et al. Cardiac effects of different tricyclic antidepressant drugs. *Brit. J. Psychiatry* 129:335 (1976).
54. Freeman, J.W. and Loughhead, M.G. Beta blockade in the treatment of tricyclic antidepressant overdosage. *Med. J. Aust.* 1:1233 (1973).
55. Lancaster, N.P. and Foster, A.R., Suicidal Attempt by Imipramine Overdosage, *Brit. Med. J.* 2:1458 (1959)
56. Curry, A.S. Seven fatal cases involving imipramine in man. *J. Pharm. Pharmacol.* 16:265 (1964).
57. Williams, R.B. and Sherter, C. Cardiac complications of tricyclic antidepressant therapy. *Ann. Int. Med.* 74:395 (1971).
58. Marshall, A. and Moore, K. Pulmonary disease after amitriptyline overdose. *Brit. Med. J.* 1:716 (1973).
59. Masters, A.B. Delayed death in imipramine poisoning. *Brit. Med. J.* 3:866 (1967).
60. Harthorne, J.W. et al, Management of Massive Imipramine Overdosage with Mannitol and Artificial Dialysis, *New Eng. J. Med.* 268:33 (1963)
61. Newton, R.W. Physostigmine salicylate in the treatment of tricyclic antidepressant overdosage. *J.A.M.A.* 231:941 (1975).
62. Lewis, S.A. and Oswald, I. Overdose of tricyclic antidepressants and deductions concerning their cerebral action. *Brit. J. Psychiatry.* 115:1403 (1969).
63. Davies, D.M. and Allaye, R., Amitriptyline Poisoning, *Lancet*, 2:543 (1963)
64. Gaultier, M. et al. The cardiotoxicity of imipramine in man and animals. *Proc. Europ. Soc. Study Drug Tox.* 6:171 (1965).
65. Sigg, E.B. et al. Cardiovascular effects of imipramine. *J. Pharm. Exp. Therap.* 141:237 (1963).
66. Sigg, E.B. Pharmacological studies with tofranil. *Can. Psych. A.J.* 4:S75 (1959).
67. Muller, O.F. et al. The hypotensive effect of imipramine hydrochloride in patients with cardiovascular disease. *Clin. Pharm. Therap.* 2:300 (1961).

68. Freyhan, F.A. Clinical effectiveness of Tofranil in the treatment of depressive psychoses. *Can. Psych. A.J.* 4:S86 (1959).
69. Malitz, S. et al. Preliminary evaluation of Tofranil in a combined in-patient and out-patient setting. *Can. Psych. A.J.* 4:S152 (1959).
70. Moir, D.C. et al. Cardiotoxicity of amitriptyline. *Lancet* 2:561 (1972).
71. Wikland, B. Deaths from arteriosclerotic heart disease outside hospitals. *Acta. Med. Scand.* 184:129 (1968).
72. Biorck, G. et al. Studies on myocardial infarction in Malmo 1935 to 1954: Morbidity and mortality in a hospital material. *Acta Med. Scand.* 159:253 (1957).
73. Vedin, J.A. Sudden Death: Identification of high risk groups. *Am. Heart J.* 86:124 (1973).
74. Wikland, B. Medically unattended fatal cases of ischemic heart disease in a defined population. *Acta. Med. Scand.* Suppl. #524 (1971).
75. Fulton, M. et al. Sudden death and myocardial infarction. *Circulation* (Suppl. 4) 40:182 (1969).
76. Bates, R.J. et al. Cardiac rupture—challenge in diagnosis and management. *Am. J. Cardiol.* 40:429 (1977).
77. Boston Collaborative Drug Surveillance Study. Adverse Reactions to the Tricylic Antidepressant Drugs. *Lancet* 1:529 (1972).
78. Biggs, J.T. et al. Tricyclic antidepressant overdose. Incidence of symptoms. *J.A.M.A.* 238:135 (1977).
79. Shader, R.I. and Di Mascio, A. *Psychotropic Drug Side Effects.* Williams and Wilkins, Baltimore (1970).
80. Wood, C.A. et al. Management of tricyclic antidepressant toxicities. *Dis. Nerv. Sys.* 37:459 (1976).
81. Duvoisin, R.C. and Katz, R. Reversal of central anticholinergic syndrome in man by physostigmine. *J.A.M.A.* 206:1963 (1968).
82. Munoz, R.A. and Kuplic, J.R. Large overdose of tricyclic antidepressants treated with physostigmine salicylate. *Psychosomatics* 16:77 (1975).
83. Granacher, R.P. and Baldessarini, R.J. Physostigmine. Its use in acute anticholinergic syndrome with antidepressant and antiparkinson drugs. *Arch. Gen. Psych.* 32:375 (1975).
84. Baum, T. et al. Observations on models used for the evaluation of antiarrhythmic drugs. *Arch. Internat. Pharmacodyn.* 193:149 (1971).
85. Brown, T.C.K. Sodium bicarbonate treatment for tricyclic antidepressant arrhythmias in children. *Med. J. Aust.* 2:380 (1976).
86. Bell, D.B. and Schaff, J. Fatal reaction to tranylcypromine (parnate). *Hawaii Med. J.* 22:440 (1963).
87. Marra, J.P. et al. Suicide by the ingestion of tranylcypromine. *J.A.M.A.* 192:1104 (1965).
88. Bacon, G.A. Successful suicide with tranylcypromine sulphate. *Am. J. Psychiatry* 119:585 (1962).
89. Jacobziner, H. and Raybin, H.W. Accidental Chemical poisoning. Hydralazine hydrochloride, mercury, tranylcypromine, and permanganato intoxication. *N.Y. State J. Med.* 63:1210 (1963).
90. Mattell, G. and Thorstrand, C. A case of fatal nialamid poisoning. *Acta Med. Scand.* 181:79 (1967).
91. Doyle, J.T. et al. Factors related to suddenness of death from coronary disease: Combined Albany-Framingham studies. *Am. J. Cardiol.* 37:1073 (1976).
92. Kuller, L. et al. Epidemiologic study of sudden and unexplained death due to arteriosclerotic heart disease. *Circulation* 34:1056 (1966).
93. Bainton, C.R. and Peterson, D.R. Deaths from coronary heart disease in persons 50 years of age and younger. A community wide study. *New Eng. J. Med.* 268:569 (1963).

94. Reynertson, R.H. and Tzagournis, M. Clinical and metabolic characteristics. Effects on mortality in coronary disease. *Arch. Int. Med.* 132:649 (1973).
95. Oxman, H.A. et al. Identification of the patients at highest risk for sudden death within 5 years following their first myocardial infarction (abstract). *Am. J. Cardiol.* 31:150 (1973).
96. Donlon, P.T. and Tupin, J.P. Successful suicides with thioridazine and mesoridazine: A result of probable cardiotoxicity. *Arch. Gen. Psychiatry.* 34:955 (1977).
97. Joubert, P.H. and Olivier, J.A. Fatal suicidal ingestion of thioridazine. *Clin. Toxicol.* (Suppl. 2) 7:133 (1974).
98. Kannel, W.B. et al. Precursors of sudden coronary death: Factors related to the incidence of sudden death. *Circulation* 51:606 (1975).
99. Chiang, B.N. et al. Predisposing factors in sudden cardiac death in Tecumseh, Mich. *Circulation* 41:31 (1970).
100. Fisher, S.D. and Tyroler, H.A. Relationship between ventricular premature contractions on routine electrocardiography and subsequent sudden death from coronary heart disease. *Circulation* 47:712 (1973).
101. Hagstrom, R.M. et al. The risk of sudden death following myocardial infarction. *Arch. Environ. Health* 15:450 (1967).
102. Spiker, D.G. and Biggs, J.T. Tricyclic Antidepressants. Prolonged Plasma Levels after Overdose. *J.A.M.A.* 236:1711 (1976).
103. Fuge, C.A., Treatment of Poisoning by Antidepressant Drugs, *Brit. Med. J.* 4:108 (1967)
104. Gard, H., et al, Qualitative and Quantitative Studies on the Disposition of Amitriptyline and other Tricyclic Antidepressant Drugs in Man as it Relates to the Overdosed Patient, *Clin. Toxicol.* 6:571 (1973)

APPENDIX

The Histopathologic Study of The Atrioventricular Node, The His Bundle And Its Branches.

Because of the growing realization that sometimes an anatomical defect involving infra-atrial conducting and pacemaker tissues can be the sole explanation for the occurrence of a seemingly mystifying sudden death, it is important to be aware of technical methods which permit detailed examinations of these particular structures. One such method is the one described by Lev et al in 1951[1] and later modified by Shanklin and Laite in 1963.[2]

The following is the technique devised by Lev et al. "The heart is opened at autopsy in the conventional way. The heart, its chambers packed with cotton, is fixed for 6 to 24 hours in 4% formaldehyde solution. The parietal and inferior walls of both atria and ventricles are then cut away, leaving the septal wall of the chambers intact. The pars membranacea is observed carefully, as well as the Eustachian valve, the coronary sinus, the central fibrous body, the muscle of Lancisi and the Crista Supraventricularis. This gives the general location and direction of the atrioventricular node, the His bundle, and the right bundle branch."

"Cut #1 is made along a line about 5 to 12 mm below the moderator band to produce an angle of about 45 degrees with the line of the Crista. Cut #2 is made at right angles to cut #1 and passes through the junction of the Eustachian valve and the limbus. Cut #3 is made at right angles to the second cut, passing though the base of the aorta. Cut #4 is made just lateral to the moderator band at right angles to the third cut. This leaves a rectangle of tissue containing all of the desired structures with the exception of the lower aspect of the left bundle branch fasciculi. Cut #5 is made at right angles to the baseline passing through the middle of the pars membranacea. Cut #6 is made at right angles to the baseline passing through the muscle of Lancisi.

Cut #7 is made at right angles to the baseline dividing the remainder of the tissue into several blocks. (blocks 3 and 4). Every 20th section is saved through block #1 and every 40th section thereafter. These sections are stained with hematoxylin and eosin. No other stains are necessary to identify the various structures but the elastic and reticulum stains may be used as aids in the identification of the right branch. Altogether, this method yields from 150 to 200 sections of this portion of the adult heart."

However, the method introduced by Lev et al possessed certain disadvantages. Thus, the large number of microscope slides and cover slips entailed a fairly large expenditure of money, the problem of storage of these numerous slides created certain difficulties and there was an inordinate amount of time consumed by technical help because of the extensive number of sections which were involved.

Because of these considerations, Shanklin and Laite advocated that in conjunction with the method of semiserial sectioning described by Lev et al, a simpler means of examining and storing the cut sections of the heart would be to modify the film strip and plastic spray method originally introduced by Pickett and Sommer and adapt it to the type of histopathologic study originally devised by Lev et al.

Accordingly, they employed a Bausch and Lomb dissecting microscope and an x-ray viewbox for low-powered scanning of the film strips in anatomic sequence and then as they moved the film along the stage of the microscope, they marked with ink dots those areas they wished to examine more closely with the aid of a standard optical microscope. In their experience, little difficulty was encountered in tracing the conduction tissues on appropriately stained hematoxylin and eosin preparations, but they found that the best definition of these structures was achieved by the use of the Masson stain and by the PAS-hematoxylin and eosin technique. Moreover, they confirmed that, in several instances, such semiserial sectioning of the nodal and conducting tissues had disclosed abnormalities which were able to clarify clinical events ordinary methods of postmortem examination had been unable to explain.[3-18] Furthermore, as Shanklin and Laite had observed, the film strip technique eliminated the expense of large numbers of microscope slides and cover slips and simplified the storage of the stained tissues. Additional detailed information regarding this modification of the technique introduced by Lev et al can be obtained by consulting the original report by Shanklin and Laite.

REFERENCES

1. Lev, M. et al. A method for the histopathic study of the atrioventricular node, bundle and branches. *Arch. Pathol. Lab. Med.* 52:73 (1951).
2. Shanklin, D.R. and Laite, M.B. Pickett-Sommer film strip technique. *Arch. Path.* 75:91 (1963).

3. Gault, J.H. et al, Fatal familial cardiac arrhythmias: Histologic observations on the cardiac conduction system. *Am J. Cardiol.* 29:548 (1972).
4. Schwartz, C.J. and Walsh, W.J. The Pathologic Basis of Sudden Death. *Progr. Cardiovasc. Dis.* 13:465 (1971).
5. James, T.N. Pathology of small coronary arteries. *Am. J. Cardiol.* 20:679 (1967).
6. James, T.N. Sudden death in young athletes. *Ann. Int. Med.* 67:1013 (1967).
7. James, T.N. et al. Pathology of the cardiac conduction system in Marfan's syndrome. *Arch. Int. Med.* 114:339 (1964).
8. James, T.N. An etiologic concept concerning the obscure myocardiopathies. *Progr. Cardiovasc. Dis.* 7:43 (1964).
9. James, T.N. and Sherf, L. Fine structure of the His bundle. *Circulation* 37:1049 (1968).
10. Thung, N. et al. Hypoxia as the cause of hemorrhage into the cardiac conduction system, arrhythmia, and sudden death. *J. Thorac. Cardiovasc . Surg.* 44:687 (1962).
11. James, T.N. On the cause of syncope and sudden death in primary pulmonary hypertension. *Ann. Int. Med.* 56:252 (1962).
12. James, T.N., et al. Observations on the pathophysiology of the long Q-T syndromes with special reference to the neuropathology of the heart. *Circulation* 57:1221 (1978).
13. Hudson, R.E.B. The human conducting system and its examination. *J. Clin. Pathol.* 16:492 (1963).
14. James, T.N. Morphology of human atrioventricular node, with remarks pertinent to its electrophysiology. *Am. Heart J.* 62:656 (1961).
15. Frink, R.J. and James, T.N. Normal blood supply of the human His bundle and proximal bundle branches. *Circulation* 47:8 (1973).
16. Lie, J.T. and Titus, J.L. Pathology of the myocardium and the conduction system in sudden coronary death. *Circulation* 52:53 (Suppl. 3) (1975).
17. Schwartz, C.J. and Gerrity, R.G. Anatomical pathology of sudden unexpected coronary death. *Circulation* 52:18 (Suppl. 3) (1975).
18. Frink, R.J. et al. Non-obstructive coronary thrombosis in sudden cardiac death. *Am. J. Cardiol* 42:48 (1978).

APPENDIX

Tricyclic Antidepressant Poisoning: Therapeutic Aspects

Left untreated, the usual hallmarks of tricyclic antidepressant intoxication such as variable levels of coma with or without convulsions, peripheral anticholinergic effects (mydriasis, urinary bladder atony, dry mouth, sinus tachycardia), delayed intraventricular conduction, and hypotension can be expected to be followed by a cardiac arrest due to circulatory collapse and life threatening ventricular tachyarrhythmias. Consequently, as soon as the presence of tricyclic antidepressant poisoning is suspected, it is imperative to admit the patient to an Intensive Care Unit. There, base line studies such as an electrocardiogram, chest x-ray, blood electrolyte levels, blood chemistry levels, arterial blood gas levels and pH can be obtained; afterward, cardiac activity should be monitored constantly and the usual grouping of vital signs should be checked at suitable intervals.

As yet, there is no specific antidote for tricyclic antidepressant poisoning, but despite this circumstance, most patients will recover when those responsible for their care will use promptly, measures designed to achieve the following therapeutic objectives: (a) to attenuate the adverse cerebral effects directly related to the anticholinergic property of the tricyclic antidepressant drug; (b) to control and prevent, insofar as possible, recurrent convulsive episodes; (c) to facilitate the excretion of the tricyclic antidepressant and its metabolites; (d) to eliminate insofar as possible, the possibility of further absorption of residual portions of the drug which might still be remaining in the gastrointestinal tract; (e) to maintain an adequate respiratory exchange and thereby avoid any intercurrent anoxia or respiratory acidosis; (f) to employ those pharmacologic agents which could have a salutory effect on the heart, circulation, electrolyte distribution, and acid-base balance.

Inasmuch as it is the central anticholinergic effect of tricyclic antidepressant compounds which can account for the coma and any associated nonconvulsive neurologic or psychiatric phenomena in patients who have swallowed an overdose of these drugs, physostigmine currently can be considered a basic remedy in instances of tricyclic antidepressant poisoning. This drug is a powerful inhibitor of cholinesterase and because it can traverse the blood brain barrier, it can exert this particular effect within the brain substance as well as at peripheral sites of the body.

A recently discovered preparation with a similar mode of action is galanthamine, but its effectiveness and possible side effects in sufficient numbers of patients with tricyclic antidepressant poisoning still have not been investigated. Galanthamine is a phenantridine derivative of the snowdrop flower which grows wild in Bulgaria and because it is hydrolysis-resistant, it can produce a reversal of cholinesterase activity longer lasting than the reversal produced by the usual dose of physostigmine. Thus, its discovery seems to be a promising development but, as yet, its use must be deferred until more information concerning its possible adverse effects can be established. Such considerations cannot be overlooked inasmuch as it is known already that physostigmine can produce certain undesirable effects in patients who not only are unconscious but who, in addition, exhibit evidences of cardiac conduction defects resulting from tricyclic antidepressant intoxication. Moreover, it is acknowledged that physostigmine should be prescribed with caution for patients with respiratory distress or for patients with a history of bronchial asthma. Correspondingly, it would be prudent to avoid its use in patients with a history of diabetes, coronary artery disease, various abnormalities of the gastrointestinal tract, or glaucoma.

Other common side effects of physostigmine which are particularly undesirable in the unconscious patient with tricyclic antidepressant intoxication are vomiting and hypersalivation. Therefore, a decision to employ this drug in such patients should not be made unless two conditions are met. The first is to inform the hospital personnel in the Intensive Care Unit of the nature of the various untoward reactions to physostigmine which can occur; the second is to instruct them to be prepared to administer promptly a suitable antidote if the use of one is required. The most effective drug for this purpose is atropine sulphate; the dose can be predicated on the amount of physostigmine given just before the side effect occurred. In this connection, it should be noted that 0.5 mg of atropine, by injection, will counteract each mg of physostigmine which had been administered. However, some observers have suggested that an anticholinergic drug which does not cross the blood brain barrier would be a more desirable antidote in such circumstances. Thus, instead, propantheline has been recommended to reverse the untoward peripheral cholinergic effects of physostigmine.

Nevertheless, despite the awareness that there may be disadvantages to the use of physostigmine in patients who require treatment for an episode of tricyclic antidepressant intoxication, there is now a substantial body of data to indicate that many of them will benefit from its use. The recommended initial dose is 2 mg, given by intramuscular or *slow* intravenous injection (rapid intravenous injections may produce seizures). If no toublesome cholinergic signs appear following the administration of this test dose, and if no clinical change is noted within 15 to 30 minutes, an additional 1 or 2 mg dose of physostigmine should be given. This treatment should be continued until the patient's clinical status improves or cholinergic toxicity is seen. Pulse, mental status, and bowel motility seem to show the most rapid clinical change, usually within a few minutes, whereas changes in pupillary diameter or response to light may be extremely slow. Additional doses of physostigmine may be needed in intervals of 30 minutes to 2 hours. Currently, this must be given by injection but the short duration of action of physostigmine also provides an added margin of safety. If, after this method of administration of physostigmine has restored consciousness but has not abolished any residual agitation, diazepam can be given; the initial recommended dose of diazepam is 40 to 50 mg orally or less if it must be administered parenterally. If the patient remains agitated after these doses of diazepam have been administered, additional doses of 10 mg every 4 hours may be prescribed. Clearly, the use of major tranquilizers which possess anticholinergic actions should be avoided.

Moreover, the development of convulsive episodes in patients with tricyclic antidepressant intoxication, sometimes can lead to more serious complications inasmuch as they can increase the workload of a heart which already may have been poisoned by the drug overdose. Therefore, it is important that they be controlled as soon as possible, by means of appropriate anticonvulsant drugs. Clearly, those which produce further cerebral depression would not be suitable; thus, it would be hazardous to employ a barbiturate preparation in these circumstances. Also, some authors have disapproved the use of paraldehyde because, in large doses, this drug can depress both respiration and the circulation.

Consequently, the preferable preparation would seem to be either parenteral diazepam or a curare alkaloid. However, the curare derivative must be given with the patient's ventilation controlled by adequate devices and it should be administered only by physicians skilled in its use. Thus, a benzodiazepine preparation would seem to be the anticonvulsant drug of choice in patients with tricyclic antidepressant intoxication. Also, since convulsions in such patients may be secondary to anoxia and not necessarily the result of cerebral excitation induced by the tricyclic antidepressant overdose, it is advisable that supportive measures be employed to assure adequate respiratory exchange in all patients with tricyclic antidepressant intoxication who are also comatose. Thus, if they are deemed necessary, the placement of a pharyngeal airway or the introduction of a cuffed endotrachial tube into the larynx should not be delayed if, from the outset of the hospitalization, there is any suggestion of the presence of a ventilatory impairment. However, ordinarily, their use would not be mandatory if there is no clinical evidence of serious respiratory depression or if the values of the arterial blood gases do not indicate the presence of hypoxemia and/or respiratory acidosis. Undoubtedly, intermittent suctioning of the major airways would be advisable if there is any evidence of retained secretions. In general, proper attention to this problem should preclude the need for a tracheostomy.

Moreover, it would be pertinent to this discussion to review which methods can be employed in patients with tricyclic antidepressant intoxication to remove any residual amounts of the "poison" from the gastrointestinal tract. Thus, some observers have suggested that forced emesis should be the initial procedure when the patient has been admitted to the hospital shortly after the overdose of the drug has been swallowed.

To accomplish this purpose, the posterior pharynx can be stimulated mechanically with the examiners finger; also, a similar result can be obtained by the instillation into the stomach through a gastric tube of a strong solution of salt or mustard. Although 10 or 20 cc of syrup of ipecac, administered to a conscious patient, would be equally effective in promoting emesis, the action of this preparation has a latent period of 20 minutes or longer. Moreover, inasmuch as the emetic action of ipecac depends on gastrointestinal absorption, it cannot be used in conjunction with other measures designed to minimize the absorption of the overdose of tricyclic antidepressant compounds the patient had consumed.

Emesis can be achieved also by the intravenous injection of 0.01 mg of apomorphine per kg of body weight but, generally, forced emesis is to be avoided in patients with tricyclic antidepressant intoxication who exhibit signs of cerebral depression or who are convulsing.

Alternatively, the portions of the "poison" remaining in the gastrointestinal tract can be removed by gastric lavage. In general, this method of removal of the overdose is safer to use particularly in unconscious patients, because it will prevent the complications which might ensue if vomitus might be aspirated.

During gastric lavage, the patient should be prone with the head and shoulders lowered and turned slightly toward the left side; however, sometimes, a more productive lavage return can be achieved by moving the patient from left to right during the lavage procedure. With a mouth gag in place, a size #30 gastric tube is passed into the stomach. If central nervous system function is depressed, and introduction of the tube produces retching, it is wise to introduce a cuffed endotracheal airway into the larynx before the gastric tube is forced into the stomach.

Once this is accomplished, the gastric contents should be withdrawn repeatedly with the same large syringe attached to the gastric tube. Between aspirations, a lavaging solution consisting merely of 200 cc of isotonic saline between each aspiration is repeatedly instilled and withdrawn until the aspirate becomes clear. It is imperative that such gastric lavage should not be delayed inasmuch as its efficacy quickly decreases as the interval increases between the time of drug ingestion and time the stomach is evacuated.

After gastric lavage has been completed, it would be appropriate to insert, through the gastric tube, lodged in the stomach or upper small intestine, a charcoal slurry which can prevent systemic absorption of any tricyclic antidepressant which may have entered the small intestine by way of an enterohepatic pathway. The benefits to be expected from this form of therapy can be judged from the results of in vitro studies and from findings in patients who were admitted to the hospital following the ingestion of megadoses of a tricyclic antidepressant, as well as in patients who were consuming customary doses of this drug. Thus, the in vitro studies demonstrated that 1 gm of activated charcoal in 10 cc of gastric juice bound 95% of 10 mg of amiptripyline or its metabolite, nortriptyline, which were added to this mixture.

Moreover, the importance of this observation is enhanced by human data which indicate that each of the major metabolites of amitriptyline or imipramine, as well as the respective parent compounds, normally are secreted into the gastric juice in considerable quantities. Equally meaningful was the discovery that during the first 24 hours following the respective admissions of several patients with tricyclic antidepressant intoxication, much larger amounts of the drug could be removed by gastric lavage than were excreted in the urine.

Data of this sort are especially impressive inasmuch as two groups of investigators have shown already that when a customary dose of radioactively tagged imipramine was administered to patients, an average of 40% of the radioactivity was detected in the urine during the ensuing 24 hours. Moreover, other studies in rats have shown that whereas biliary excretion of nortriptyline can be as high as 55% of the administered dose, only a small percentage was extractible from the feces; thus, it was evident that most of the drug was absorbed from the small intestine. Clearly, then, these various observations would seem to substantiate the position of those who have recommended the use of an activated charcoal slurry to "detoxify" patients with tricyclic antidepressant intoxication.

Moreover, since considerable absorption of a tricyclic antidepressant can take place in the small intestine where it returns after it has moved from the stomach and into the liver (the enterohepatic pathway), it would be a rational procedure to speed the downward passage of the activated charcoal slurry with its adsorbed poison along the remainder of the intestinal tract. Therefore, the last instillation of the charcoal slurry should be followed by the instillation into the stomach of a solution containing 10 to 30 gm of sodium sulphate. The effectiveness of these "detoxifying" measures can be judged also by data which have shown that if treatment with activated charcoal is begun 2 to 3 hours after ingestion of the overdose of a tricyclic antidepressant, it may be possible to remove up to 30 percent of the ingested dose during the first 24 hours with a combination of gastric lavage and the instillation of an activated charcoal slurry. In this same connection, it is noteworthy that others have observed that giving activated charcoal every 4 to 6 hours for the first 24 to 48 hours after ingestion of the tricyclic antidepressant overdose may require as much as 100 gm of activated charcoal, if the amount to be adsorbed is as much as 4 gm.

To prepare a slurry of activated charcoal which can pass through the gastric tube, the proportions should be 20 to 30 gm of activated charcoal and this amount should be mixed with 4 to 6 ounces of water. Thus, an appropriate dose during the first 24 hours would be 100 to 200 cc of such an activated charcoal slurry, instilled every 2 hours.

Concurrently, with the administration of the charcoal slurry, it would be appropriate to utilize some additional means of promoting the elimination of the tricyclic antidepressant compound from the body fluids and tissues. Ordinarily, it would be expected that either hemodialysis or peritoneal dialysis could accomplish this purpose but because repeated studies have shown that 90% of a tricyclic antidepressant compound reaching the blood stream tends to become bound to plasma proteins, it generally is agreed that dialysis is of little benefit in connection with the management of tricyclic antidepressant intoxications. This view has been confirmed also by observations which have indicated that when dialysis has been employed in such a situation, the dialysate contains almost negligible amounts of the compound responsible for the intoxication.

On the other hand, forced diuresis, using simultaneously an osmotic diuretic such as mannitol perorally along with infusions of isotonic saline solutions, still is regarded by some authorities as an effective means of promoting the excretion of a tricyclic antidepressant and its metabolites from the body. Admittedly, the level of the parent tricyclic antidepressant compound in the blood in instances of tricyclic antidepressant intoxication is extremely low and sometimes entirely undetectible, but this finding does not necessarily exclude the possibility that mannitol which increases the renal plasma flow, the glomerular filtration rate and the extent of urine flow, cannot promote the elimination from the body of certain metabolites which may be more important than the parent compound in the production of the symptomatology characteristic of an episode of tricyclic antidepressant poisoning.

It should be recognized also that if mannitol is to be effective, large doses of this hexahydric alcohol must be administered. The loading dose should be

25 to 50 gm; thereafter 10 to 20 gm per hour should be given. The adequacy of the amount administered can be judged by the urine output; urine volumes of up to 1 liter per hour should be achievable with the use of this treatment plan. Also, aside from the simultaneous intravenous infusion of sizeable quantities of normal saline solution, it might be advantageous to inject along with the saline infusion, 40 mg of furosemide, in order to further increase urine output. However, it should be appreciated that if mannitol is employed in this manner, great care must be exercised to supply sufficient water and electrolyte needs at the same time. Moreover, there are dangers associated with osmotic diuresis in the presence of congestive heart failure, shock, or renal failure.

It should be realized also that an improvement in the clinical state of patients with tricyclic antidepressant intoxication who, therefore, have been treated with osmotic diuresis need not be ascribed exclusively to an enhanced renal excretion of the "poison." Conceivably, the benefits of this procedure, at least in some instances, can be related to a reduction of the cerebral edema which, supposedly, is an associated occurrence in many patients who have consumed an overdose of a tricyclic antidepressant.

Unquestionably, the complications which are most likely to have an adverse effect on the survivability of patients with tricyclic antidepressant intoxication are anoxia, abnormalities of acid base balance, hypotension, and major ventricular arrhythmias. Consequently, it should be the responsibility of those involved in the care of tricyclic antidepressant overdosed patients to monitor them continuously, particularly during the first five days of their hospitalization, and to institute appropriate corrective measures as soon as any of these alarming developments are detected.

However, inasmuch as there is still an inadequate understanding of the pathogenesis of such arrhythmias in patients with tricyclic antidepressant poisoning, the treatment of this particular cardiotoxic effect would require, at least, the maintenance of proper ventilatory function and also the correction of any abnormalities with respect to the serum electrolytes or the acid base balance. Various antiarrhythmic drugs also have been recommended but their efficacy still remains to be proven. Moreover, certain studies would suggest that drugs with a quinidine-like action are especially contraindicated. Certain observers in France and Australia as well as a few in the United States tend to favor the infusion of solutions of molar sodium lactate or sodium bicarbonate and there seems to be a sound basis for their use.

Sustained hypotension with the patient supine, even though the cardiac rhythm is not irregular, is considered by some to be another ominous finding and thus a result of a tricyclic antidepressant overdose which should be treated not only aggressively, but in a well organized manner as well. In this connection, the recommendations that the hemodynamic status of the patient be established before treatment of the hypotension is begun would seem to be a highly cogent suggestion.

Accordingly, when it would seem likely that sustained hypotension is the forerunner of circulatory collapse, a Swan-Ganz catheter should be placed in the pulmonary artery and the following measurements should be made: arterial and mixed venous blood gases in terms of their respective concentration and partial pressures; the pH of the arterial blood; the level of the pulmonary arterial pressure; the level of the left atrial (wedge) pressure; and the cardiac output. Then, if the left atrial pressure is found to be low, volume expansion with intravenous infusions should be the first measure to be employed. If, on the other hand, the left atrial pressure is above 18 mm of mercury and the cardiac output and peripheral resistance are found to be low, then an agent to increase cardiac contractility is indicated. For this purpose, a variety of preparations which produce a positive inotropic effect can be employed but dopamine would seem to be the substance most likely to achieve this desired effect without producing any untoward reactions.

REFERENCES

Arieff, A.I. and Friedman, E.A. coma following *non narcotic drug overdosage:* Management of 208 adult patients Am. J. Med. Sci. 296:405 (1973)

Bailey, R.R. et al. Hemodialysis and Forced Diuresis for Tricyclic Antidepressant Poisoning. Brit. Med. J. :238 (1974).

Baker, A.B. Treatment of poisoning by antidepressants. Brit. Med. J. 4:50 (1967).

Baraka, A. and Harik, S. Reversal of central anticholinergic syndrome by gallanthamine. J.A.M.A. 238:2293 (1977).

Bigger, J.T. et al. Is physostigmine effective for cardiac toxicity of tricyclic antidepressant drugs? J.A.M.A. 237:1311 (1977).

Bigger, J.T. et al. The effects of tricyclic antidepressants on the heart and blood pressure. Pract. Cardiol. 1:65 (1978).

Brown, T.C.K. Sodium bicarbonate treatment for tricyclic antidepressant arrhythmias in children. Med. J. Aust. 2:380 (1976).

Brown, T.C.K. et al. The use of sodium bicarbonate in the treatment of tricyclic antidepressant-induced arrhythmias. Anaesth. Intensive Care 1:203 (1973).

Burks, J.S. et al. Tricyclic antidepressant poisoning. Reversal of coma, choreoathetosis, and myoclunus by physostigmine. J.A.M.A. 230:1405 (1974).

Crammer, J.L. Treatment of poisoning by antidepressants. Brit. Med. J. 4:50 (1967).

Crammer, J. and Davies, B. Activated charcoal in tricyclic drug overdose. Brit. Med. J. 1:527 (1962).

Crocker, J. and Morton, B. Tricyclic antidepressant drug toxicity. J. Clin. Toxicol. 2:397 (1969).

Davis, J.M. et al. Overdosage of psychotropic drugs. A review (Part II). Dis. Nerv. Sys. 29:246 (1968).

Duvoisin, R.C. and Katz, R. Reversal of central anticholinergic syndrome in man by physostigmine. J.A.M.A. 206:1963 (1968).

Freeman, J.W. and Loughhead, M.G. Beta blockade in the treatment of trycyclic antidepressant overdosage. Med. J. Aust. 1:1233 (1973).

Gard, H. et al. Qualitative and quantitative studies on the disposition of amitriptyline and other tricyclic antidepressant drugs in man as it relates to the management of the overdosed patient. *Clin. Toxicol.* 6:571 (1973).

Granacher, R.P. and Baldessarini, R.J. Physostigmine: Its use in acute cholinergic syndrome with antidepressant and antiparkinson drugs. *Arch. Gen. Psych.* 32:375 (1975).

Harthorne, J.W. et al. Management of massive imipramine overdosage with mannitol and artificial dialysis. *New Eng. J. Med.* 268:33 (1963).

Holinger, P.C. and Klawans, H.L. Reversal of tricyclic overdosage-induced central anticholinergic syndrome by physostigmine. *Am. J. Psych.* 133:9 (1976).

Jefferson, J.W. A Review of the Cardiovascular Effects and Toxicity of Tricyclic Antidepressants. *Psychosom. Med.* 37:160 (1975).

Manoguerra, A.S. and Weaver, L.C. Poisoning with tricyclic antidepressant drugs. *Clin. Toxicol.* 10:149 (1977).

Marshall, L.J. and Green, V.A. Propranolol and diazepam for imipramine poisoning. *Lancet* 2:1249 (1968).

Moccetti, T. et al. Cardiotoxicity of tricyclic antidepressants. *Schweiz. Med. Wehnsehr.* 101:1 (1971).

Munoz, R.A. and Kuplic, J.R. Large overdose of tricyclic antidepressants treated with physostigmine salicylate. *Psychosomatics* 16:77 (1975).

Newton, R.W. Physostigmine salicylate in the treatment of tricyclic antidepressant overdosage. *J.A.M.A.* 231:941 (1975).

Noble, J. and Mathew, H. Acute poisoning by tricyclic antidepressants: Clinical features and management of 100 patients. *J. Clin. Toxicol.* 2:403 (1969).

Rumack, B.H. Anticholinergic poisoning: Treatment with physostigmine. *Pediatrics* 52:449 (1973).

Slovis, T.L. et al. Physostigmine therapy in acute tricyclic antidepressant poisoning. *J. Clin. Toxicol.* 4:451 (1971).

Snyder, B.D. et al. Reversal of amitriptyline intoxication by physostigmine. *J.A.M.A.* 230:1433 (1974).

Steel, C.M. et al. Clinical effects and treatment of imipramine and amitriptyline poisoning in children. *Brit. Med. J.* 3:663 (1967).

Wood, C.A. et al. Management of tricyclic antidepressant toxicities. *Dis. Nerv. Sys.* 37:459 (1976).

APPENDIX

The Management of Acute Cardiac Arrest

Most authorities experienced with the use of life support measures now agree that the initial treatment for a witnessed sudden cardiac arrest in persons not yet connected to a cardiac monitor should be started as promptly as possible at the scene of the arrest. Undoubtedly, it would be desirable to be certain, from the outset, whether the cardiac arrest was due to cardiac standstill, electromechanical dissociation, or a chaotic type of ventricular arrhythmia but, obviously, when such an accident occurs away from an intensive care unit, it would be impractical to wait for instrumental aids which could provide such information before beginning the use of those procedures commonly categorized as basic life support measures. Thus, when a psychiatric patient, with or without a previous history of heart disease, suddenly has become unresponsive, apneic, asphygmic, and there is inaudibility of the heart sounds and dilatation of the pupils, the overriding imperative at that moment is to promptly apply the principles of cardiopulmonary resuscitation (CPR); simultaneously, instructions should be given to arrange for the rapid transportation of the victim to a facility where advanced life support intervention can be provided

Alternatively, if a portable defibrillation unit is immediately available, it should be the first modality to be employed inasmuch as there is no longer any dispute that the use of even a portable defibrillator within seconds after a witnessed cardiac arrest has occurred should increase materially the incidence of recovery from such a catastrophe. However, it should be recognized that such a high success rate can be anticipated only if the cardiac mechanism associated with the cardiac arrest is ventricular fibrillation. Moreover, experience has shown that in order to abolish an acute cardiac arrest by the use of a defibrillator unit, the highest available energy should be employed at the outset, using an anteroposterior placement of the electrodes to the chest; otherwise, if lesser shock levels are used and fail to effect electrical reversion, valuable seconds have been dissipated.

However, if a portable defibrillator is not immediately available, it is the obligation of any health professional who has witnessed an acute cardiac arrest, to carry out the following missions which collectively are the basic principles of cardiopulmonary resuscitation (CPR). One of these principles is to maintain adequate pulmonary ventilation; another is to restore the movement of the blood stream throughout the body and thus insure adequate perfusion of such vital structures as the heart, lungs, and brain; the third is to prevent irreversible anoxic brain damage.

Moreover, with respect to cardiopulmonary resuscitation, it must be recognized, from the outset, that delayed or improper coordination of the requisite techniques can be one important factor responsible for either a total failure of survival or survival complicated by persistent brain damage. Persistent anoxic brain damage can result from the following set of circumstances: (1) delayed onset of CPR; (2) possible ineffectiveness of cardiac massage in relation to the neurological signs during resuscitation; 3) too frequent periods of interruption of cardiac massage; 4) lack of supplementary measures to improve the circulatory state once spontaneous cardiac action has been restored. *Thus, it should be evident that the salvageability of persons with an acute cardiac arrest is dependent largely on the rapid response to this type of emergency by personnel already familiar with the principles of CPR.*

Still to be properly evaluated is the advantage to be gained by noting the response to a blow to the precordial area immediately before chest compression is initiated in instances of acute cardiac arrest. It is known that a "precordial thump" can generate a small electrical stimulus in a heart that is still reactive and, thus, in an occasional instance, the preliminary use of such a precordial thump may be effective in restoring a heart beat in cases of ventricular asystole and in reversing ventricular tachycardia or ventricular fibrillation of recent onset. However, generally it is agreed that a precordial thump is of little value in connection with the treatment of acute cardiac arrest and therefore it cannot be expected to be a reliable substitute for external cardiac compression.

Inasmuch as the immediate predecessor of ventricular fibrillation of whatever cause is usually ventricular tachycardia that occurs during the vulnerable period of the ventricle, it is only during this brief intervening period of ventricular tachycardia that a cardioplegic ventricular arrhythmia can be expected to respond favorably to the ultralow energies generated by a blow to the chest. In delivering the precordial thump, an adherence to the following rules is mandatory; 1) deliver a sharp, quick single blow with the bottom fleshy part of the fist; 2) the target should be the mid-portion of the sternum; 3) the distance traversed by the fist should be 8 to 12 inches; 4) deliver the thump within the first minute afer the cardiac arrest has occurred.

On the other hand, the time lost by resort to thump-version may counter the benefits to be achieved by immediate defibrillation or other efforts designed to support the circulatory apparatus. Thus, when there is a lack of immediate response to precordial thump in the form of spontaneous breathing and a return of pulsations in the carotid artery, CPR should be started at once; correspondingly then, the rescuer should not perform additional chest thumps before doing so.

With respect to cardiopulmonary resuscitation (CPR) it is a cardinal principle that external cardiac compression always must be accompanied by additional measures designed to provide ventilation of the lungs by artifical means. Compression of the sternum during external cardiac massage produces some ventilation as well, but the volumes are insufficient for adequate oxygenation of the blood.

Moreover, to assure the entry of air into the lungs, the first act of the rescuer, or an assistant, should be the maintenance of an open airway. This can be accomplished easily and quickly by tilting the victim's head backward as far as possible while the victim is lying supine on the floor. To perform the head tilt, the rescuer places one hand beneath the victim's neck and the other hand on his forehead. Then the rescuer lifts the neck with one hand and tilts the head backward by pressure with his other hand on the forehead. This maneuver, which should be performed rapidly and expeditiously, extends the neck and lifts the tongue away from the back of the throat. Anatomical obstruction of the airway caused by the tongue dropping against the back of the throat thereby is eliminated. Once this is accomplished, the head must be maintained in this position by an assistant at all times throughout the resuscitation procedures.

If the head tilt is unsuccessful in opening the air passage adequately, additional forward displacement of the lower jaw may be required. This can be accomplished by a triple maneuver in which the rescuer places his or her fingers behind the angle of the victim's jaw and 1) forcefully displaces the mandible forward while 2) tilting the head backward and 3) using his or her thumbs to retract the lower lip to allow breathing through the mouth as well as through the nose. The jaw thrust maneuver is performed best when the rescuer or an assistant takes a position at the top of the victim's head. Then, while an assistant maintains the head and jaws in this position, the rescuer can begin external cardiac compression. In addition, the assistant assumes the responsibility for performing mouth to mouth ventilation intermittently while the rescuer applies rhythmic compression to the thorax in order to maintain an adequate circulation (external cardiac massage).

In some cases, mouth-to-nose ventilation is more effecive than mouth-to-mouth ventilation. The former is recommended when it is impossible to open the victim's mouth, when it is impossible to ventilate through the mouth, when the victim's mouth is seriously injured, when it is difficult to achieve a tight seal around the mouth, and when, for some other reason, the assistant rescuer prefers the nasal route.

For the mouth-to-nose technique, the assistant rescuer keeps the vicim's head tilted back with one hand on the forehead and uses the other hand to lift the victim's lower jaw; this maneuver should seal satisfactorily the lips and thereby prevent the dissipation of the air-stream being forced into the nasal passages.

Properly performed, mouth-to-mouth or mouth-to-nose breathing should result in rhythmic visible expansion of the chest. The victim is then allowed to exhale passively, and the rescuer should be able to see the chest fall when the victim exhales. When mouth-to-nose ventilation is used, it may be necessary to open the victim's mouth or to separate the lips to allow the air to escape during exhalation; sometimes, because of an undue relaxation of the soft palate and the resulting nasophyaryngeal obstruction, the egress of air through the nasal passages will be impeded. In terms of timing, the cycle of forced respiration should be repeated approximately every 5 seconds at least, whether the artifical ventilation consists of mouth to mouth breathing or mouth to nose breathing.

Moreover, the rescuer should not look for foreign bodies in the upper airways unless their presence is either known or strongly suspected. Such suspicion is justified if the first attempts to provide artificial ventilation are unsuccessful, in terms of expanding rhythmically the chest wall during inspiration. Then, if there is such evidence of obstruction of the air passages, the rescuer's fingers should sweep through the pharyngeal area for the purpose of removing any obstructing material. Modifications of the Heimlich procedure, also described in the Appendix, may be used for the same purpose and if these fail to clear the airway, an emergency tracheostomy may be necessary.

Logistically, artificial ventilation must be closely coordinated with proper external cardiac compression. However, it must be recognized that external cardiac massage consists of the rhythmic application of pressure over only the lower half of the sternum and not over the xiphoid process. Such intermittent pressure applied to the sternum compresses the heart against the vertebral column and produces a pulsatile artificial circulation. Although the carotid artery blood flow resulting from external cardiac compression usually is only one quarter to one third of normal, experience has shown that this amount is adequate to maintain adequate perfusion of the heart and of the brain. To avoid the application of pressure to the xiphoid process, the rescuer places the heel of his hand on the lower half of the sternum about 1 to 1½ inches away from the tip of the xiphoid and toward the victim's head, while kneeling along side the victim's body.

Then while the rescuer kneels alongside the body of the victim, the shoulders are brought directly over the victim's chest while keeping arms straight and exerting pressure almost vertically downward to depress the lower sternum. The compression must be rhythmic and timed so that there are 60 compressions per minute or 1 compression per second. Moreover, within this time frame, the rescuer relaxes briefly after each compression of the sternum. However, the heel of the rescuer's hand should not be removed from the chest during the relaxation phase; thus, between each compression, the rescuer's hand merely returns to its resting position and remains in place over the sternum. *Experience has shown also that effective compression is achieved only if, during the downward movement, the heel of the hand not in contact with the sternum simultaneously pushes against the dorsum of the hand which is in place against the sternum.*

Under no circumstance should compression be interrupted for more than 5 seconds; it should be stopped only if spontaneous cardiac activity has been restored and the victim is fully awake. When there are two rescuers, optimum ventilation and circulation are achieved by quickly "interposing" one inflation after each five chest compressions without any pause in compression (5:1 ratio). One rescuer performs external cardiac compression while the other one remains at the patient's head, keeps it tilted back, and continues exhaled-air ventilation. Interposing the breaths without any pause in compression is important, since every interruption in cardiac compression results in a drop of blood flow and blood pressure to zero. A single rescuer must execute both artificial ventilation and artificial circulation using a 15:2 ratio, i.e. two quick lung inflations after each 15 chest compressions.

The reaction of the pupils should be checked during cardiopulmonary resuscitation since the behavior of the pupil provides one of the best clues to the overall status of the patient. A pupil which constricts when exposed to light indicates adequate oxygenation and blood flow to the brain. If the pupils remain widely dilated and do not react to light, serious brain damage is imminent or has occurred; dilated but reactive pupils are less ominous. During CPR the carotid or femoral pulse should be palpated periodically in order to check the effectiveness of the external cardiac compression or the return of a spontaneous heart beat. In this connection, it is more desirable to note the pulsations in the carotid artery rather than in the femoral or radial arteries.

Some complications can occur from the use of cardiopulmonary resusciation but these can be avoided if the following rules are observed: 1) the rescuer must never compress over the xiphoid process at the tip of the sternum. This bony prominence extends over the abdomen and undue pressure on it may cause laceration of the liver, which can be lethal; 2) in order to avoid any bony fractures, the rescuer must never touch the patient's ribs when compressing; at all times the heel of the hand must be kept in the middle of the patient's chest over the lower half of the sternum. For the same reason, sudden jerking movements must never be used to compress the chest; the compression action should be smooth, regular, and uninterrupted with 50% of the cycle compression, and 50% of the cycle relaxation. 3) Compression of the abdomen and the chest simultaneously also should be avoided because otherwise the liver may be bruised or even ruptured. *A maximum sense of urgency must continue throughout the resuscitation procedures.* Cardiopulmonary resuscitation must never be interrupted for more than 5 seconds at a time for any purpose. However, the longer it is necessary to continue cardiopulmonary resuscitation, the less likely it is to succeed. Even under optimum circumstances, deterioration is progressive during heart-lung resuscitation and the sense of urgency must be preserved until all efforts to restore cardiac activity are abandoned.

Clearly, when it is evident that no benefit can be expected from cardiopulmonary resuscitation, this procedure should not be initiated, Thus, when it is known or can be determined with a degree of certainty that cardiac arrest already had been present for more than 5 or 6 minutes, there is no known intervention which can be expected to restore cardiac activity. If there is a question of the extent of the arrest in terms of time, the patient should be given the benefit of the doubt and resuscitation procedures should be started; however; cardiopulmonary resusciatation is not indicated in a patient who is known to be in the terminal stage of an incurable condition.

The decision to stop cardiopulmonary resuscitation is a medical one and depends upon an assessment of the cerebral and cardiovascular status. However, it is generally agreed that the persistence of deep unconsciousness, the absence of spontaneous respiration, and the persistence of fixed dilated pupils for 15 to 30 minutes are indications of cerebral death and therefore, further resuscitative efforts usually are futile. Correspondingly, cardiac death may be assumed when there is no return of electrocardiographic activity after 10 to 15 minutes of continuous cardiopulmonary support, or even before this time, if there is evidence of electromechanical dissociation.

External cardiac compression machines are adjuncts which may be used when prolonged resuscitation or transportation of the patient is required. However, they should be designed to approximate the performance of the manual methods already mentioned. Moreover, experience has shown that it is always advisable to start CPR with the manual method first, instead of relying on mechanical methods which may not be immediately available during the early critical phase of an acute cardiac arrest.

Correspondingly, attempts at reoxygenation by exhaled-air methods or by inhalation of room air or oxygen via a suitable mask should always precede attempts at tracheal intubation. Moreover, inasmuch as intubation of the trachea should be considered only if trained personnel for such a procedure are available, it would be best to postpone it until the victim has received already the benefits of basic life support measures and is still alive on arrival at the Intensive Care facility. Once the victim has reached such a unit, appropriate judgements can be made with respect to respiratory assists, drug therapy, as well as the use of a defibrillatory device or an artificial pacemaker.

REFERENCES

Basic life support. *J.A.M.A.* 227:833 (Suppl.) (1974).
Johnstone, R.E. Cardiopulmonary resuscitation. *J.A.M.A.* 228:977 (1974).
Kouwenhoven, W.B. and Langworthy, O.R. Cardiopulmonary resuscitation: An account of 45 years of research. *J.A.M.A.* 226:877 (1973).
Loeb, H.S. Cardiac arrest. *J.A.M.A.* 232:845 (1975).
Shapter, R.K. et al. Cardiopulmonary resuscitation: Basic life support. *Clinical Symposia* (Ciba) 26:4 (1974).
Statement by the Ad Hoc Committee on Cardiopulmonary Resuscitation of the Division of Medical Sciences, National Academy of Sciences-National Research Council. *J.A.M.A.* 198:138 (1966).
Stephenson, H.E. *Cardiac Arrest and Resuscitation* C.V. Mosby Co., St. Louis, Missouri (1964).
Tobin, J.R. Cardiac Emergencies, Part I. *Postgrad. Med.* (1966).

APPENDIX

Emergency Treatment Of Alimentary Strangulation

In all probability, food choking occurs during inspiration, when there is a greater likelihood for a bolus of unmasticated food to be sucked into the laryngeal orifice. The exact incidence of this complication in either the general population or in psychiatric patients is unknown but it has been estimated to be the sixth leading cause of accidental death; its victims have been numbered by certain authorities to exceed those accidentally killed by firearms or airplane accidents. However, regardless of any disagreements regarding its precise incidence, it certainly can be expected that, in the years ahead, the frequency of such fatalities gradually will diminish. This decline can be anticipated inasmuch as it has been amply confirmed that the use of a simple maneuver, originally devised by Heimlich, can successfully abort sudden deaths due to alimentary strangulation.

In the past, it was customary to attempt manual removal of the obstructing bolus of food but, almost invariably, such efforts failed to achieve the desired result. Autopsy findings, in instances of alimentary strangulation, generally have shown that the bolus of food had either lodged in the back of the throat, beyond the reach of the rescuer's finger or had entered the trachea and thus had occluded the major airways. Recently, an instrument for removing food from the back of the throat has been designed by Eller and Haugen but because a device of this sort almost never is available when the emergency has arisen, it has proven to be of limited value in reducing fatalities of this sort.

The principles of the Heimlich procedure are based not on an empirical approach; instead, they evolved from carefully conducted animal experiments. In connection with such investigations, a cuffed endotracheal tube with the lumen plugged by a rubber stopper was inserted under direct vision through the mouth into the larynx of four beagle hounds, each anesthetized with thiamylal given intravenously. The cuff was then distended with 3 to 4 cc of air, causing total obstruction of the trachea; the purpose was to simulate a bolus of food caught in the human larynx.

Each animal treated in this manner immediately developed respiratory distress as evidenced by spasmodic paradoxical respiratory movements of the chest and diaphragm. Subsequently, the palm of the experimenter's hand was pressed deeply and firmly upward into the abdomen of the animal, a short distance below the rib cage, thereby pushing against the diaphragm. Following this procedure, the endotracheal tube (bolus) "popped out" of the trachea. After several labored respirations, the dog then resumed his normal breathing. The experiment was repeated more than 20 times in each of these animals, and, regularly, the same result was achieved.

Thereafter, the usual clinical situation in man was simulated by inserting a bolus of raw hamburger into the dog's larynx until the respiratory passage was totally occluded. Likewise, in such a setting, abdominal pressure was applied and, in each instance, after one or two compressions, the bolus promptly was ejected from the larynx; seconds afterward, normal respiratory exchange was established.

Therefore, Heimlich has recommended that when the rescuer is confronted with a case of alimentary strangulation, the rescuer should stand behind the victim, wrapping both arms around the waist but avoiding a crushing "bear hug"; the correct method is to place a single fist above the navel just below the rib cage and then make a series of quick upward thrusts against the upper abdominal wall until the obstructing substance is dislodged (Figure 1).

When the victim is sitting, the rescuer stands, behind the victim's chair and performs the maneuver in the same manner. When the victim has collapsed and is lying prone, a variation of this maneuver can be followed. In such a situation. The rescuer kneels astride the victim's hips and places the heel of one hand (the bottom hand) on the abdomen slightly above the navel and below the rib cage; the other hand then covers the bottom hand while a series of quick upward thrusts are made against this part of the victim's abdomen. Quick upward thrusts should be employed because experience has shown that such a practice enhances the possibility that the obstructing material in the trachea will be expelled. If vomiting should occur, the victim should be placed in the lateral decubitus position and all foreign material should be removed from the mouth in order to prevent an aspiration pneumonia.

As Heimlich explained, his procedures proved to be successful in 16 persons when traditional methods of rescue, such as reaching into the throat to remove the object or slapping the victim on the back were attempted but

TO SAVE A CHOKING VICTIM

The basic technique

The Heimlich maneuver uses air in the lungs to force an obstruction out of the airway. To move the air you have to apply sudden pressure below the rib cage, which forces the diaphragm up and compresses the lungs. The basic technique (above) begins with a fist. Note the knob formed by the thumb and index finger—that's what helps push the diaphragm upward. Place your fist thumbside against the abdomen, slightly above the navel and below the rib cage. Then grasp your fist with your free hand and press into the abdomen with a quick upward thrust. Do this while standing or kneeling behind a standing or sitting victim with your arms wrapped around his waist (right). Repeat this procedure several times if necessary.

proved to be unsuccessful. In most of these instances, the asphyxiating bolus was felt by the tip of the finger but it could not be removed until it was ejected by the abdominal pressure maneuver, which has been described. Thus, a familiarity with the Heimlich procedure should be a basic requirement with respect to all personnel who are responsible for the care of psychiatric patients but especially for those patients who show signs of regressive behavior.

REFERENCES

Heimlich, H.J. A life-saving maneuver to prevent food-choking. *J.A.M.A.* 234:398 (1975).
Heimlich, H.J., The Heimlich Maneuver: Prevention of death from choking on foreign bodies. *J. Occup. Med.* 19:208 (1977).
Special Report of Physicians Medical Practice Committee of the American College of Physicians: "Emergency Relief of the Obstructed Airway." *Bull. Amer. Coll. Phys.* 5:12 (1977).

Index

acetaldehyde, excess, 53
acetaldehyde dehydrogenase, availability of, in alcoholics, 70
Addiction Research Foundation of Ontario, Canada, 44
adrenal cortical steroids, 183
adrenergic activity and sudden death, 274-275
adrenergic blocking agents, 125
  use of, 266-267
adrenomedullary secretions, excess, 29
adult respiratory distress syndrome, 59, 60
adynamic ileus, 149, 291
alcohol sensitivity, ethnic differences in, 44
alcohol withdrawal syndrome, 63
alcoholic fatty liver disease, coronary arteriosclerosis and acute alcoholism in chronic alcoholics, 69
alcoholic myocardiopathy, 60, 75-80
  associated ECG changes in, 76
  associated physiologic changes in, 76
  diagnosis of, 76
  earliest symptoms of, 76
  electron microscopic findings in, 77-78
  gross physiologic findings in, 79
  pathogenesis of, 79-80
  postmortem histochemical findings in, 78-79
alcoholic psychosis, 22
alcoholism, chronic, and fatal hyperpyrexia, 158
aldehyde infusions, effects of, 246-247
alimentary strangulation, emergency treatment of, 339-342
American College of Cardiology, 232
anger, effect of on heart rate systolic blood pressure, 33
angina pectoris
  drug effects on, 33
  and sudden death, 31-33
  symptoms of, 32
anginal syndrome, 71

angiophraxis, chronic, 17
anhidrotic febrile illness, 154
antabuse. *See* disulfiram
anticonvulsants combined with chlorpromazine, 131-132
antiparkinsonian drugs, contributory effects of, 158
apnea, 291
arrhythmogenic thanatoid syncope, prodomes of, 253
arteries, extramural, chronic angiophraxis of, 17
artherosclerotic coronary disease, 17
asphyxia, obstructive, 89-101
asphyxia, acute, emergency treatment of, 96
asthma, fatal, 96-100
  postmortem findings, 97, 98
ataractics, 130
atherosclerotic coronary artery, 15
atherosclerotic coronary lesions in cirrhotic patients, 74
atherosclerotic stenosis, 136
atrioventricular node, His bundle and branches, histopatholgic study of, 317-319
atrocious eating habits, 90, 92

bangungut syndrome, 118-119
barbiturates combined with chlorpromazine, 132-133
barium enema, 143
basic electrolyte disorder, 52
basophilic degeneration, 113
  of the myocardium, 112
behavior, change in general, and sudden death, 22
Bell's Mania, 166, 167, 171. *See also* exhaustive mania, acute beta blocking agents, 271, 276
  effect of on anginal symptoms, 33

biochemical lesion, 57
Boston Collaborative Drug Study, 303
brain syndrome, chronic, 15, 16, 22, 25, 129
breathlessness and sudden death, 22

cafe coronary, 89-91
Canadian Medical Association Journal, 131
cardiac anomalies, congenital, 12
cardiac arrest
  acute, 12, 13
    management of, 331-337
    symptoms of, 13
  arrhythmogenic, 28-31
cardiac arrhythmia, 22
  congenital, 268
  fatal familial, 259-260
cardiac compression
  external, 333
  interruption of, 335
cardiac hypertrophy, 112, 113, 115
cardiac tamponade, acute, 18
cardiogenic shock, 28
cardiopulmonary resuscitation (CPR), 331-337
  principles of, 331
  urgency, maximum sense of, 336
cardiorrhexis, 18
cardiotoxic effect, 230
carotid or femoral pulse, palpated, 335
catecholamine activity, 296
catecholamines, 30, 124
  excessive accumulation of, 154
  release of, 48
chest pains as rare symptom, 21-23
chlorpromazine
  administration, effects of, 55, 209-210
  overdose of, 155
chlorpromazine therapy after lobotomy, 137-138
choking victim, to save a, 341
cholinesterase activity, reversal of, 322
ciliary activity in the major air passages, effect of phenothiazines on, 129
coronary arteriography, 72
coronary arteriosclerosis and fatty liver as risk factors, 44-49
coronary artery, extramural, thromvotic obstruction of, 17
coronary artery disease, occlusive, 12
coronary circulation, occlusive disease of, 68-69

coronary heart disease, 17
coronary insufficiency, acute, 17
coronary microcirculation, 284, 285
coronary sclerosis with acute posterolateral myocardial infarction, 23
coronary stenosis, progressive, 18
coronary thrombosis, acute, 17, 18
countershock therapy, 276, 288
crib deaths, 127
cyanosis and sudden death, 22
cytologic alterations, 203, 204

defibrillation unit, portable, 331
delayed repolarization syndrome, 234
delirium tremens, 55, 60-63
  defined, 61
  hyperactivity and restraint stress, 61
delerium tremens, potassium depletion and cardiac arrhythmias, 63-68
depolarization of left ventricle, abnormal, 114
diuresis, forced, 326
dilantin therapy combined with chlorpromazine, 136-137
disulfiram, effects of, 53-54

ECG anomaly, inherited, sudden death, and congenital hearing defect, 260-265
  ECG findings, 260-261
  familial features, 260
  genesis of, 261
ECG changes forecasting sudden cardiac arrest, 229-230
ECG findings, significance of, 184-185
ECG responses to pharmacolgic agents, 273
ECG results, 242-244
electrocardiogram
  intersyncopal, 265, 268
  "resting," 262, 263, 270, 271
  "resting" intersyncopal, 261, 264, 265, 266, 269
  synsyncopal, 265, 270
electrocardiographic consideration in sudden death, 229-252
electrocardiographic survey, 25-28
electrolyte abnormalities, 310-312
electrolyte disturbance and ventricular arrhythmias in alcoholics, 49-52
emotional stress and sudden death, 30
emotionality and syncopal attacks, 263

epilepsy
  cryptogenic, 123
  grand mal, 128
  idiopathic, 132, 133
  patients with, 128
  petit mal, 128
  post-lobotomy, 123
  psychomotor, 131
epinephrine, 33
epinephrine and amarin, effects of, 244
epinephrine and propiophenone, effects of, 244
epinephrine, injected and petroleum ether, inhaled, effects of, 246
ergotamine tartrate administration, 238-239
etiologies, combination, 212-215
exhaustive mania, acute, 165-176
  typical attack of, 165-173
exhaustive psychosis, 171. See also exhaustive mania, acute
exhaustive syndrome, 168

familial heart disease, 12
familial syncope, 267-268
family data, 257-259
fat embolism syndrome, 57-60
fatal catatonia. See exhaustive mania, acute
fatal reaction. See wet lung syndrome
fatal syncope, 12, 262, 263, 269
fatty liver syndrome, alcohol induced, 41-49
  conclusions, 43-44
  epidemiologic surveys, 42-44
  postmortem findings, 42
femoral or carotid pulse, palpated, 335
focal myocytolysis, 212, 215
forensic science laboratory, 161
forced respiration, cycle of, 334

gallop rhythm, 22
gastro-esophageal sphincter mechanism, function of, 129
glottal-esophageal reflux, 129-130
glottal spasm, 129
grand mal seizure, 127

haloperidol, 64
heart, 29
heart failure, congestive, 76

heart sounds, faint, 22
heat stroke, 153
  clinical features of, 154
Heimlich procedure, 334
  principles of, 339-341
  victim lying prone, 340
  victim sitting, 340
heroin, "loading" dose of, 192
heroin abuser, myocardial necrosis in, 221-222
heroin intoxication. See wet lung syndrome
"heroin lung," 190
hostility, high levels of and sudden death, 33-34
hyperpyrexia
  and calming drugs, 62
  effects of, 61
  fatal, 153-164
    nomenclature, 153
    risk factors in, 155-162
  malignant thermogenic anhidrotic, 157, 158. See also Siriasis fatal, non-exertional variety of, 158, 159
  malignant thermogenic hyperhidrotic, 154
  pharmacogenic, malignant postmortem data on, 159
hypertrophy, left ventricular, 115
hypocalcemia, 235
  electrocardiographic counterpart of, 236
hypoglycemia
  in development of myocardial necrosis, 48
  fatal vs. symptomatic, 48
  induced, 60
  spontaneous, 46
  and sudden death, 45-49
hypoglycemia episode, alcohol-induced, 46-49
hypokalemia, 64, 229, 235
hypokalemia-like effect, 230
hypomagnesemic chronic alcoholic, 67
hypoventilatory hypoxemia, 193
hypoxemia
  as etiologic factor, 186
  drug-induced, 186
  and wet lung syndrome, 196-197

ileus, adynamic, 149, 291
inherited hearing deficit, and sudden death syndrome, 254
inherited susceptibility to sudden death, 253-280
  chromosome studies, 254

clinical features, 253-255
family history, 254
mode of inheritance of, 255
postmortem examination, 54
intracranial disease, effects of, 210-211
  method, 210
  findings, 210-211
  conclusions, 211
intracranial pressure and pulmonary edema, 124
intravascular coagulopathy
  hyperpyrexia-produced, 159
  management of, 159-160
intravascular lipid deposits, scoring of, 57
intravenous narcotism, acute. See wet lung syndrome
involutional melancholia, 22

jaw thrust maneuver, 333

kinetics and cardioplegic ventricular arrhythmia, disordered, 49

lesion
  acute, 18
  biochemical, 57
  silent, 23
  stenotic, 17
lethal catatonia, 167, 168, 171, 173
  similarity to delirium tremens, 61
lipodystrophy of the liver, 62
liquor and painless myocardial infarction, 26-27
lithium treatment, effects of, 241-242
liver disease, 193-195
liver pathology, resulting from serum or viral hepatitis, 194-195
lobotomy and combined chlorpromazine and anticonvulsant therapy, 133

magnesium depletion, role of, 65-68
magnesium depletion therapy, 67
manic depressive psychosis, 22
megacolon
  clinical features of, 143
  enemata in, use of, 143-144
  fatal, 141-155

in the insane, 142, 143, 146, 147
  localization of, 142
  pathogenesis of, 141-142
  pathologic features of, 142
  phenothiazine, effects of, 149-150
  semantic liberties of, 147
  surgical considerations in, 146-147
methadone, 183-185
  effect, 185
microscope, dissecting, 318
mitochondrial adenosine triphosphate, generation of, 203
monoamine oxidase inhibitors, 56-57
  and tricyclic antidepressant, synergism between, 161
mouth-to-mouth breathing, 334
mouth-to-nose breathing, 334
myocardial cytokalipenia, and ventricular arrhythmias, 204
myocardial hypoxia, 117
  zonal type of, 29
myocardial infarction
  acute, 16, 17, 18, 22
    symptoms of, 21
  athoracodynic acute, 23
  healed, relationship to sudden death, 27
  painless, 23, 24
myocardial ischemia, 70
myocardial necrosis, 203-233
  experimental methods in, 203-205
  in heroin abuser, 221-222
  hypoglycemia in development of, 48-49
myocardial rupture, 18
  prevention, 20
myocardiopathy, 12, 114
  alcoholic, 60, 75-80
  hypertrophic, 117
myocardium, basophilic degeneration of, 112
myofibrillary degeneration, 211-212
  pathologic features of, 211-212
myoglobinuria, 159
myonecrotic lesion, acute, 29

narcotic addiction, 177-207. See also wet lung syndrome
narcotic addicts, death rate among, 179
narcotism. See wet lung syndrome
neurogenic risk factors, 255-259
  hemodynamic studies of, 256
  histologic studies of, 256-257

neurologic manipulation, results of, 255-256
neurologic risk factors, 255-259
nicotine, effects of, 193
nonfatal syncope, 269

orthopnea and sudden death, 22
oxygen consumption by the myocardium, alcohol-induced, 71
oxygen at high pressure, adverse effects of, 135
oxygen wasting hormones, release of, 30

pallor and sudden death, 22
paraldehyde, 55
paretic neurosyphilis, 22
PAS-hematoxylin and eosin technique, 318
PAS methods, 113
PAS positive, diastase-resistant material, 110
PAS and positive Schiff reactions, 112
periodic acid-Schiff (PAS) technique, 111
petechial hemorrhages, 167
petroleum ether, inhaled and injected epinephrine, effects of, 246
pharmacogenic hypopyrexia, pathogenesis of, 162
phenothiazine(s)
  derivatives and cerebrotropic drugs, effects of, 54
  effects of, 215-221
  and T-wave abnormalities, 230-231
phenothiazines in sudden death role of, 281-298
phenothiazine-related deaths, alleged, 107-111
  histologic studies, 109-111
phenothiazine therapy, 16
  adverse effects of, 128
physiogenic seizure, 268
physiologic derangements in convulsive episode, 125-126
physostigmine
  antidote for, 322
  contraindications, 322
pigment deposits, 106
postconvulsive asphyxia, 281
postictal fatalities, 123-144
potassium depletion, 64
potassium therapy, contraindications to, 237-238
precordial thump, 332
prinzmetal angina, 74

procedure, 25-26
programmed meditation, results from, 276-277
prolapsed mitral valve syndrome, 12
promazine, effects of, 54-55
propoxyphene, effects of, 56
pseudo-epilepsy, 268
pseudo-epileptic prodromes, 286
pseudo-epileptic syndrome and inherited repolarization anomaly, combination of, 267
pseudo-pneumonic syndrome, 24-25
  manifestations of, 24-25
psychiatric diagnosis of decedents, 22
psychic shock, 167
psychotropic agents, 155-162, 281-316
pulmonary capillaries, role of endothelial damage of, 189
pulmonary capillary porosity, increased, 189
pulmonary edema, 123
  acute
    drug-induced, 179, 180
    pathologic features of, 181-183
  arterial oxygen tension values in, 187
  arterial pH values in, 187
  carbon dioxide tension values in, 187
  catecholamine activity, role of, 190
  drug-induced, 180
  heroin-induced, 186
  hypoxia and pulmonary vessel contractility, 191
  immunologic abnormalities, 190
  increased permeability of pulmonary capillaries in, 186-189
  methadone-induced, 183-185
  neurohumoral influences, 190
  pathogenesis of, 124-125
  postictal, 123
  vasoactive amines, actions of, 191-193
pump failure, 28, 30
  marginal, 24

Q-T interval, lengthening of, 115
Q-T interval syndromes, 234
"quinidine-like" effect, 230
quinidine and thioridazine, cardiac effects of, 240

rapid eye movements (REM) sleep, 117, 119, 127, 276, 277

and ventricular ectopia, 276-277
Regional Poisoning Center (Edinburgh), 300
repolarization anomaly, inherited, 268
repolarization anomaly and pseudoepileptic syndrome, inherited, combination of, 267
restraint stress, 168, 296
   adverse effects of, 169-173
   effects of on pigs, 205-209
   histologic findings, 207
   macroscopic findings, 207
   method and procedure, 206
   results, 206-207
risk-factors, in fatal hyperpyrexia, 155-162
Romano-Ward syndrome, 265-274
   electrocardiographic data (Garza), 271-272
   pharmacologic studies (Garza), value of, 272

seizure activity, metabolic and biochemical correlates of, 126-218
seizure diathesis, 123
seizure prone, 260
seizure threshold, phenothiazine effects on, 130
seizures, pentylene tetrazol-induced, 125
   cardiac irregularities and, 125
serum potassium level and U-wave enlargement, 233-238
schizophrenic reaction, 22
   chronic, 15, 16, 17
sick sinus syndrome, 12
singultus and sudden death, 22
sinus tachycardia, 116
siriasis, 153, 154
sleep apnea syndrome, 104
   fatal, 127
S-T segment deviations, and sudden death, 229
S-T and T-wave changes, nonspecific, 116
staining methods, 111
status epilepticus, 123, 133
stenotic lesion, 17
street heroin, 177, 179
structural cardiac abnormalities, 68-80
sudorific activity, 162
   sudden interruption of, 154
sudden death, 62
   and adrenergic activity, 274-275
   angina pectoris and, 31-33
   causes of, 12
   emotional stress and, 30
   high levels of hostility and, 33-34
   manifestations of, 22
   tricyclic antidepressants in, 302-312
   weak spells and, 22
   witnessed
      expected, 12
      unexpected, 12
sympathetic outflow, surgically induced, 242
sympatheticomimetic aldehydes, accumulation of, 48
synchronous sleep, 127-128
syncopal attacks and emotionality, 263
syncopal prodromes, 286
syncope, 262, 269, 291
   arrhythmogenic thanatoid, 253
   familial, 267-268
   fatal, 262, 263, 269
   nonfatal attacks, 260, 269
   thanatoid, 262, 263, 264, 276
synsominal deaths, 11, 103-126
   genetic predisposition to, 104-105
syphilitic cardiovascular disease, 16

T-wave abnormalities, 115
   drug-induced, 230-233
   intermittent abnormality of, 116
tachyphagia, 90
teleorentgenogram, 143
thanatoid syncope, 262, 263, 264, 276
therapeutic management, 270-271
thioridazine, 64
   and chlorpromazine, effects of on seizure frequency, 134-136
   effects of, 282-298
   and T-wave abnormalities, 231
tracheal intubation, 336
tricyclic antidepressant poisoning, hallmarks of, 321
   no specific antidote for, 321
   therapeutic aspects, 321-328
tricyclic antidepressants in sudden death
   additional electrocardiographic surveys, 306-308
   customary doses in coronary patients, effects of, 302-303
   electrocardiographic findings, 304-305
   megadoses, effects of, 300
   role of, 298-312

salvage rate, 309-310
single megadose on the heart, effect of, 303-304
typical symptoms, 26

U-wave prominence and arrhythrogenic cardiac arrest, 242-244

valsalva maneuver, 124, 127
ventricular arrhythmia, possible physiologic mechanisms for, 298
ventricular asystole, 332
ventricular ectopia and REM sleep, 276-277
　close temporal relationship between, 277
ventricular fibrillation, 29, 54
ventricular hypertrophy, 12
ventricular premature contractions, repeated, and sudden death, 229
ventricular repolarization, 106
　inherited, 105-107
　nonfatal hereditary abnormal, 263
ventricular tacharrhythmia, evaluation of persistent, 272-273
visceral congestion
　terminal, 105, 106
　widespread, 104, 123

Weak spells and sudden death, 22
wet lung syndrome, 57, 177-207
　alcohol as risk factor in, 180-181
　anoxic brain damage, severe pneumonia and, 197
　characteristics of, 192
　defined, 177-178
　effect on electrocardiogram, 184
　hypoxemia and respiratory acidosis and, 196-197
　methadone-induced, 184
　persistent hypoxemia as risk factor in, 181
　therapeutic choices for, 180
　toxicologic and postmortem findings, imperfect correlation between, 195-196